Biomedical and Clinical Engineering for Healthcare Advancement

N. Sriraam
Ramaiah Institute of Technology, India

A volume in the Advances in Bioinformatics and Biomedical Engineering (ABBE) Book Series

IGI Global
DISSEMINATOR OF KNOWLEDGE

Published in the United States of America by
IGI Global
Medical Information Science Reference (an imprint of IGI Global)
701 E. Chocolate Avenue
Hershey PA, USA 17033
Tel: 717-533-8845
Fax: 717-533-8661
E-mail: cust@igi-global.com
Web site: http://www.igi-global.com

Library of Congress Cataloging-in-Publication Data

Names: Sriraam, N., 1974- editor.
Title: Biomedical and clinical engineering for healthcare advancement / N. Sriraam, editor.
Description: Hershey, PA : Medical Information Science Reference, [2020] | Includes bibliographical references. | Summary: "This book examines advances in healthcare applications driven by the adoption of new technologies and novel algorithms"-- Provided by publisher.
Identifiers: LCCN 2019022165 | ISBN 9781799803263 (hardcover) | ISBN 9781799803270 (ebook)
Subjects: MESH: Biomedical Enhancement | Biomedical Technology | Biomedical Engineering | Nanotechnology
Classification: LCC R858 | NLM W 82 | DDC 610.285--dc23
LC record available at https://lccn.loc.gov/2019022165

This book is published in the IGI Global book series Advances in Bioinformatics and Biomedical Engineering (ABBE) (ISSN: 2327-7033; eISSN: 2327-7041)

British Cataloguing in Publication Data
A Cataloguing in Publication record for this book is available from the British Library.

All work contributed to this book is new, previously-unpublished material.
The views expressed in this book are those of the authors, but not necessarily of the publisher.

For electronic access to this publication, please contact: eresources@igi-global.com.

Advances in Bioinformatics and Biomedical Engineering (ABBE) Book Series

ISSN:2327-7033
EISSN:2327-7041

Editor-in-Chief: Ahmad Taher Azar, Prince Sultan University, Riyadh, Kingdom of Saudi Arabi and Benha University, Egypt

MISSION

The fields of biology and medicine are constantly changing as research evolves and novel engineering applications and methods of data analysis are developed. Continued research in the areas of bioinformatics and biomedical engineering is essential to continuing to advance the available knowledge and tools available to medical and healthcare professionals.

The **Advances in Bioinformatics and Biomedical Engineering (ABBE) Book Series** publishes research on all areas of bioinformatics and bioengineering including the development and testing of new computational methods, the management and analysis of biological data, and the implementation of novel engineering applications in all areas of medicine and biology. Through showcasing the latest in bioinformatics and biomedical engineering research, ABBE aims to be an essential resource for healthcare and medical professionals.

COVERAGE

- DNA Structure
- Protein Structure
- Structural Biology
- Data Analysis
- Drug Design
- Robotics and Medicine
- Genetics
- DNA Sequencing
- Molecular Engineering
- Data Mining

IGI Global is currently accepting manuscripts for publication within this series. To submit a proposal for a volume in this series, please contact our Acquisition Editors at Acquisitions@igi-global.com or visit: http://www.igi-global.com/publish/.

The Advances in Bioinformatics and Biomedical Engineering (ABBE) Book Series (ISSN 2327-7033) is published by IGI Global, 701 E. Chocolate Avenue, Hershey, PA 17033-1240, USA, www.igi-global.com. This series is composed of titles available for purchase individually; each title is edited to be contextually exclusive from any other title within the series. For pricing and ordering information please visit http://www.igi-global.com/book-series/advances-bioinformatics-biomedical-engineering/73671. Postmaster: Send all address changes to above address.

Titles in this Series

For a list of additional titles in this series, please visit:
https://www.igi-global.com/book-series/advances-bioinformatics-biomedical-engineering/73671

Attractors and Higher Dimensions in Population and Molecular Biology Emerging Research and Opportunities
Gennadiy Vladimirovich Zhizhin (Russian Academy of Natural Sciences, Russia)
Engineering Science Reference • copyright 2019 • 232pp • H/C (ISBN: 9781522596516) • US $165.00 (our price)

Computational Models for Biomedical Reasoning and Problem Solving
Chung-Hao Chen (Old Dominion University, USA) and Sen-Ching Samson Cheung (University of Kentucky, USA)
Medical Information Science Reference • copyright 2019 • 353pp • H/C (ISBN: 9781522574675) • US $275.00 (our price)

Medical Data Security for Bioengineers
Butta Singh (Guru Nanak Dev University, India) Barjinder Singh Saini (Dr. B. R. Ambedkar National Institute of Technology, India) Dilbag Singh (Dr. B. R. Ambedkar National Institute of Technology, India) and Anukul Pandey (Dumka Engineering College, India)
Medical Information Science Reference • copyright 2019 • 340pp • H/C (ISBN: 9781522579526) • US $365.00 (our price)

Examining the Causal Relationship Between Genes, Epigenetics, and Human Health
Oscar J. Wambuguh (California State University – East Bay, USA)
Medical Information Science Reference • copyright 2019 • 603pp • H/C (ISBN: 9781522580669) • US $295.00 (our price)

Expert System Techniques in Biomedical Science Practice
Prasant Kumar Pattnaik (KIIT University (Deemed), India) Aleena Swetapadma (KIIT University, India) and Jay Sarraf (KIIT University, India)
Medical Information Science Reference • copyright 2018 • 280pp • H/C (ISBN: 9781522551492) • US $205.00 (our price)

For an entire list of titles in this series, please visit:
https://www.igi-global.com/book-series/advances-bioinformatics-biomedical-engineering/73671

IGI Global
DISSEMINATOR OF KNOWLEDGE

701 East Chocolate Avenue, Hershey, PA 17033, USA
Tel: 717-533-8845 x100 • Fax: 717-533-8661
E-Mail: cust@igi-global.com • www.igi-global.com

Table of Contents

Detailed Table of Contents

Recent advancement in wearable technology has created a huge impact in healthcare delivery and clinical diagnosis. Remote access of physiological, vital parameters from patients and improvement in their day-to-day quality of life were the significant indicators due to this availability of wearable technology. Though wearable physiological monitoring systems for long-term monitoring of Electro cardiogram (ECG) were developed at high-cost involvement, there is a huge need for such technology for resource-constrained settings, at a low cost. This chapter suggests a wearable ECG monitoring system by making use of single channel textile sensors for screening of cardiac episodes. The proposed Cardiac signal framework (CARDIF) with chest textile-based sensors ensures the required qualitative signal for clinical assessment and the evaluation of fidelity measures confirms its suitability for early screening of cardiac episodes. The proposed CARDIF framework involves low-cost design without sacrificing the required clinical diagnosis requirement and can be extended for long-term, continuous monitoring in resource-constrained settings.

Minimally invasive otorhinolaryngology surgery uses a system that consists of an endoscope, microscope, high-resolution display, and several surgical tools to perform procedures of the Ear, Nose and Throat (ENT) up to the upper Oesophagus. The complexity, and number of systems used, forces the surgeon to focus on multiple factors rather than exclusively on the procedure. This chapter focuses on the development of a system integrating the endoscopic feed with a Mixed Reality (MR) headset. For that, the visual data stream from an endoscopy system is integrated with an MR head-mounted device. An application was developed using Unity, Visual Studio, and Windows 10 SDK. The application also had the ability to access pre-operative images through its Graphical User Interface, and was integrated with the endoscopic feed wirelessly over a local area network. The application was tested in an educational abdominal phantom. The goal was to streamline the surgeon's focus more on the patient and to provide access to pre-operative images for in-procedure comparison at their fingertips.

This chapter aims to provide an overview of recent studies in the field of biomedical nanotechnology, which is described as the combination of biology and nanotechnology. The field includes innovations such as the improvement of biological processes at the nanoscale, the development of specific biomaterials, and the design of accurate measurement devices. Biomedical nanotechnology also serves areas like the development of intelligent drug delivery systems and controlled release systems, tissue engineering, nanorobotics (nanomachines), lab-on-a-chip, point of care, and nanobiosensor development. This chapter will mainly cover the biomedical applications of nanotechnology under the following titles: the importance of nanotechnology, the history of nanotechnology, classification of nanostructures, inorganic, polymer and composite nanostructures, fabrication of nanomaterials, applications of nanostructures, the designs of intelligent drug delivery systems and controlled release systems, bioimaging, bioseparation, nano-biomolecules, lab-on-a-chip, point of care, nanobiosensor development, tissue engineering and the future of biomedical nanotechnology.

We don't doubt for a moment that we are conscious, but what is 'Consciousness'? Understanding consciousness, its nature, and characteristics has remained a hard problem for several centuries. While philosophers, neuroscientists, physicists, psychologists, and psychiatrists grapple with this hard problem, clinicians are in need of a practical way to 'measure' consciousness (or its surrogate). Determining whether a patient is conscious or not, and measuring the degree of consciousness, could be critical and potentially life-saving in a clinical scenario. In this chapter, we will review recent scientific approaches for modelling and measuring consciousness, and their clinical applications with an emphasis on a host of issues (theoretical, philosophical, methodological, technological, & clinical) and challenges that need to be satisfactorily and convincingly addressed going forward.

The term chronic kidney disease (CKD) refers to the malfunction of the kidney and its failure to remove toxins and other waste products from blood. Typical symptoms of CKD include color change in urine, swelling due to fluids staying in tissue, itching, flank pain, and fatigue. Timely intervention is essential for early recognition of CKD as it affects more than 10 million people in India. This chapter suggests a decision tree-based data mining framework to recognize CKD from Non chronic kidney disease (NCKD). Data sets derived from open source UCI repository was considered. Unlike earlier reported work, this chapter applies the decision rules based on the clustered data through k-means clustering process. Four cluster groups were identified and j48 pruned decision tree-based automated rules were formatted. The performance of the proposed framework was evaluated in terms of sensitivity, specificity, precision, and recall. A new quantitative measure, relative performance, and MCC were introduced which confirms the suitability of the proposed framework for recognition of CKD from NCKD.

Electromyogram (EMG) signals are commonly used by doctors to diagnose abnormality of muscles. Manual analysis of EMG signals is a time-consuming and cumbersome task. Hence, this chapter aims to develop an automated method to detect abnormal EMG signals. First, authors have applied the improved eigenvalue decomposition of Hankel matrix and Hilbert transform (IEVDHM-HT) method to obtain the time-frequency (TF) representation of motor unit action potentials (MUAPs) extracted from EMG signals. Then, the obtained TF matrices are used for features extraction. TF matrix has been sliced into several parts and fractional energy in each slice is computed. A percentile-based slicing is applied to obtain discriminating features. Finally, the features are used as an input to the classifiers such as random forest, least-squares support vector machine, and multilayer perceptron to classify the EMG signals namely, normal and ALS, normal and myopathy, and ALS and myopathy, and achieved accuracy of 83%, 80.8%, and 96.7%, respectively.

Infant cries are referred as the biological indicator where infant distress is expressed without any external stimulus. One can assess the physiological changes through cry characteristics that help in improving clinical decision. In a typical Neonatal Intensive Care Unit (NICU), recognizing high-risk and low-risk admitted preterm neonates is quite challenging and complex in nature. This chapter attempts to develop pattern recognition-based approach to identify high-risk and low-risk preterm neonates in NICU. Four clinical conditions were considered: two Low Risk (LR) and two High Risk (HR), LR1- Appropriate Gestational Age (AGA), LR2- Intrauterine Growth Restriction (IUGR), HR1-Respiratory Distress Syndrome (RDS), and HR2- Premature

Rupture of Membranes (PROM). An overall cry unit of 800 (n=20 per condition) was used for the proposed study. After appropriate pre-processing, Bark Frequency Cepstral Coefficient (BFCC) was estimated using three methods. Schroeder, Zwicker and Terhardt; and Transmiller; and a non-linear Support Vector Machine (SVM) Classifier were employed to discriminate low-risk and high-risk groups. From the simulation results, it was observed that sensitivity specificity and accuracy of 91.47%, 91.42%, and 92.9% respectively were obtained using the BFCC estimated for classifying high risk and low risk with SVM classification.

Breast Cancer (BC) is the leading cause of death in women, worldwide. The Eastern Cooperative Oncology Group (ECOG) Performance Status (PS) of BC can be studied using HRV measures. The main purpose of this chapter is to give an insight to clinicians via HRV measures with respect to age to make them understand the PS of patients. Data from 114 BC patients was segregated into two age groups, G1 (20 to 40 years) and G2 (41 to 75 years). The 5-minute electrocardiogram of the subjects was taken and HRV measures were extracted. One-way ANOVA with Posthoc Tukeys' HSD test was done. Triangular Index, Ratio of standard deviation of poincare plot perpendicular to the line of identity to the standard deviation along line of identity, Detrended Fluctuation Analysis descriptors, Approximate Entropy, Sample Entropy and Correlation Dimension significantly decreased from ECOG0 to 4 and from G1 to G2. The sympathetic activity increased with vagal withdrawal as age advanced.

In this chapter, motor imagery (MI) based brain-computer interface (BCI) is introduced incorporating the explanation of key components required to design a practical BCI device. Its application to the medical and nonmedical sector is discussed in detail.

In the experimental study, a feature extraction method using time, frequency, and phase analysis of Motor imagery EEG is presented. For the classification of MI task, EEG signals are decomposed using a dual-tree complex wavelet transform (DTCWT) and then time, frequency, and phase features are extracted. The validation of the proposed method is conducted using BCI competition IV dataset 2b. A Support vector machine (SVM) classifier is used to perform the classification task. Performance of the proposed method is compared with the standard feature extraction methods. The proposed scheme achieved a larger average classification accuracy of 82.81% which is better than that obtained by other methods.

Retinal disease/condition examination is one of the significant areas of the medical field. A variety of retinal abnormality assessments based on fundus image-assisted trials are widely proposed by the researchers to examine the parts of the retina. Recently, traditional and soft computing-based approaches are executed to inspect the optic disc and the blood vessels of the retina to discover disease/damages. This work implements (i) A two-phase methodology based on Jaya Algorithm (JA) and Kapur's Entropy (KE) thresholding and level-set segmentation for the optic disc evaluation and (ii) JA-based Multi-scale Matched Filter (MMF) for the blood vessel assessment. During this analysis, various benchmark datasets such as RIM-ONE, DRIVE, and STARE are considered. The experimental study substantiates that JA-assisted retinal picture examination offers better results than other related existing methodologies.

Malignant melanoma has caused countless deaths in recent years. Many calculation methods have been created for automatic melanoma detection. In this chapter, based on the traditional concept of shape signature and convex hull, an improved boundary description shape signature is developed. The convex defect-based signature (CDBS) proposed in this paper scans contour irregularities and is applied to skin lesion classification in macroscopic images. Border irregularities of skin lesions are the predominant criteria for ABCD (asymmetry, border, color, and diameter) to distinguish between melanoma and nonmelanoma. The performance of the CDBS is compared with popular shape descriptors: shape signature, indentation depth function, invariant elliptic Fourier descriptor (IEFD), and rotation invariant wavelet descriptor (RIWD), where the proposed descriptor shows better results. Multilayer perceptron neural network is used as a classifier in this work. Experimental results show that the proposed approach achieves significant performance with mean accuracy of 90.49%.

Preface

The constantly changing landscape of current practices in healthcare creates a need for knowledge resources that will empower professionals, academic educators, researchers, and industry consultants all over the globe. *Biomedical and Clinical Engineering for Healthcare Advancement* is a dynamic reference source that will meet these needs by exploring the latest coverage on all aspects of healthcare applications driven by the adoption of new technologies from different fields, covering topics such as telemedicine applications, artificial intelligence, image-guided surgery, medical imaging techniques, and bionics.

This reference source is arranged into 11 chapters contributed by global experts, drawing on their experiences, observations, and research surrounding bioimaging, biosensors, and robotics. A brief description of each chapter can be found in the following paragraphs.

In Chapter 1: "A Wearable ECG Monitoring System for Resource-Constrained Settings" proposed by Uma Arun (M.S. Ramaiah Institute of Technology, India) and Natarajan Sriraam (M.S. Ramaiah Institute of Technology, India) provide a summary of how recent advancements in wearable technology have created a huge impact in healthcare delivery and the ability for clinicians quickly to diagnose patients. They discuss how wearable monitors will help doctors for early screening of cardiovascular diseases by making wearable textile gel less sensors.

In "ENT Endoscopic Surgery and Mixed Reality: Application Development and Integration" proposed by Elmer Gomes Ataide (Otto-von-Guericke-Universität, Germany), Holger Fritzsche (Otto-von-Guericke-Universität, Germany), Marco Filax (Otto-von-Guericke-Universität, Germany), Dinesh Chittamuri (Otto-von-Guericke-Universität, Germany), Lakshmi Potluri (Otto-von-Guericke-Universität, Germany), Axel Boese(Otto-von-Guericke-Universität, Germany) and Michael Friebe (Otto-von-Guericke-Universität, Germany) explore the idea of a minimally invasive otorhinolaryngology surgery that uses a system consisting of an endoscope, microscope, high-resolution display and several surgical tools to perform procedures of the ear, nose and throat (ENT). The authors propose the development of a system integrating the endoscopic feed with a mixed reality (MR) headset with the goal to streamline the surgeons focus on the patient and to provide access to pre-operative images for in-procedure comparison at their fingertips.

In "Biomedical Nanotechnology: Why 'Nano'?" by Pinar Çakir Hatir (Istanbul Arel University, Turkey) will examine recent studies in the field of biomedical nanotechnology, which is described as the combination of biology and nanotechnology. Mainly, the author will look at the biomedical applications of nanotechnology and how it is being used in a healthcare setting.

In "Measuring Consciousness in the Clinic" by Nithin Nagaraj (Indian Institute of Science) will review recent scientific approaches for modelling and measuring consciousness, and their clinical applications with an emphasis on a host of issues (theoretical, philosophical, methodological, technological and clinical) and how these challenges must be addressed moving forward.

In "A Decision Tree on Data Mining Framework for Recognition of Chronic Kidney Disease" by Ravindra B. V. (Manipal Academy of Higher Education, India), Sriraam N (M. S. Ramaiah Institute of Technology, India) and Geetha M (Manipal Academy of Higher Education, India) emphasize the classification of chronic kidney disease (CKD) and non-chronic kidney disease (NCKD) using datamining framework and evaluate how the two diseases are different from one another and require different treatments. Additionally, they present new data and frameworks that will be able to help physicians recognize the differences between the two diseases sooner than ever before.

In "Classification of EMG Signals Using Eigenvalue Decomposition-Based Time-Frequency Representation" by Rishi Sharma (Institute of Advanced Technology, India), Mohit Kumar (Vel Tech Rangarajan Dr. Sagunthala R & D Institute of Science and Technology, India) and Ram Pachori (Indian Institute of Technology, India) will explore electromyogram (EMG) signals and explain how clinicians use this test for the diagnosis of abnormality in the muscle. As manual analysis of EMG signals is incredibly time consuming the authors provide an overview of an automated method they have created which detects abnormal EMG signals.

In "Identification of High Risk and Low Risk Preterm Neonates in NICU: Pattern Recognition Approach" by S. Tejaswini (M. S. Ramaiah Institute of Technology, India), Sriraam N. (Ramaiah Institute of Technology, India) and Pradeep G. C. M. (Ramaiah Medical College and Hospital, India) observe an automated means of detecting infant cries in a neonatal intensive care unit (NICU) is proposed and how the infants use their cries to express distress to physicians is exploited. The authors evaluate the infants cries to develop a pattern recognition approach that will identify whether a neonate is currently at low risk (LR) or high risk (HR) condition.

In "Effect of Age on Heart Rate Variability Analysis in Breast Cancer Patients: Heart Rate Variability in Breast Cancer" by Reema Shukla (Birla Institute of Technology, India), Yogender Aggarwal (Birla Institute of Technology, India),

Rakesh Sinha (Birla Institute of Technology, India) and Shreeniwas Raut (HCG Abdur Razzaque Ansari Cancer Center, India) examine breast cancer (BC) and how it is leading cause of death among women. The authors main purpose is to provide clinicians with data on heart rate variability (HRV) and how that affects treatment for women who have been diagnosed with breast cancer.

In "Introduction to Motor Imagery-Based Brain-Computer Interface: Time, Frequency, and Phase Analysis-Based Feature Extraction for Two Class MI Classification" by Nitesh Malan (Banaras Hindu University, India) and Shiru Sharma(Banaras Hindu University, India) present different aspects of a motor imagery (MI) based brain-computer interface (BCI) system. This includes how a BCI system would be used in varying healthcare situations.

In "A Study on the Examination of RGB Scale Retinal Pictures Using Recent Methodologies" by A. Swarnalatha (St. Joseph's College of Engineering, India), V. Rajinikanth (St. Joseph's College of Engineering, India), Palani Thanaraj k. (St. Joseph's College of Engineering, India), V. Rajinikanth (St. Joseph's College of Engineering, India), A. Sheryl Oliver (St. Joseph's College of Engineering, India) and M. Esther Hannah (St. Joseph's College of Engineering, India) identify how new soft-computing advances can help clinicians inspect the optic-disc and the blood vessels of the retina to discover disease and damage that they were previously unable to detect.

In "Classification of Skin Lesion Using (Segmentation) Shape Feature Detection" by Satheesha T. Y. (Independent Researcher, India), Sushmita Udupa (Nagarjuna College of Engineering and Technology, India) and Guru Raj Murthugudde (Sri Venkateswara College of Engineering, India) investigate malignant melanoma and how new developments in convex defect-based signature (CDBS) can help physicians detect and classify skin lesions as melanoma or nonmelanoma faster than ever before.

The wide-ranging coverage of this publication provides insight to a greater understanding of all topics, research, and discoveries pertaining to clinical engineering in healthcare. Furthermore, the contributions included in this publication will be instrumental in the development of knowledge offerings in this field. This academic reference will motivate readers to further contribute to the recent findings in this vast field, creating possibilities for additional research and discovery into the future of innovation.

Chapter 1
A Wearable ECG Monitoring System for Resource-Constrained Settings

Uma Arun
Center for Medical Electronics and Computing, M. S. Ramaiah Institute of Technology, India

Natarajan Sriraam
https://orcid.org/0000-0003-3790-3900
Center for Medical Electronics and Computing, M. S. Ramaiah Institute of Technology, India

ABSTRACT

Recent advancement in wearable technology has created a huge impact in healthcare delivery and clinical diagnosis. Remote access of physiological, vital parameters from patients and improvement in their day-to-day quality of life were the significant indicators due to this availability of wearable technology. Though wearable physiological monitoring systems for long-term monitoring of Electro cardiogram (ECG) were developed at high-cost involvement, there is a huge need for such technology for resource-constrained settings, at a low cost. This chapter suggests a wearable ECG monitoring system by making use of single channel textile sensors for screening of cardiac episodes. The proposed Cardiac signal framework (CARDIF) with chest textile-based sensors ensures the required qualitative signal for clinical assessment and the evaluation of fidelity measures confirms its suitability for early screening of cardiac episodes. The proposed CARDIF framework involves low-cost design without sacrificing the required clinical diagnosis requirement and can be extended for long-term, continuous monitoring in resource-constrained settings.

DOI: 10.4018/978-1-7998-0326-3.ch001

INTRODUCTION

Cardiovascular diseases (CVDs) tops the foremost reason for death all over the world according to the survey reported by World Health Organization (WHO).In 2018 million people died due to CVDs, Stroke and coronary heart diseases contribute significantly for the cause of death. Hence there is a huge need to monitor cardiac activities continuously and to identify the potential risk at an earlier stage. Wearable technology and computing showed a promising clinical diagnosis tool due to its ability to monitor the physiological vital parameter continuously as well as for long-term monitoring.

For Biomedical research community, design and developing ubiquitous physiological monitoring system for resource constrained settings is quite challenging. Electrocardiogram (ECG) signals are considered as the vital biomarker to assess and monitor the cardiac activities. Heart and circulatory system disorders are the major causes of death all over the world according to World Health Organization (WHO) (Kirstein .T. et al.,2002). The main reasons are obesity, intensive consumption of salty and oily foods, stress, lack of exercise and genetic factors. The number of cardiologists per patient having heart disease is very less. Due to this, the heart-related diseases increase and mortality rate is very high. Long-term monitoring and consistent medical observation could help in reducing mortalities (Rantanen et al., 2001). Keeping in mind the importance of heart rate variability towards assessing the cardiovascular-pulmonary functionalities, wearable mode gains its importance for home centric applications.

The development of gel less textile-based electrodes gained importance in the recent years for wearable computing applications due to its rapid conductive properties between the skin surfaces and less prone to artifacts motion. The selection of textile materials for such application merely depends on the material's durability, reusability and launder ability (Grancaric et al., 2017).

In recent years, many wearable physiological monitoring systems are being used for real-time healthcare monitoring. The wearable systems combine high-tech components and wearable devices. The smart wearable system includes sensors, actuators and communication equipment. Early detection of vital conditions of patients is possible using these wearable healthcare systems (Norstebo et al., 2003)

Electrocardiogram is a bio-signal from which the electrical action of the heart is observed. ECG measurements are performed using Ag/AgCl electrodes.(Constant .J et al.,1997) (Uma Arun et al.,2016). But these electrodes are not used directly as contact cannot be maintained with skin (Pola & Vanhala). So, conductive gel was applied to patients before attaching Ag/AgCl electrodes. These electrodes create an itching sensation on the skin during long-term usage. Other issues were that the disposable electrodes could not be reused, and preparation of the skin was time-consuming (Ocha et al., 2008)

All these problems were avoided by using textile electrodes which ensured continuous and long-term monitoring with repeatability. The textile electrodes were designed by making use of conductive yarn with a fabric material (Ueno et al., 2007). They acted as a capacitor along with skin and sensor. The conductivity was improved by skin humidity and body sweat. The textile electrode materials are typically synthetic, for example, polyester or polyamide. They endure abrasion very well, absorb moisture only a little and dry fast. The textile electrodes are good for long time measurement, because they do not irritate skin. In addition, they are light weight, ductile and washable. The impedance of electrode-skin interconnection, is 1-5 $M\Omega/cm^2$ for textile electrodes. (Kannaian et al., 2013)

This specific pilot study proposes a wearable ECG monitoring system for resource-constrained settings. A cardiac signal framework referred as CARDIF is proposed which comprises of textile-based conductivity sensor with an analog front end amplifier and a reconfigurable real time processor. Single channel lead I configuration was considered. The performance of the proposed wearable system was evaluated qualitatively and quantitatively.

RELATED BACKGROUND

A brief review on wearable sensors for remote health monitoring was reported (Majumdar et al., 2017). Winokar et al. (2013) have designed a low power wearable ECG monitoring for long-term continues cardiac activities assessment. The five electrodes user driven wearable system confirms its suitability for clinical usage after the experimental study evaluation results.

Gjoreski et al. (2014) proposed a system that makes use of ECG sensor and accelerometer for Telehealth application. The user's typical day-to-day activities were assessed to recognize the vital parameters such as heart rate and respiratory rate and accelerometer data were Correlated with cardiac episodes .The robustness of the proposed system was evaluated quantitatively and qualitatively.

A mobile phone-based, ultra-low-power remote ECG monitoring has been proposed (Hadizadeh et al., 2019).The proposed work emphasized on removal of motion artifacts by appropriate signal processing algorithm. A lightweight, wearable ECG system was designed. For the wearable system-mobile phone interface, appropriate design considerations for BLE were taken into account with factors such as minimum and maximum connection interval, slave latency and connection supervision timeout multiplier were calculated. The system was found to be robust during the experimental study where hear signals were assessed during intense physical activities. Attempts are under consideration towards detection of arrhythmia for the proposed wearable mobile phone applications.

A smart multiple-patient remote monitoring with IOT framework was proposed (Spano et al., 2016). ECG prototype sensor with low energy, low cost solutions was suggested for smart home integrated applications. The IOT platform with the smart home grid configuration found to be quite durable and realizable for real-time patient remote monitoring applications.

A specific methodology has been proposed to improve the quality of synthesized ECG for wireless ECG monitoring applications (Tomasic et al., 2013).The fidelity and statistical measures confirms the suitability of synthesized ECGs with that of target 12-lead ECGs. The study further confirms that much focus need to be given in the quality of ECGs rather on the wireless body electrode positions.

Valchinov et al. (2014) have presented a wearable ECG system for health and sports monitoring. Dry Contact electrode was used for recording of ECGs.

Shih-Hong et al. (2017) have proposed a Wearable, Wireless Multi-parameter monitoring system to evaluate the cardiopulmonary functionalities. The study integrated the walking functionalities with real-time physiological parameters. The results showed the dynamic changes which were found suitable towards developing assistive tools.

Rossi et al. (2015) have designed a low power bio impedance module for wearable system. For impedance measurement, breathing and cardiac activities were considered and the testing was performed. The simulation results showed the suitability of the proposed module for wearable applications.

STUDY DESIGN

In the present study, knit jersey conductive fiber material was used as textile conductive sensor. The fabric was made of 63% cotton, 35% silver yarn and 2% spandex. The proposed material is very soft, matte and perfect wearable with double sided interfacing. This conductive fabric had different resistance in each direction. It had 46Ω per foot across the rows and 460Ω per foot across the columns. The textile material which had less impedance was made to contact with the skin. Two numbers of 5”x2” rectangle pieces were joined by keeping the low impedance side outside and high impedance side inside. Then, a medical-grade button was snapped in between the textile material, so that the button would not make any contact with the skin. The textile material provided a contact with the skin on one side. On the other side, the snapped medical-grade button was connected to the sensor. It was stitched using a conductive thread and attached with a Velcro to form a wrist band.

Three wrist bands of same size were stitched and attached to right arm, right wrist and left arm. Figure 1 shows the implementation of textile electrode as a wrist band.

The skin-electrode contact impedance measurement was done. The arrangement of textile and disposable electrodes for the measurement of contact impedance is shown in Figure 2. All the contact impedance was lying below 5 MΩ, which was necessary for the textile material to be used as the sensing electrode. So, the textile material could be used as an electrode on par with disposable electrode.

Figure 1. Textile electrodes

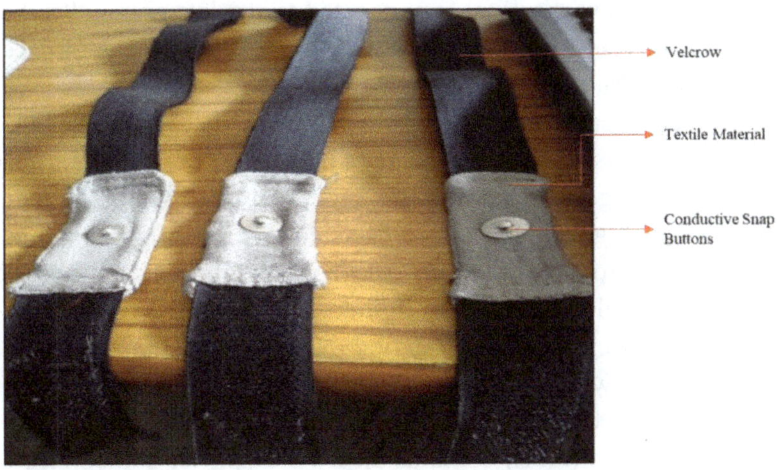

Figure 2. Arrangement of textile electrode and disposable electrodes

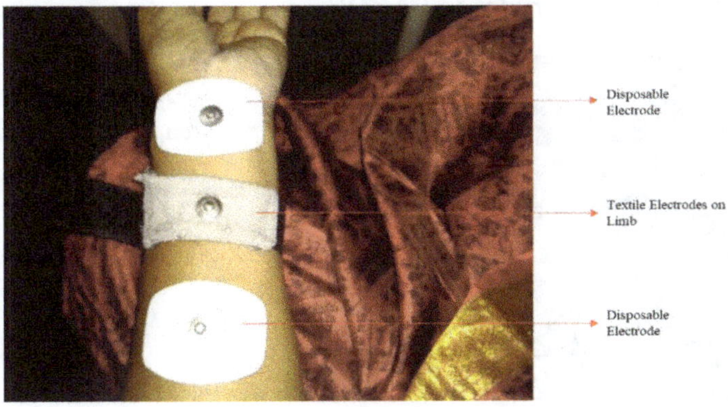

CHEST ELECTRODES

The textile electrodes were connected in the chest as shown in the Figure 3. Here right chest was connected to –ve terminal and left chest was connected to the +ve terminal with right abdomen acts as a reference. This arrangement of the electrodes were in accordance with the Einthoven's triangle. The two chest electrodes were interconnected by a Velcro and the lower one was connected by another adjustable Velcro.

LIMB ELECTRODES

The textile electrodes were connected in single channel in the limb .The entire setup is shown in the Figure 4 for lead I, where the right arm is connected to –ve terminal of the electrode. The +ve terminal is connected to the left arm and right wrist is connected to the reference. The arrangement of the electrodes were in accordance with the Einthoven's triangle.

The arrangement of cardiac signal recording framework (CARDIF) block diagram with textile electrode is shown in the Figure 5. In the CARDIF setup an analog front end (AFE) and reconfigurable input output processor was used.

The output of analog front end was connected to a reconfigurable input/output real time embedded processor. The processor was connected to a host computer through USB and wireless. It was configured in Lab VIEW platform to acquire analog signal and process it. It was a digital data and stored in MS-Excel format. The signal processing was implemented using Lab VIEW virtual instrumentation block sets with the real time processor.

The analog front end (AFE) contains an ECG amplifier and connected to the textile electrodes to measure ECG signal.

Figure 3. Textile chest electrodes in CARDIF

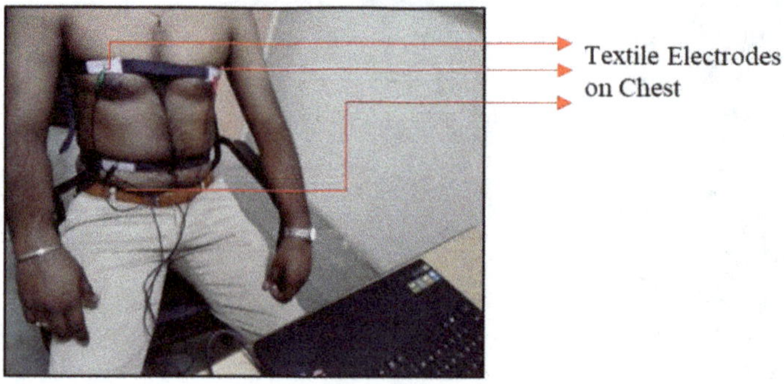

Figure 4. Set up of limb electrodes in Lead I configuration

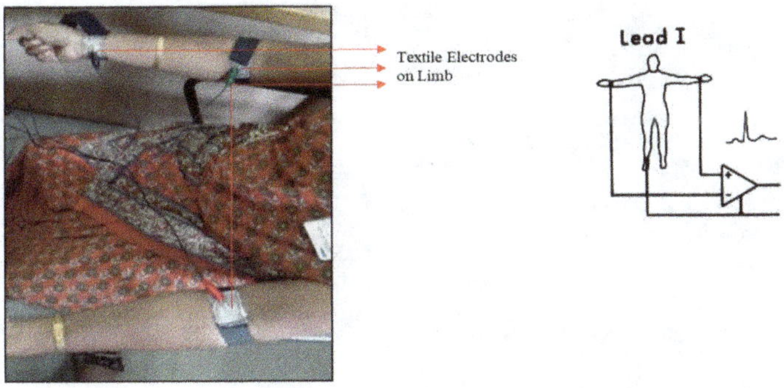

Specifications of Sensor Node-Analog Front End:

Offset ~1.00 V (±0.3 V)
Gain 1 mV body potential / 1 V sensor output

The processor was wired with the system to display the parameters. The output ECG waveform was also displayed simultaneously. The signals were stored in a thumb drive for further processing.

Data was collected from 68 healthy male and female subjects of 18 to 50 years with BMI of 23.11 Kg/m^2 (average). In addition, the physical examination was done for all subjects to know the health condition .The subjects accepted voluntarily for ECG recording and given the written consent form. The subjects were instructed before to avoid alcohol and smoke within the past 24 hours of ECG recording. The subjects with obesity and female with pregnancy or phase of menstrual cycle were excluded from the experiment. The ECG data was recorded for thirty minutes by using CARDIF in sitting condition. Due ethical clearance was obtained from Ethical Board of M. S. Ramaiah Medical College before the commencement of the study. The experiment setup is shown in Figure 6.

Figure 5. CARDIF block diagram

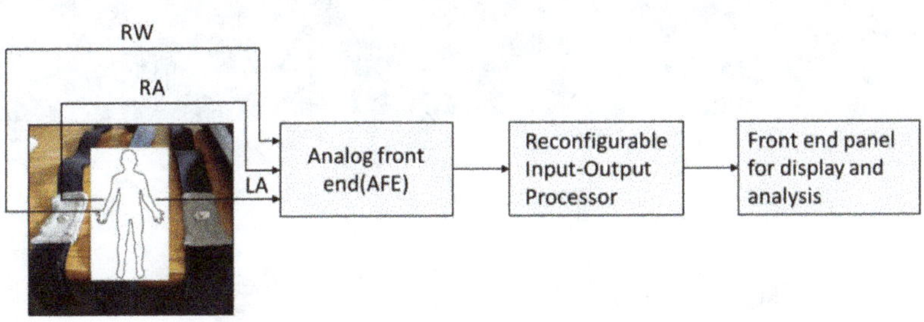

Figure 6. Experiment Setup of CARDIF

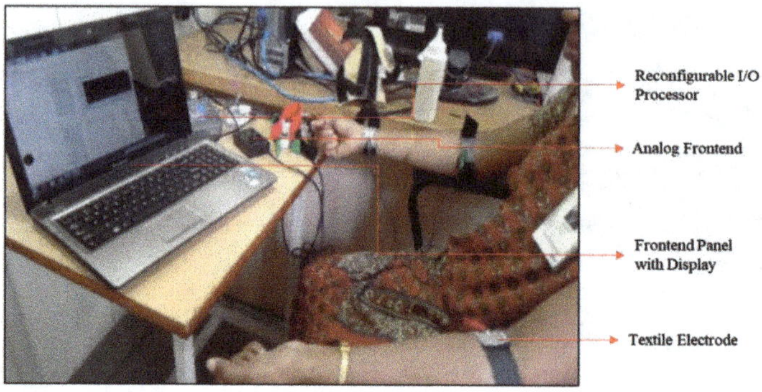

QUALITATIVE AND QUANTITATIVE ASSESSMENTS

The qualitative assessment was done from the visual inspection of the ECG output, available in the front panel of the display and analyzer. The ECG output available is shown in Figure 7.

Baseline wander is a low frequency artifact in the ECG that arises from breathing, electrically charged electrodes and subject movement. The original or raw ECG and after application of baseline wandering removal on raw ECG are shown in Figure 8.

Figure 7. ECG ouput from front panel display and analyser

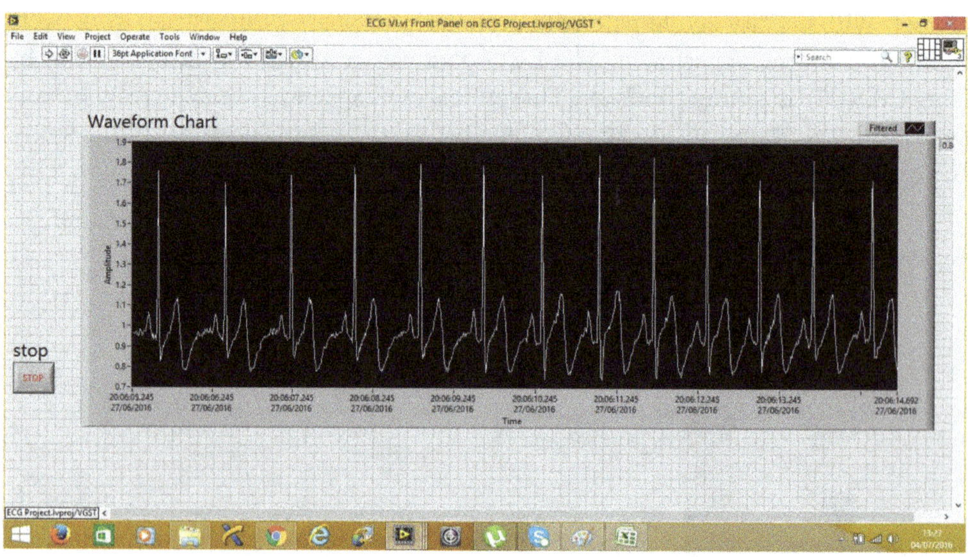

Figure 8. Raw ECG before and after baseline wandering process

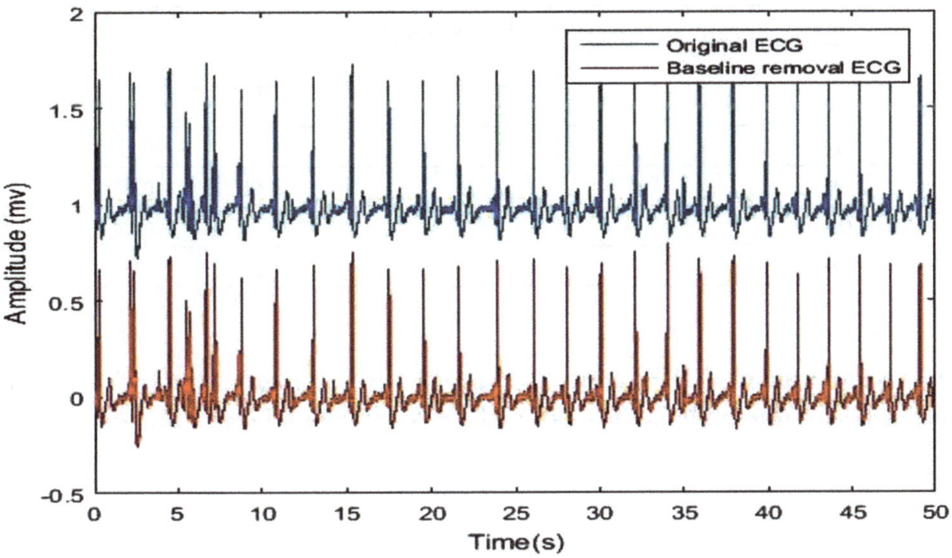

The performance of the textile limb and chest electrodes were compared by finding the parameters for the cardiovascular system using MAT LAB. Different important parameters were estimated from chest and limb as shown in Table 1. BPM is nothing but, number of beats per minute, SNR is the signal to noise ratio in dB and RR interval is the difference between the two consecutive R waves in seconds. The result shows that there was improvement in signal to noise ratio when using chest electrodes as compared to the ratio obtained using limb electrodes.

The duration of various components of ECG such as P, QRS, T, PR, QT and RR from Ag/AgCl electrode and textile electrodes were reported in Table 2.

PSD is the power spectral density plotted against frequency. A sample waveform of ECG output and PSD are shown in Figure 9 and 10.

The quantitative assessment was done by statistical analysis of the ECG signal obtained from both limb and chest electrodes. The procedure was done for the same

Table 1. Results of textile limb and chest electrodes

Parameter	Limb Electrode	Chest Electrode
BPM	80.96	83.06
SNR in dB	-20.08	-25.32
RR Interval (sec)	0.65	0.81

Table 2. Values of components of ECG from Ag/AgCl electrode and textile electrodes

Wave	Reference Electrode (Ag/AgCl)	Textile Electrodes
P	0.06 s	0.04 s
QRS	0.06 s	0.05 s
T	0.14 s	0.16 s
PR	0.12 s	0.10 s
QT	0.36 s	0.32 s
RR	0.84 s	0.68 s

subjects from the CARDIF set up. The box plot was drawn for the BPM and RR interval taken from both the methods and are shown in Figures 11 and 12.

Figure 9. ECG

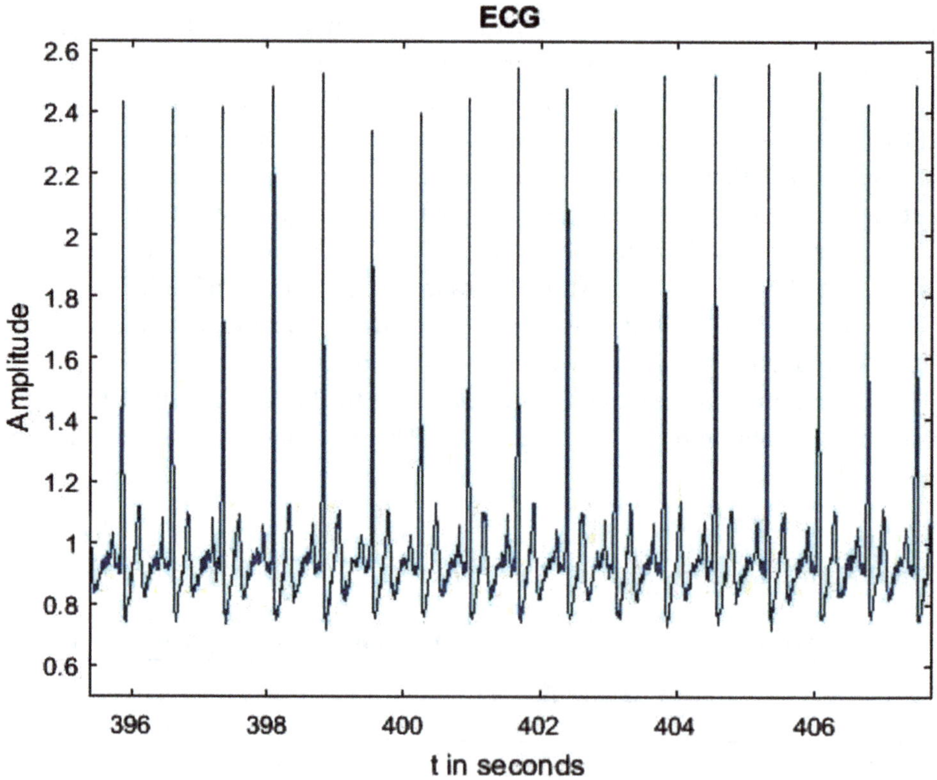

Figure 10. PSD

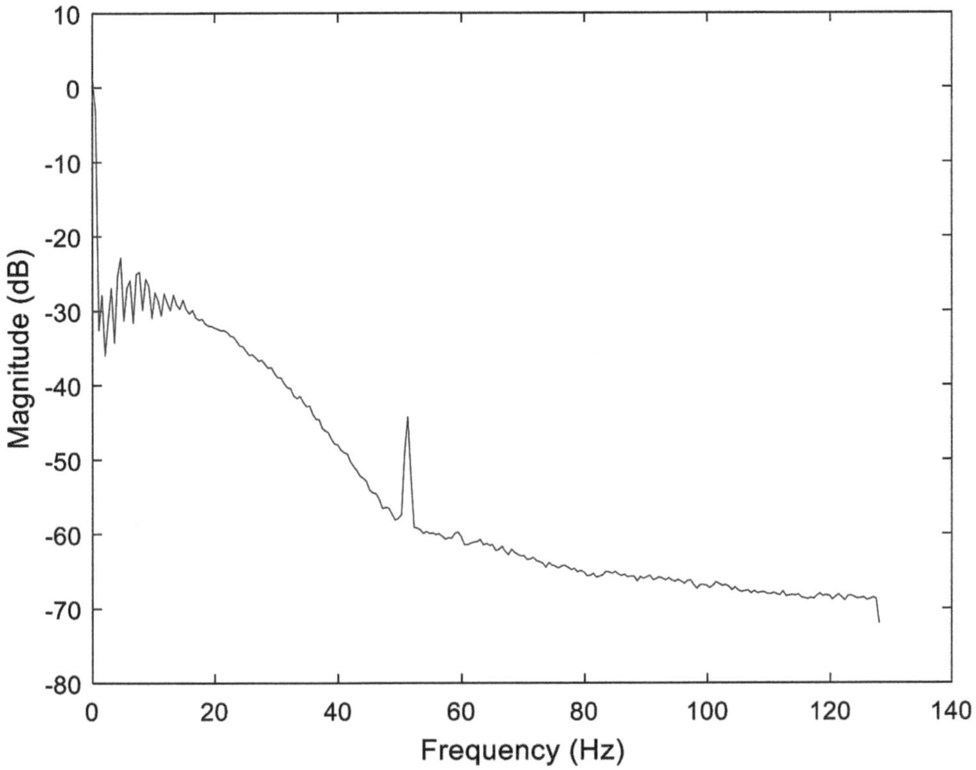

The result shows that the BPM obtained when using chest electrodes are same as compared to the BPM obtained using limb electrodes. And the RR interval obtained from both the methods were within the standard values.

DISCUSSION

Suresh et al (2012) have developed a low cost 3 lead wireless wearable ECG devices for mobile applications. The complexity of design methods includes usage of wet surface electrodes, blue tooth enabling function, limited storage functionalities of the microcontroller. The design proposed by Spano et al.,(2016) with low power wearable settings suffered severely in terms of design, cost involvement and access of digital data remotely without losing the diagnostic requirement. The arrangement of real time electrocardiogram signals obtained using textile based electrodes by T. Kannaian et al .,(2013)was complex and not a portable system. In Textile based inductive sensor, proposed by Sun Ok Gi et al. (2015), a non-contact sensor was

Figure 11. Box plot of BPM from chest and limb

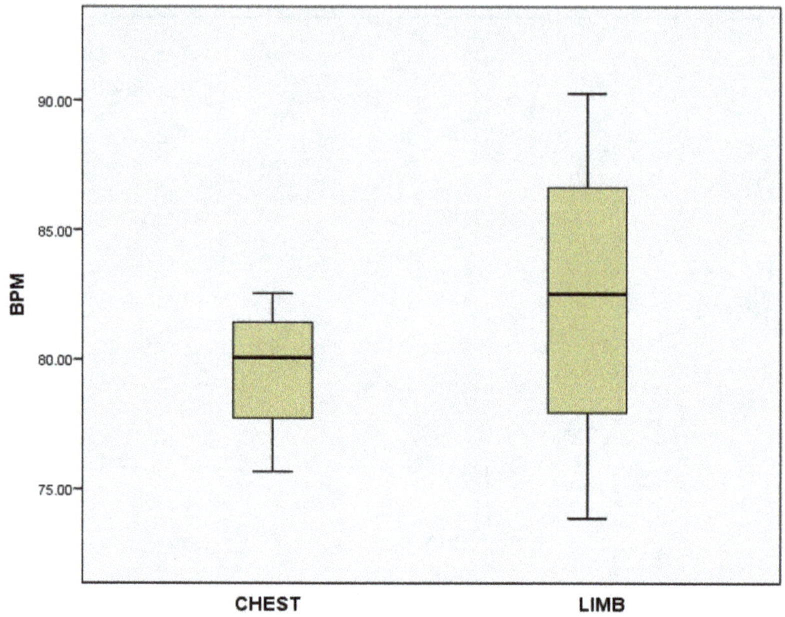

Figure 12. Box plot of RR Interval from chest and limb

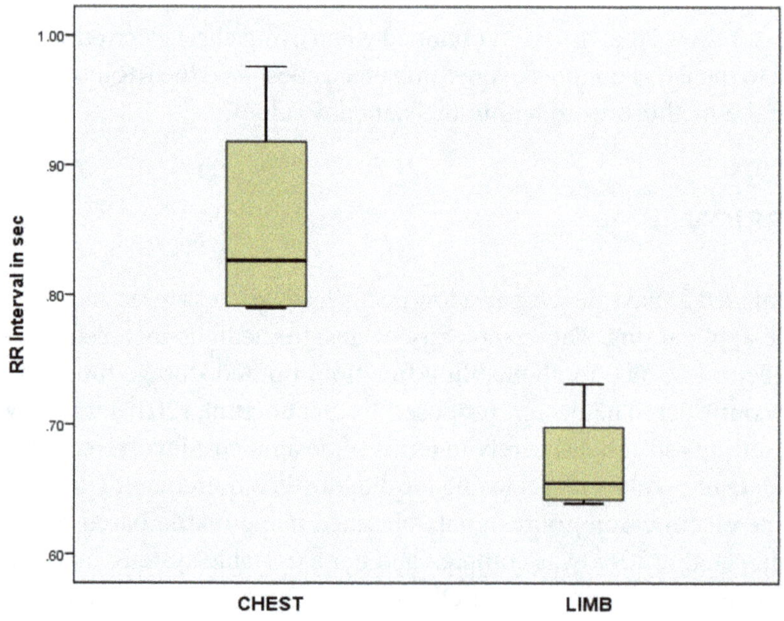

used with magnetic induced conductivity principle. There was a time lag between the ECG signal taken from coil compared to the signal taken from the other sensor. The proposed method was found to be very simple, portable and no time lagging for the data acquisition. Hence it can be used in resource-constrained settings. Clinical validation using the current set up is undergoing which provides better scope for introducing this proposed modality on resource-constrained settings for screening.

CONCLUSION

Development of wearable technology to provide quality healthcare delivery has taken up good shape in recent years. This specific study showed a pilot work on design and development of single channel textile-based sensors for continuous recordings of ECG. The proposed setup referred as "CARDIF" comprised of wearable textile sensors with a front-end amplifier and real time processor to collect the ECG recordings continuously. The single channel chest and limb recordings were assessed qualitatively and quantitatively. The results were quite promising and can be extended to resource-constrained settings for early screening of cardiac episodes through analysis of continuous ECG recordings.

ACKNOWLEDGMENT

This research work was supported by the Department of Bio-Technology (DBT), Government of India. (Grant Number: BT/PR14751/MED/32/422/2015)

REFERENCES

Akbulut, F. P., & Akan, A. (2018). A smart wearable system for short term cardiovascular risk assessment with emotional dynamics. *Measurement, 128*, 237–246. doi:10.1016/j.measurement.2018.06.050

Alesanco, A., & Garcıa, J. (2010). Clinical Assessment of Wireless ECG Transmission in Real-Time Cardiac Telemonitoring. *IEEE Transactions on Information Technology in Biomedicine, 14*(5), 1144–1152. doi:10.1109/TITB.2010.2047650 PMID:20378476

Arun, U., Sriraam, N., & Avvaru, S. (2016, October). Study and investigation of continuous cardiac monitoring using vernier EKG with myRIO processor. In 2016 International Conference on Circuits, Controls, Communications and Computing (I4C) (pp. 1-4). IEEE.

Castelletti, S., Dagradi, F., Goulene, K., Danza, A. I., Baldi, E., Stramba-Badiale, M., & Schwartz, P. J. (2018). A wearable remote monitoring system for the identification of subjects with a prolonged QT interval or at risk for drug-induced longQT syndrome. *International Journal of Cardiology, 266*, 89–94. doi:10.1016/j.ijcard.2018.03.097 PMID:29887480

Constant, J. (1997). *Essentials of Learning Electrocardiography: A Complete Course for the Non-Cardiologist.* New York, NY: Parthenon Pub Group.

Di Rienzo, M., Vaini, E., & Lombardi, P. (2018). Development of a smart garment for the assessment of cardiac mechanical performance and other vital signs during sleep in microgravity. *Sensors and Actuators. A, Physical, 274*, 19–27. doi:10.1016/j.sna.2018.02.034

Fung, E., Järvelin, M. R., Doshi, R. N., Shinbane, J. S., Carlson, S. K., Grazette, L. P. ... Peters, N. S. (2015). Electrocardiographic Patch Devices and Contemporary Wireless Cardiac Monitoring. *Frontiers in Physics, 6*, 149. doi:10.3389/fphys.2015.00149 PMID:26074823

Fuhrhop, S., Lamparth, S., & Heuer, S. A. (2009). Textile Integrated Long-Term ECG Monitor with Capacitively Coupled Electrodes. *Proc. of the IEEE BioCAS* (pp. 21–24). 10.1109/BIOCAS.2009.5372095

Gjoreski, H., Rashkovska, A., Kozina, S., Lustrek, M., & Gams, M. (2014). Telehealth using ECG sensor and accelerometer. In *Proceedings of the 2014 37th International Convention on Information and Communication Technology, Electronics and Microelectronics (MIPRO).* doi:10.1109/mipro.2014.6859575

Grimnes, S., & Martinsen, G. (2008). *Bioimpedance and Bioelectricity Basics.* London, UK: Academic Press.

Hadizadeh, E., Rabbani, R., Azizi, Z., Barekatain, M., Hakhamaneshi, K., Khoram, E., & Fotowat-Ahmady, A. (2019). Ultra Low-Power System for Remote ECG Monitoring.

Kannaian, T., Neelaveni, R., & Thilagavathi, G. (2013). Design and development of embroidered textile electrodes for continuous measurement of electrocardiogram signals. *Journal of Industrial Textiles, 42*(3), 303–318. doi:10.1177/1528083712438069

Kirstein, T., Cottet, D., Grzyb, J., & Tröster, G. (2002, October). Textiles for signal transmission in wearables. In *Proc. ACM of First Workshop on Electronic Textiles (MAMSET 2002)*, San Jose, CA.

Li, S.-H., Lin, B.-S., Wang, C.-A., & Yang, C.-T. (2017). Design of wearable and wireless multi-parameter monitoring system for evaluating cardiopulmonary function. *Medical Engineering & Physics*, *47*, 144–150. doi:10.1016/j.medengphy.2017.06.009 PMID:28684215

Li, S.-H., Lin, B.-S., Wang, C.-A., Yang, C.-T., & Lin, B.-S. (2017). Design of wearable and wireless multi-parameter monitoring system for evaluating cardiopulmonary function. *Medical Engineering & Physics*, *47*. doi:10.1016/j.medengphy.2017.06.009

Majumder, S., Mondal, T., & Deen, M. (2017). Wearable sensors for remote health monitoring. *Sensors, 17*(1), 130. doi:10.339017010130

Norstebo, C. A. (2003). Intelligent Textiles, Soft Products. *Journal of Future Materials.*

Ocha, V., Seromenho, R., Correia, J., Mascioletti, A., Picano, A., & Goncalves, G. (2008). Wearable computing for patients with coronary diseases. *Proc. of the IEEE Int. Conf. Automation, Quality Testing, Robotics*, 3, pp. 37–42. doi:10.100710916-015-0272-9

Pola, T. & Vanhala, J. (2007). Textile Electrodes in ECG Measurement. In 2007 3rd International Conference on Intelligent Sensors, Sensor Networks and Information.

Rantanen, J., Vuorela, T., Kukkonen, K., & Ryynänen, O. (2001). Improving human thermal comfort with smart clothing. *Proceedings of the 2001 IEEE Systems, Man and Cybernetics Conference*.10.1109/ICSMC.2001.973012

Rossi, S., Pessione, M., Radicioni, V., Baglione, G., Vatteroni, M., Dario, P., & Della Torre, L. (2015). A low power bioimpedance module for wearable systems. *Sensors and Actuators. A, Physical.* doi:10.1109/ICSMC.2001.973012

Spano, E., Di Pascoli, S., & Iannaccone, G. (2016). Low-Power Wearable ECG Monitoring System for Multiple-Patient Remote Monitoring. *IEEE Sensors Journal*, *16*(13), 5452–5462. doi:10.1109/JSEN.2016.2564995

Susurla, S., Krishna Kumar, R., & Kamakoti, V. (2012). Portable Low Cost 3 Lead Wireless Wearable ECG Device. *IFMBE Proceedings*, *39*. doi:10.1007/978-3-642-29305-4_349

Tomasic, I., Frljak, S., & Trobec, R. (2013). Estimating the Universal Positions of Wireless Body Electrodes for Measuring Cardiac Electrical Activity. *IEEE Transactions on Biomedical Engineering*, *60*(12), 3368–3374. doi:10.1109/TBME.2013.2276291 PMID:23925363

Ueno, A., Akabane, Y., Kato, T., Hoshino, H., Kataoka, S., & Ishiyama, Y. (2007). Capacitive sensing of electrocardiographic potential through cloth from the dorsal surface of the body in a supine position: A preliminary study. *IEEE Trans. Biomed. Eng.*, *54*(4), 759–766.

Valchinov, E., Antoniou, A., Rotas, K. & Pallikarakis, N. (2014). Wearable ECG System for Health and Sports Monitoring. doi:10.13140/2.1.2281.4406

Webster, J. G. (1998). *Medical Instrumentation: Application and Design*. New York, NY: John Wiley & Sons.

Winokur, E. S., Delano, M. K., & Sodini, C. G. (2013). A wearable cardiac monitor for long-term data acquisition and analysis. *IEEE Transactions on Biomedical Engineering*, *60*(1), 189–192. doi:10.1109/TBME.2012.2217958

Xu, P. J., Zhang, H., & Tao, X. M. (2008). Textile-structured electrodes for electrocardiogram. *Textile Progress*, *40*(4), 183–213. doi:10.1080/00405160802597479

Zhang, J., Cao, Y., Qiao, M., Ai, L., Sun, K., Mi, Q., ... Wang, Q. (2018). Human motion monitoring in sports using wearable graphene-coated fiber sensors. *Sensors and Actuators A. Physica A*, *274*, 132–140.

Zou, C., Qin, Y., Sun, C., Li, W., & Chen, W. (2017). Motion artefact removal based on periodical property for ECG monitoring with wearable systems. *Pervasive and Mobile Computing*, *40*, 267–278.

Chapter 2
ENT Endoscopic Surgery and Mixed Reality:
Application Development and Integration

Elmer Jeto Gomes Ataide
Otto-von-Guericke-Universität, Germany

Holger Fritzsche
Otto-von-Guericke Universität, Germany

Marco Filax
Otto-von-Guericke Universität, Germany

Dinesh Chittamuri
Otto-von-Guericke Universität, Germany

Lakshmi Sampath Potluri
Otto-von-Guericke Universität, Germany

Michael Friebe
https://orcid.org/0000-0002-8624-0800
Otto-von-Guericke Universität, Germany

ABSTRACT

Minimally invasive otorhinolaryngology surgery uses a system that consists of an endoscope, microscope, high-resolution display, and several surgical tools to perform procedures of the Ear, Nose and Throat (ENT) up to the upper Oesophagus. The complexity, and number of systems used, forces the surgeon to focus on multiple factors rather than exclusively on the procedure. This chapter focuses on the development of a system integrating the endoscopic feed with a Mixed Reality (MR) headset. For that, the visual data stream from an endoscopy system is integrated

DOI: 10.4018/978-1-7998-0326-3.ch002

with an MR head-mounted device. An application was developed using Unity, Visual Studio, and Windows 10 SDK. The application also had the ability to access pre-operative images through its Graphical User Interface, and was integrated with the endoscopic feed wirelessly over a local area network. The application was tested in an educational abdominal phantom. The goal was to streamline the surgeon's focus more on the patient and to provide access to pre-operative images for in-procedure comparison at their fingertips.

INTRODUCTION

Otorhinolaryngology or Ear Nose and Throat (ENT) Endoscopic surgery is a procedure that allows for the examination of the middle ear, nasal passage and openings to the sinus and the upper section of the oesophagus through the nasal and oral cavities. ENT Endoscopic surgery benefit the patient in terms of minimal invasiveness as only the natural orifices (Ear, nose and throat) are used. This causes less pain in patients and decreases the amount of time taken for them to heal from the surgical procedure (Sher 1986). ENT endoscopy is a form of image guided minimal invasive surgery for observation, manipulation and resection resulting in minimal trauma and faster patient recovery (Reuter 1999). As per iData Research Inc. in the year 2018 there were close to 23.8 million Endoscopic surgeries performed in the United States. An ENT Endoscopic surgery is performed with the aid of an endoscope, microscope, high resolution display and endoscopic tools. There is little integration between these instruments, which makes navigation cumbersome. The high-resolution display provides a rather limited field of view of the patient anatomy and its placement causes the surgeon to divert attention from the patient to the screen. (Nicolau 2011). Additionally, this involves the constant movement of the surgeon's head and can cause discomfort as the number of procedures a day increases. Image guided surgeries often require the surgeon to have ready access to the patient's pre-operative images. Currently this is achieved by accessing the images on an individual system located within the surgical suite. The introduction of an integrated system that reduces the stress on surgeons and enables the access of pre-operative images could prove to be beneficial as well as time-efficient. These are some of the pains or unmet clinical needs that were observed during surgery visits and clinical input. Mixed reality (MR) in the surgical suite could be a solution to address these issues. Mixed reality helps bridge the gap between the unmodelled real world and a virtual modelled environment (Fullum, 2009) (Figure 1). It allows

Figure 1. Simplified representation of a 'Virtuality Continuum' depicting the position of AR
(Milgram 1994)

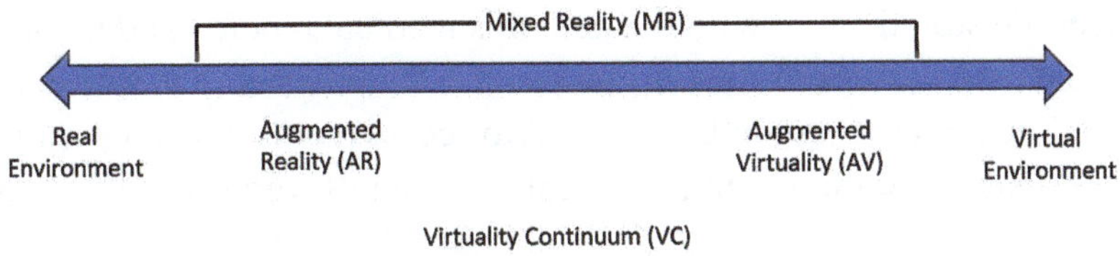

for seamless integration of virtual objects into the real world. The virtual aspect has the capability to react to human movements and gestures (Rodrigues 2017).

The introduction of MR in the health sector is not recent, but is gaining increased researchers' interest now. One of the first instances of its use could be a surgical simulator proposed and developed by Satava (1993). The developed application was meant to be a training tool for surgeons to practice surgeries before performing them on actual patients. Khor et. al. (2016) discussed that augmented reality (AR), virtual reality (VR) and mixed reality have all become vital components of today's surgical workflow. These technologies have proposed uses in terms of anatomical evaluations in medical education, broadcasting and recording surgery, telementoring and remote education of medical professionals. They also stated that this technology comes with its own set of limitations. AR, VR and MR devices have limited usage due to their shorter battery lives and lower computational capacities that may result in latency in video feeds during surgeries in addition to lack of privacy and confidentiality. Sielhorst et al. (2004) provided a review of visualization of medical images using MR. Prior work has also described the use of AR with a see-through, head-mounted display to render ultrasound images directly onto a patient's body[10]. Philip J. Edwards et al. (2004) in their work analyzed the use of AR in surgical guidance for microscope-assisted guided interventions. It was found that AR surgical guidance particularly with respect to depth perception is clinically effective and improves the outcome of the procedure. AR has also been used to improve laparoscopic partial nephrectomy. The system developed was able to navigate and superimpose virtually created images and real-time images in porcine renal units (Teber et al., 2009).

The presented literature suggests that AR, VR and MR are tools that enhance surgical performance in various aspects. During ENT endoscopic surgeries the surgeon is subjected to long hours in the surgical suite. Endoscopic surgeries comprise of a large number of tools that the surgeon has to use in addition to which he has to look at the patient as well as the screen on which the endoscopic feed is displayed. This tends to be a tiring and painstaking process and results in the surgeon being fatigued after some time. Pre-operative images play a vital role in surgical planning and the surgery itself. Sometime it so happens that the surgeon needs to go back and refer to his initial plans made with the help of these pre-operative images. E.g. tumor location, location of the incision, region to be excised, etc. As mentioned, these images are stored along with the patient's medical records and are accessible through a separate system in the surgical suite. This means that if and when the surgeon needs to refer to these images, he has to access them on this separate system. Through the analysis of these unmet clinical needs and several surgical visits it was concluded that the development of an application that integrates a mixed reality headset and an endoscopic system while also providing the possibility to access patient pre-operative images directly through this application could serve as a solution to the problem statement.

This article speaks about the approach and the steps taken to achieve a successful integration between an endoscopic system and an MR headset and enable the surgeon with the ease of access to patient pre-operative images during an ENT endoscopic surgery and improve overall surgical efficiency. The work presented herein is a result of the clinical need expressed by the surgeons and their input has been a valuable aspect to the project's design and development.

METHODS

This work employed the Biodesign innovation process to carry out the complete development (Figure 2). The Biodesign process dictates that in order to carry out efficient medical device development three key iterative steps need to be followed. a) Identify Unmet Clinical Needs, b) Invent concepts and solutions and c) Implement these concepts and solutions to address the unmet clinical needs (Krummel et al.,

Figure 2. The Biodesign process for innovating medical technologies

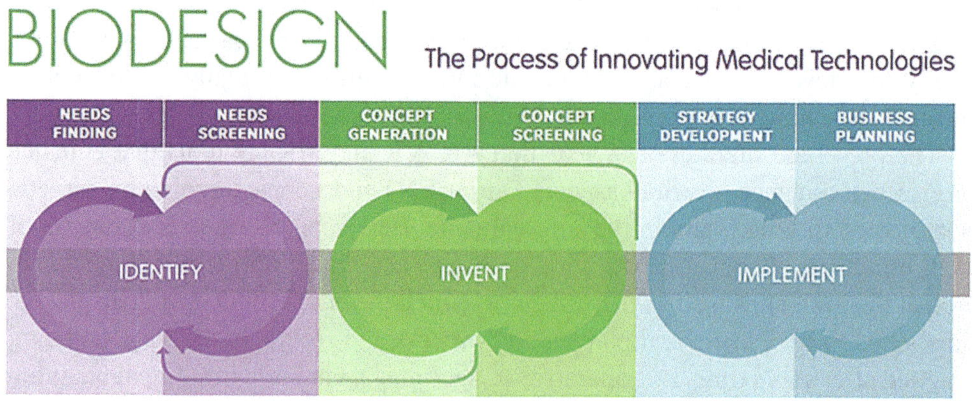

2017). For the identification of the unmet clinical needs experienced by the surgeons, surgical visits to the ENT department were conducted. This was repeated multiple times to get a better understanding of the pains experienced by the surgeon. The pains experienced by the surgeons were used to define the sequence of events for the application. This together with the input of the surgeons formed the basis of the invention step. The implementation is seen through the application development and testing that was carried out.

Surgical Visits

Over the course of two months various surgeries were witnessed. A few of which were acoustic neuroma, spasmodic dysphonia and papillary carcinoma (residual tumour removal). These procedures were performed using an endoscopic system and certain pains were highlighted during their courses. In the acoustic neuroma surgery, the surgeon had to excise a tumour developed on the vestibulocochlear nerve. Due to the near microscopic nature of this procedure, the surgeon had to constantly move between performing the surgery and looking at the screen (Figure 3). This was stated to be the main pain of the surgeon.

The spasmodic dysphonia procedure consists of injecting the vocal folds with a Botox solution in order to improve the speech of the patient. Here the surgeon uses an endoscope and a syringe containing the Botox solution. It was noted that the presence of multiple tools during the procedure diverted the surgeon's attention from the display at times. During the removal of the residual papillary carcinoma, the surgeon needed to refer to pre-operative images. In order to do this the surgeon

Figure 3. Placement of the endoscopy display screen in an awkward position during an ENT Endoscopy procedure

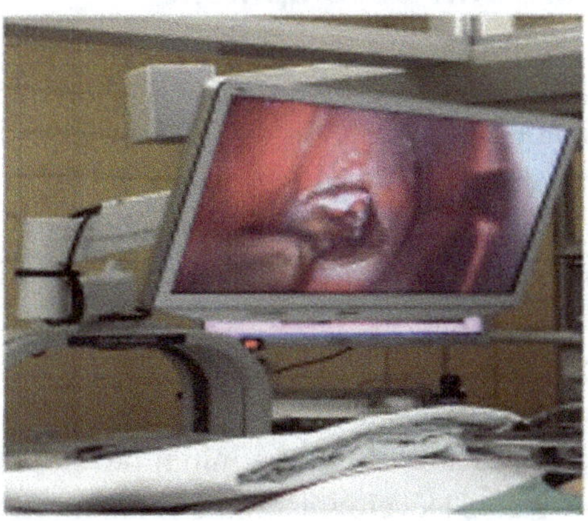

sometimes had to move from his position near the patient and to an additional system in the surgical suite to access the patient's records and view these images. The surgeon stated that in all cases, the option of an MR based heads-up display of the procedure with the access to patient pre-operative images would benefit the surgeon and subsequently with this the patient. These surgery visits helped to understand the need for such a system and aided in the design and development of the system architecture for the application and integration of the endoscopic system with an MR headset.

The integration of the endoscopic system with an MR headset was achieved using the following steps.

- Definition of the sequence diagram and use case diagram
- System architecture and development
- Integration of the MR headset with the endoscopic system

Definition of Sequence of Events

The surgical visits provided the authors with a list of requirements to be used to define the sequence of all possible events that take place (Figure 4).

The initiation of the application is done via its deployment in the MR headset. The application verifies the connection with endoscopic tower through the Stream Catcher. The video stream from the endoscopic tower is displayed on the MR headset through the application when all the connections are intact.

A screenshot can be taken of a desired frame and will be saved in a designated folder. The pre-operative images are imported into the application by clicking on the "PoI button". This would enable the user (surgeon) to compare the real-time image feed with the pre-operative images.

System Architecture and Development

The Mixed Reality application works on a Holographic feature in the Headset. The application is a combination of a Virtual Environment (VE) and a Graphical User Interface (GUI) and was designed and built using Visual Studio & Unity (Integrated Development Environment). The Application was built into a single package as an individual application file with the help of visual studio's built in solution for local machine and remote devices. The VE was developed in Unity and the functionality script was written using C# in Visual Studio and with the help of Windows 10 SDK (Software Development Kit) to enable its features on the MR device.

The Mixed Reality Tool Kit enabled the initial development of a holographic application in Unity Integrated Development Environment (IDE) supporting spatial mapping and understanding. The environment was designed with a selection of a solid black background. The environment helps the user to place the field of view in a fixed position according to the real-world coordinates. The MR headset spatially maps the surrounding environment using a polygonal mesh feature. A 3D holographic plane is represented in the environment and is accessible with the help of the GUI.

Figure 4. Sequence diagram of events

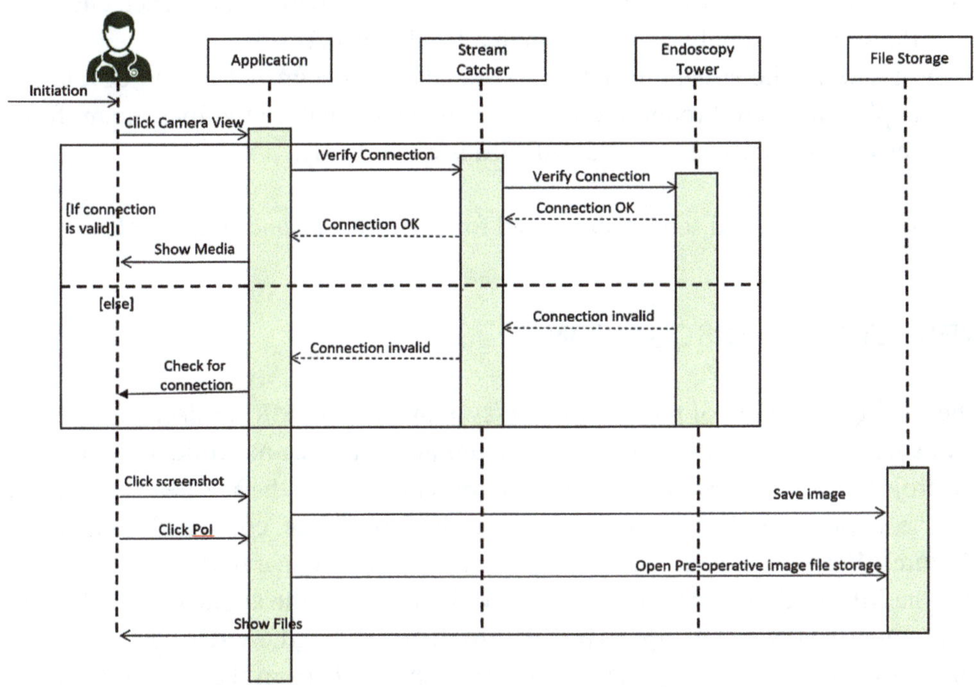

Figure 5. Integration process of endoscopic system with the MR headset

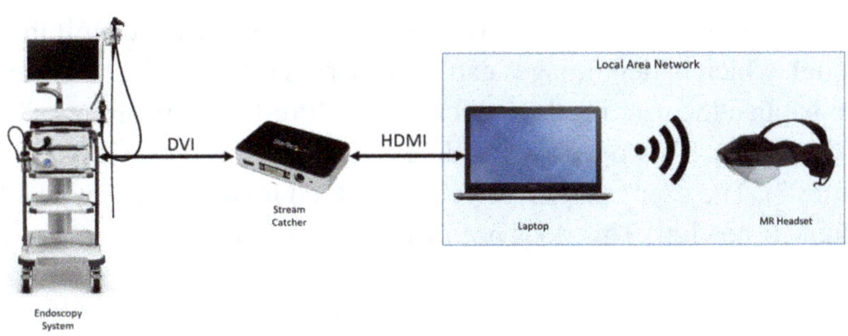

Integration of the MR Headset With the Endoscopic Tower

The integration of the MR headset with the endoscopic tower was performed as follows (Figure 5):

Step 1: The video stream output of the endoscopic tower was set to DVI. The endoscopic tower was connected to the Stream Catcher using a DVI cable.
Step 2: The Stream Catcher was connected to a Laptop using an HDMI cable.
Step 3: The Stream Catcher application settings were changed so that the system protocol was set to HTTP Live Streaming (HLS).
Step 4: The stream button was clicked to initiate the video stream hence enabling the stream of a public URL through a local area network.
Step 5: The public streaming URL generated was recognized by the developed application and through the local area network enables the live stream from the endoscopic system to the MR headset wirelessly.

The application and setup were tested for performance and functionality.

RESULTS AND DISCUSSION

The initial integration of the endoscopic system with the MR headset was carried out using a stream catcher, a laptop and a unique local area network. This enabled the projection of the view from the endoscopic camera onto the MR headset display.

The application is accessed and controlled by voice commands and hand Gestures. Voice commands and hand gestures are the input parameters that are built into the MR headset functionalities. The Main feature of the application is that the endoscopic feed from the surgical procedure is displayed on the MR heads-up display through Unity by accessing the public streaming URL from the Stream Catcher. The endoscopic camera view is seen through the MR headset display. In addition to this, a feature to acquire a screenshot of desired areas is added to the application and can be accessed and controlled via gestures and voice commands.

For the in-procedure comparison of pre-operative images, we built in an access panel through which patient images can be imported into the MR heads up display. For this to happen the user needs to click on the "Pre-Operative Images" button in the GUI (Figure 6). This opens up a file explorer in a system within the surgical suite (Figure 7). The user can then select the desired images that they would like to view in the MR headset. This does not influence the endoscopic view of the user.

Figure 6. Developed application GUI depicting feed from endoscopic system during testing in an educational abdominal endoscopy phantom

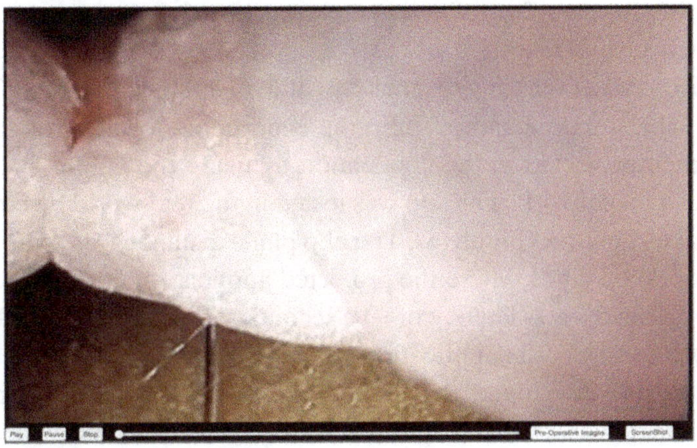

Testing

The initial development and integration with an MR headset was tested at the Innovation Laboratory for Image Guided Therapies Chair of Catheter Technologies (INKA) in Magdeburg, Germany. Initial tests were conducted on an abdominal endoscopy phantom used for educational training along with the Olympus

Figure 7. Developed application GUI depicting access to a file explorer containing pre-operative images during testing in an educational abdominal endoscopy phantom

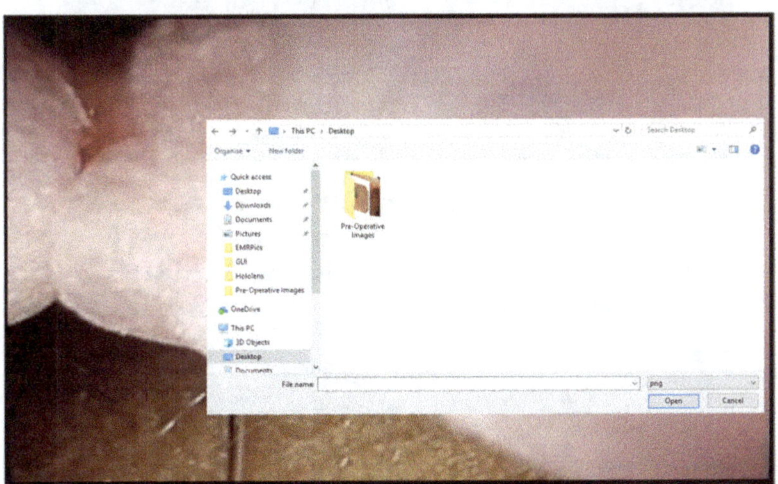

endoscopic system (Olympus Visera). The testing was carried out by students and the development team. Additionally, the application was tested for performance, functionality, interoperability, reliability and security using the Microsoft guidelines for Mixed Reality App Testing.

For the MR headset the target frame rate of the stream was set to 60 frames per second (fps). The stream acquired from the endoscopic tower through the stream catcher was then projected in the application by using the public URL through a common local area network. The app was tested in the real world by employing the environmental test matrix (Figure 8). The clip plane distance was set to 0.85 meters which is the ideal distance where the projected application is viewed comfortably through the MR headset. A latency of ~10 seconds was experienced when viewing the endoscopic stream in the application.

The application developed was functional and appropriately rendered the endoscopic camera view with the option to access files located elsewhere providing the user with effortless access to pre-operative images during the surgery.

CONCLUSION AND FUTURE OUTLOOK

The initial integration of the endoscopic system with a Mixed Reality Headset was possible. The endoscopic view could be integrated with the MR headset. The integration of the MR headset with the endoscopic tower was carried out by first

Figure 8. Example of an environmental test matrix used for the testing of the MR application in the real-world

Category	Sub-category
Light	Brightness
	Color
	Dynamic lighting
	Hologram lighting
Sound	Ambient noise
	Ambient conversation
	Spatial audio
User Movement	Head movement
	Full body movement
	Entering holograms
Physical Environment	Clutter
	Moving items
	Distance
	Incomplete scans
	Surface types

developing the application in Unity, Visual Studio and Windows 10 SDK. The endoscopic feed is captured using the Stream Catcher that is then connected to a laptop. The feed from the Stream Catcher is manifested in the application by sharing a public URL over a local area network. The application GUI enables the user to view the endoscopic stream, capture screen shots and access pre-operative images of patients.

The streamline of the surgeon's focus on the patient and the access to pre-operative images for in-procedure comparison of medical images are the main advantages of the work done. However, there are still a few limitations that need to be addressed such as issues of latency in the endoscopic feed and surgical guidance.

Further testing and refinement of the current application needs to be carried out to address the issue of latency of the endoscopic feed in the application. This could be achieved by using a laptop/computer system with higher computational capabilities or a better internet connection. Testing in a clinical setup would be crucial in improving the overall performance and customizing the application as per the surgeons' need.

Future work would also be to enable the import of medical images that consist of segmented regions of abnormal tissue. Providing the surgeon with a map of the areas that have been investigated with highlighted areas of importance is a feature that would be implemented as well. This would act as a surgical guidance feature and hence aid the surgeon in locating and comparing diseased regions with ease and improve quality of care.

ACKNOWLEDGMENT

We would like to thank all of our clinical partners at the University Clinic Magdeburg, our Cooperation partners from the industry and especially for the support of the state Saxony-Anhalt. There are no conflicts to be reported. This paper does not cover a study and or a program that involves or requires ethical approval.

This research was financially supported by the Federal Ministry of Education and Research (BMBF) in context of the 'INKA' project (Grant Number 03IPT7100X and by EFRE funding in context of the ego.-INKUBATOR program (ZS/2016/09//81061/ IK 01/2015)).

REFERENCES

Bajura, M., & Fuchs, H. (1992). Merging virtual objects with the real world: seeing ultrasound imagery within the patient. In *proceedings of the 19th annual conference on computer graphics and interactive techniques.* (pp. 203-210), New York, NY. 10.1145/133994.134061

Edwards, P. J. & Gleeson, M. (2004). Clinical experience and perception in stereo augmented reality surgical navigation. *Medical imaging and augmented reality lecture notes in computer science, 3150*, 369-376.

Fullum, T., & Gunnarsson, C. (2009). Comparison of the clinical and economic outcomes between open and minimally invasive appendectomy and colectomy: Evidence from a large commercial payer database. *Surgical Endoscopy, 24*(4), 845–853. doi:10.100700464-009-0675-0 PMID:19730950

Khor, W. S., Baker, B., Amin, K., Patel, K., & Wong, J. (2016). Augmented and virtual reality in surgery- the digital surgical environment: Application, limitations and legal pitfalls. *Annals of Translational Medicine, 4*(23), 454. doi:10.21037/atm.2016.12.23 PMID:28090510

Krummel, T. M., Yock, P. G., Zenios, S. A., Brinton, T. J., Kumar, U. N., Watkins, F. T., & Makower, J. (2017). *Biodesign: The process of innovating medical technologies.* Cambridge, UK: Cambridge University Press.

Milgram, P. & Kishino, F. (1994). A taxonomy of mixed reality visual displays. *IEICE Transactions on Information Systems, E77-D.*

Nicolau, S., & Marescaux, J. (2011). Augmented reality in laparoscopic surgical oncology. *Surgical Oncology, 20*(3), 189–201. doi:10.1016/j.suronc.2011.07.002 PMID:21802281

Reuter, M. A., & Reuter, H. J. (1999). *History of Endoscopy: An Illustrated Documentation*. Stuttgart, Germany: Kohlhammer.

Rodrigues, D. G., & Weibel, N. (2017). Exploring mixed reality in specialized surgical environments. In *CHI Conference Extended Abstracts on Human Factors in Computing Systems* (pp. 2591-2598), New York, NY. 10.1145/3027063.3053273

Satava, R. M. (1993). Virtual reality surgical simulator. *Surgical Endoscopy, 7*(3), 203–205. doi:10.1007/BF00594110 PMID:8503081

Sher, A., & Thorpy, M. (1986). Endoscopic observations of obstructive sleep apnea in children with anomalous upper airways: Predictive and therapeutic value. *International Journal of Pediatric Otorhinolaryngology*, *11*(2), 135–146. doi:10.1016/S0165-5876(86)80008-8 PMID:3744695

Sielhorst, T., & Navab, N. (2004). An augmented reality delivery simulator for medical training. In *proceedings of Workshop on Augmented Environments for Medical Imaging-MICCAI Satellite Workshop*, 141, pp. 11–20.

Teber, D., & Rassweiler, J. (2009). Augmented reality: A new tool to improve surgical accuracy during laparoscopic partial nephrectomy? Preliminary in vitro and in vivo results. *European Urology*, *56*(2), 332–338. doi:10.1016/j.eururo.2009.05.017 PMID:19477580

VandenBos, G., Knapp, S., & Doe, J. (2001). Role of reference elements in the selection of resources by psychology undergraduates. Retrieved from http://jbr.org/articles.html

Chapter 3
Biomedical Nanotechnology:
Why "Nano"?

Pınar Çakır Hatır
Istanbul Arel University, Turkey

ABSTRACT

This chapter aims to provide an overview of recent studies in the field of biomedical nanotechnology, which is described as the combination of biology and nanotechnology. The field includes innovations such as the improvement of biological processes at the nanoscale, the development of specific biomaterials, and the design of accurate measurement devices. Biomedical nanotechnology also serves areas like the development of intelligent drug delivery systems and controlled release systems, tissue engineering, nanorobotics (nanomachines), lab-on-a-chip, point of care, and nanobiosensor development. This chapter will mainly cover the biomedical applications of nanotechnology under the following titles: the importance of nanotechnology, the history of nanotechnology, classification of nanostructures, inorganic, polymer and composite nanostructures, fabrication of nanomaterials, applications of nanostructures, the designs of intelligent drug delivery systems and controlled release systems, bioimaging, bioseparation, nano-biomolecules, lab-on-a-chip, point of care, nanobiosensor development, tissue engineering and the future of biomedical nanotechnology.

BIOMEDICAL NANOTECHNOLOGY

Biomedical nanotechnology, which is defined as the combination of biology and nanotechnology, includes innovations like the improvement of biological processes in nanoscale, the development of specific biomaterials, and the design of accurate

DOI: 10.4018/978-1-7998-0326-3.ch003

measurement devices. The design of intelligent drug delivery systems and controlled release systems, tissue engineering, nanorobotics (nanomachines), lab-on-a-chip (LOC), point of care and nanobiosensor development are areas that are focused on the field of biomedical nanotechnology (Gazit, 2013).

How Small is Nano?

The word "nano" comes from the Greek word "nanos" which means "dwarf". A nanometer (nm) refers to one billionth of a meter. To understand the nanoworld better, the units of measure have been defined in Table 1 (Jones, 2005). Size comparisons between very small objects and various examples have been given to clarify the nanoscale (Table 2). For example, a water molecule is about 0.2 nm, DNA is about 2 nm in diameter, proteins are about 1-10 nm, viruses are 10-100 nm, red blood cells are 6000-8000 nm, and a hair is about 100.000 nm.

The Importance of Nanoscale

The concept of "nanotechnology" covers controlling materials at the nanoscale. For instance, the textile materials can be modified to fabricate extraordinary products or drug delivery systems can be manipulated to develop intelligent drug systems. One of the most important reasons why the properties of materials are improved is the surface area-to-volume ratio. As the dimensions of a material decrease, its surface area increases while total volume remains the same (Figure 1). This phenomenon makes nanomaterials exhibit different physical and chemical properties compared to larger particles of the same material. To give an example, when the same amount of sugar cubes and granulated sugar are put in the same amount of water, it is observed that the granulated sugar dissolves much more quickly than the sugar cubes. The reason for this is that the surface area of the granulated sugar is larger than the sugar cubes allowing the granulated sugar to have more contact with the water molecules, therefore the number of sugar molecules interacting with the water molecules is

Table 1. Units of measurements

Unit	Symbol	Explanation
Meter	m	-
Millimeter	mm	1 m = 1,000 mm
Micrometer	μm	1 m = 1,000,000 μm
Nanometer	nm	1 m = 1,000,000,000 nm
Picometer	pm	1 m = 1,000,000,000,000 pm

Table 2. Size of objects

Object	Approximate average size
Tennis ball	100,000,000 nm
Ant	5,000,000 nm
Pencil tip	1,000,000 nm
Beach sand	500,000 nm
Human hair	100,000 nm
A sheet of paper	75,000 nm
A red blood cell	7,000 nm
Bacteria	5,000 nm
Viruses	50 nm
Proteins	4 nm
The diameter of the DNA helix	2 nm
A glucose molecule	1 nm
A water molecule	0.3 nm
The atomic radius of carbon	0.077 nm
The atomic radius of hydrogen	0.032 nm

higher compared to those of sugar cubes. Reducing ingredients into small pieces when cooking, to shorten the reaction time by increasing surface area to volume ratio, can be given as another example. This fact shows that the changes in micro/nanoscale have important consequences in the macro-world. Thus, nanotechnology takes advantage of this fact to gain more control over the matter.

In addition to the high surface area to volume ratio, the quantum mechanics of nanoscale materials change at the nanoscale as well. A nanomaterial does not behave like a bulk material, in the sense that its scale becomes smaller and therefore its properties change significantly. For instance, a gold bar melts at 1064°C while

Figure 1. Surface area/volume ratio

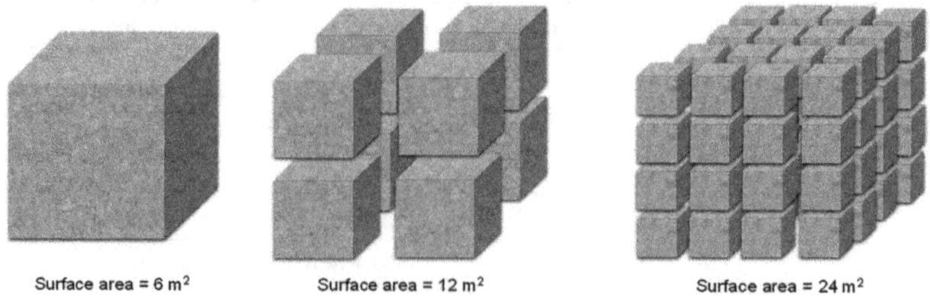

a 20 nm gold nanoparticle melts at 600°C, moreover a 1-2 nm gold nanoparticle melts at room temperature (Yadugiri, 2010). Similarly, gold nanoparticles with different particle sizes give different colors. In ancient times, people benefited from the characteristics of gold without realizing the reason behind it, and used gold nanoparticles in stained glass paintings, especially in church windows. Another example is Wootz steel, which is famous for its greatness and sharpness and is a source of pride for India. Transmission Electron Microscopy (TEM) analyses of the steel have shown that this particular steel has such good properties due to being produced from nanocomposites with carbon nanotubes and cementite wires (Srinivasan, 1997). Unfortunately, this reason was not recognized by researchers at that time. Mayan blue pigment that does not fade for centuries has indigo and white clay particles embedded in nano-sized surface grooves. Finally, local people in Central America have developed glass blades that are 3 nm in diameter and sharper than modern diamond scalpels (Eglash, 2011).

Nanotechnology has become increasingly popular in many areas such as biomedical engineering, tissue engineering, drug delivery systems, etc. For instance, within the field of drug delivery systems, targeted drug delivery systems that are designed especially for treatment of cancer are a hot topic. There are two main reasons for directing the drug molecule to the target: 1) to reduce the side effects of the drug molecule by not affecting the healthy tissue of the body 2) to increase therapeutic effect of the drug molecule by activating it on the diseased tissue. That is to say, drug targeting is not only used for therapeutic purposes but also for diagnostic purposes. For example, a fluorescence-emitting molecule or quantum dot (QD) may be incorporated into the drug delivery system to enhance the imaging sites. Likewise, a magnetic nanosystem can be used for diagnostic/therapeutic applications. Some nanosystems that can be activated by environmental factors such as changing pH, temperature, ion concentration and external factors such as light, magnetic field are attracting more and more attention. Such nanosystems are employed for many biomedical applications, particularly for the development of bioactive biomaterials to be used in tissue engineering.

Additionally, the combination of sensor technology and the nanoworld creates another diagnostic tool, namely nanobiosensor. It is an analytical device containing a biologically active element with a suitable physical transducer to generate a signal measuring as well as quantifying the number of molecules in any sample on a nanoscale. Nanobiosensors consists of two important parts; signal transduction and biorecognition element. The biorecognition components can be enzymes, antibodies, nucleic acids, proteins, microorganisms or tissues, as well as synthetic biodegradable polymer-based organic and inorganic constructs. The primary purpose of nanobiosensors is to detect any biochemical and biophysical signal associated with a particular disease at a single molecule or cell level. Another field in biomedical nanotechnology is "lab-on-a-chip"s (LOC) which refers to the micro/nanochips (circuits) on which one or more laboratory processes are performed simultaneously. LOC devices that are formed by combining microfluidic technology with nanostructures have taken on important roles in biomedical applications. The cost and process time of LOC devices, which require only a small sample volume, are significantly reduced due to the reaction speed. In this regard, LOC nanostructures are opening an important door to the point-of-care devices, a new area for diagnosis and rapid treatment applications.

THE HISTORY OF NANOTECHNOLOGY

The history of nanotechnology dates back to 1959 when Richard Feynman, a physicist, gave a speech at the California Institute of Technology titled as "There's plenty of room at the bottom" (Feynman, 1960). In his speech he talked about the problem of manipulating and controlling things on a small scale. He mentioned that even though a device, with which people can write a prayer on the head of a pin, had been invented, this was a primitive step in the direction he discussed. He emphasized that the point of miniaturization reached in those years was very inadequate, he suggested that more work should be done in this direction. It was during this very speech that, he asked the famous question that enabled scientists to enter the nanoworld: "Why cannot we write the entire 24 volumes of the Encyclopedia Britannica on the head of a pin?" If the head of a pin is magnified 25,000 times, then the area of the head of a pin becomes equal to the area of all the pages of Encyclopedia Britannica. Therefore, it is necessary to write each letter 25,000 times smaller. The resolving power of the eye is about 1/50 of a cm, which is roughly the diameter of one single dot in the encyclopedia. If the diameter of this single dot is decreased by 25,000 times, it will have enough room for around 1000 atoms. By this rough calculation, Feynman concluded that there is enough room on the head of a pin for all volumes of the Encyclopedia Britannica. "There was plenty of room at the bottom". Feynman mentioned that the nanoworld had already been discovered by biologists, however, the only thing they needed was a microscope that was 100 times more powerful than those used. He claimed that if they had more powerful imaging systems, the most important components of the nanoworld of biology, proteins, DNA and RNA and their interactions could be clarified. This fascinating speech opened the door to the world of nano. In 1973 Norio Taniguchi, a professor at the University of Tokyo, began to use the term "nano-technology" for the first time. K. Eric Drexler, an American engineer, published a book called "Engines of Creation: The Coming Era of Nanotechnology" in 1986 and created the field of "molecular nanotechnology". Drexler has adopted the idea that biological molecules can serve as nanomotor, nanomachine, nanowire, nano pump, etc. systems in nanoscale (Gazit, 2013). He wrote a hypothetical end-of-the-world scenario, *Grey goo*, in which the nanomachines self-replicate exponentially, consume all biomass, and they get out of control and take over the world.

In 1981, Gerd Binnig and Heinrich Rohrer from the IBM Research Laboratory in Zurich invented the scanning tunneling microscope (STM), which allowed scientists to see atoms and made the nanoworld visible and controllable for the first time. This invention brought Binnig and Rohrer the Nobel Prize in 1986. Immediately after that, the atomic force microscopy (AFM) was developed by IBM researchers. The development of these microscopes, which allow the observation and manipulation of atoms, has been recognized as a revolution in nanotechnology. In 1990, a team of physicists at IBM used as STM to move 35 xenon atoms and write the letters "IBM" (Eigler, 1990). This event attracted great interest as atomic level manipulation had not been possible until then.

The discovery of carbon-based nanostructures has gained momentum, as the developments in imaging systems have increased and physicists have begun to examine the nanoworld in more details. Nowadays, the building block of organic chemistry is based on carbon. Not only biomolecules such as proteins, nucleic acids, and lipids, but also many industrial products such as nylon, plastic, and Teflon are made of carbon. There are many known allotropic forms of carbon (Figure 2). In 1985, a new class of carbon allotropes, called fullerenes, was discovered. This discovery was accepted as an important step for nanotechnology and brought Curl, Smalley, and Kroto a Nobel Prize in 1996 (Reisner, 2008). The most common of the fullerene class is the buckyball (buckminsterfullerene) which is named after the Canadian Architect R. Buckminster Fuller, because of the resemblance to the architectural structure he designed. The fullerene, which consists of 60 carbons, is spherical, about 1 nm in diameter and exhibits exceptional electrical and thermal conductivity. There are allotropic clusters containing carbon in different numbers. It has also been shown that the modified fullerenes have antiviral effects. Following the discovery of carbon fullerenes, a new form of carbon nanoscale was discovered by Sumio Iijima in 1991 (Williams, 2006). This allotrope, defined as carbon nanotube (CNT), is the elongated form of the C60 fullerenes. One of its important properties is that the ratio of length to diameter is very high (1 nm diameter, 1 mm length). Carbon nanotubes can be single-walled or multi-walled. CNTs with superior mechanical and electrical properties have been regarded as the most durable material available. By isolating a single layer of graphite in 2004, an allotrope of carbon called graphene was discovered. The uniqueness of the graphene brought the scientists who discovered it the Nobel Prize in 2010. Graphene is unique because it is stronger than steel, more conductive than copper and almost invisible as it is both flexible and single-atom thick. The invisibility and conductivity of graphene

Figure 2. Allotropes of carbon

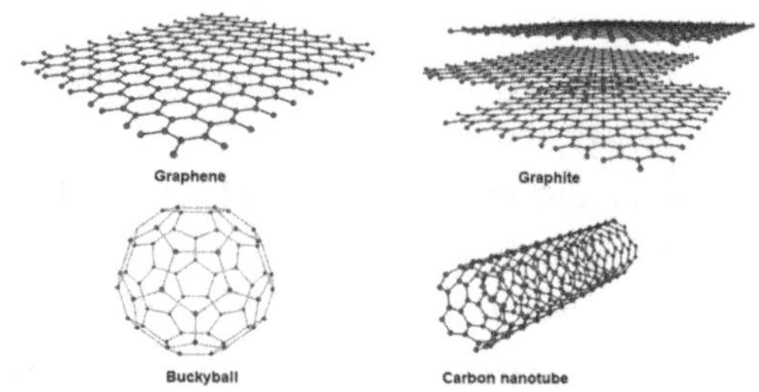

enable it to be used in many applications such as liquid crystal displays, electronic systems and solar batteries.

CLASSIFICATION OF NANOMATERIALS

Over past two decades numerous nanomaterials have been reported, thus various kinds of classifications have been created. One of the most accepted classifications based on the dimensions of nanomaterials was developed by Pokropivny (Pokropivny, 2007). According to this classification, nanomaterials are divided into four different classes based on their number of dimensions. These classes are zero-dimensional (0D), one-dimensional (1D), two-dimensional (2D) and three-dimensional (3D) nanomaterials (Figure 3). Nanoparticles, such as QD, core-shell QDs, nanocapsules belong to the class of 0D nanomaterials. They have been extensively studied in light emitting diodes (LEDs), solar cells, imaging techniques, biosensors and lasers (Tiwari, 2012).

Nanofibers, nanotubes, nanorods, nanowires and hierarchical nanostructures with a diameter of nanometer scale and with a length longer than 100 nm are called as 1D nanostructures. 1D nanostructures can be employed in many biomedical applications. Due to their porous structure and large surface area, the nanofibers can act as a skeleton mimicking the extracellular matrix for the cell attachment and nutrient transport (Xie, 2008). Nanofibers can also be functionalized by proteins, enzymes, and bioactive molecules so that they can be used in biomedical applications such as tissue engineering, the designs of intelligent drug delivery systems and controlled drug release systems. Long and hollow structures such as nanofibers are defined as nanotubes. Nanotubes, which are composed of only carbon are known as CNTs and used in many fields due to their superior mechanical, optical and electrical

Figure 3. Dimensionality classifications of nanostructures

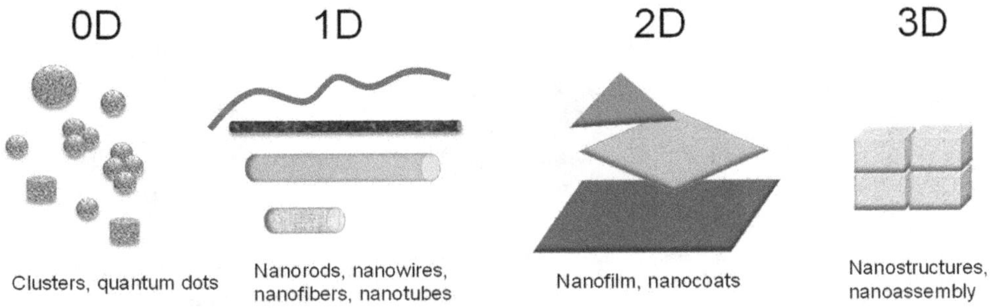

properties. CNTs are often used in biosensor design due to their unique chemical and physical properties such as high surface area/volume ratio, porous structures, small size and functionality (Wang J., 2005). Using CNTs in biosensor applications provides increased sensitivity and reduced detection limits. The high electrical conductivities of CNTs (about 100 times more than copper) allow them to be used as electrochemical transducers.

The 2D nanostructures are nanometer-thick films that they have two dimensions outside of the nanometric size range. The thicknesses of the layers, which can be in length or width in microns or larger, are smaller than 100 nm. These layers are described as nanolayers, nanofilms, nanoplates, nanosheets, nanowalls, and nanodisks.

Nanofilm structures, which are defined as 2D nanostructures, are found in nature as self-assembled structures comprised of various materials (Fakhrullin, 2014). Examples of 2D nanostructures with a thickness of up to 100 nm, which can be very large in width and length, are multi-scale organic-inorganic hybrid constructions such as biopolymer fibers, cell membranes, viruses and hard tissues. The regular nanostructures in nature are usually formed by self-assembly via Van der Waals forces, electrostatic forces or hydrogen bonds. Nowadays, because of the potential applications in biology and medicine, interest in designing 2D films similar to natural nanofilms is increasing. Ultra-thin film structures, also known as nanolayers or nanofilms, provides promising results for biosensors, antimicrobial surfaces, and drug delivery systems. The 2D nanostructures, with the desired thicknesses and properties, are mostly composed of synthetic or natural polymers. As biodegradation rates and mechanical properties can be controlled easily by molecular weights, poly (lactic

Figure 4. Types of nanostructures commonly used in biomedical applications

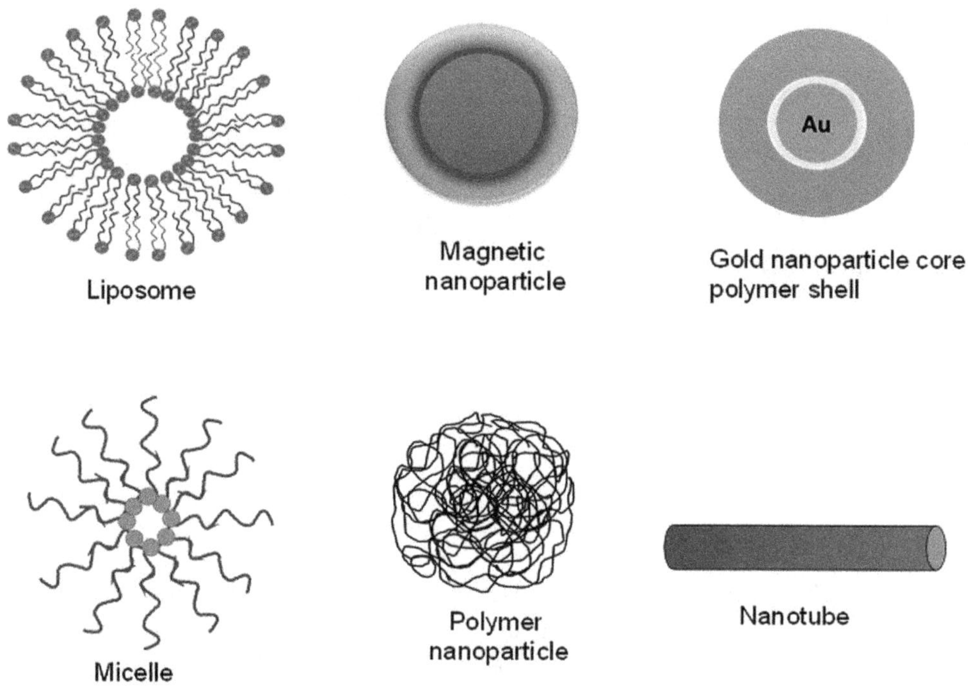

acid-PLA) and poly (lactic-co-glycolic acid-PLGA) are used for many applications. Poly (ether ester) copolymers due to their elasticity, durability and easy processability as well as biopolymers, alginate, chitosan, collagen and polysaccharide derived polymers are also preferred in a wide range of applications (Pérez-Madrigal, 2015).

Three-dimensional nanostructures are multilayer, bulk materials with a controlled structure and morphology.

Inorganic Nanostructures

Nanostructures can be classified as inorganic, organic and composite nanostructures (Zarschler, 2016).As the size of a nanostructure decreases, the surface area/ volume ratio and the number of atoms on the surface increase. The most important advantage of inorganic nanostructures such as iron oxide, silica, gold and QDs is the extraordinary optical and superparamagnetic properties they possess on the nanoscale. Inorganic nanostructures are also used as solid phase supplements in the immobilization of biomolecules such as oligonucleotides, peptides, proteins, and antibodies (Soenen, 2015).

Despite the success in vitro applications of inorganic nanoparticles in the literature, in vivo studies are limited, as extensive toxicity studies are required. Furthermore, for nanoparticles to be used in vivo, their surfaces need to be improved not only for biocompatibility but also for colloidal stability. In vivo, nanoparticles should not cause clustering, chemical degradation or agglomeration.

Polymer Nanostructures

In addition to inorganic nanostructures, polymer nanostructures are also used extensively in biomedical applications. The advantages of polymer nanostructures are their flexibility, shape, controllable size, and the fact that their surfaces can easily be modified. Some polymers, namely smart polymers, respond to environmental conditions such as pH, temperature, ion concentration, enzyme, biomolecules, magnetic fields, and light. Due to their biocompatibility, biodegradability and stability, polymers are often preferred in nanostructure design. Some of the biocompatible polymers commonly used in nanoparticle design include poly (lactic-co-glycolic acid) (PLGA), poly (ethylene glycol) (PEG), poly (N-isopropyl acrylamide) (PNIPAM), chitosan, poly (lactic acid) (PLA), poly (methyl methacrylate) (PMMA).

Hydrogels, a class of smart polymers, are cross-linked hydrophilic polymeric structures that absorb water about 20-40 times of their dry weight (Ward, 2011).

Figure 5. Schematic representation of a liposome

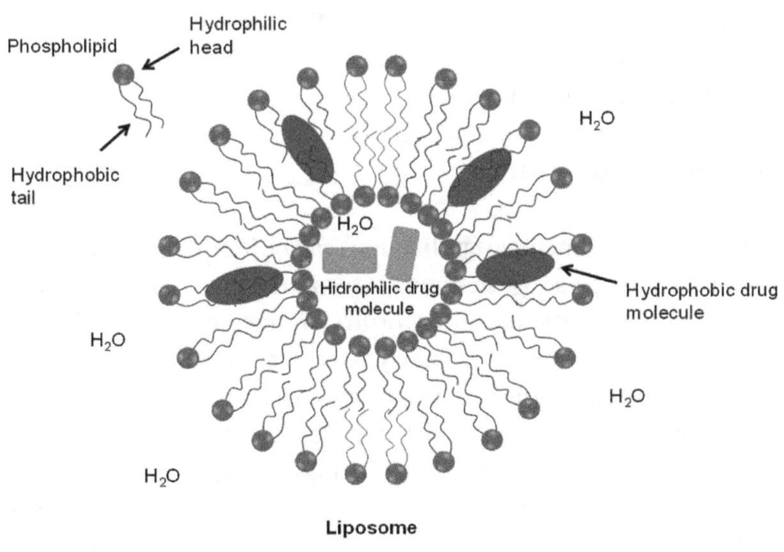

With their porous structures and hydrophilic characters, these polymers, also known as smart gels, are similar to the tissue environment, and can mimic the physical, chemical, electrical and biological properties of the tissues and can be used in biomedical applications such as drug delivery systems, controlled release systems, artificial organs, contact lenses and biosensors.

Molecularly imprinted polymers (MIPs), another intelligent polymeric nano-system, are developed as artificial enzymes and antibodies due to their biorecognition properties (Çakir, 2013). MIPs which are synthesized for the recognition of a specific molecule provide promising results for both diagnostic and therapeutic applications. MIPs can play an important role in the development of intelligent nanosystems as they can recognize biomarker molecules and react accordingly.

Another polymeric nanosystem are liposomes, which are hollow spherical nanostructures consisting of at least one lipid layer (Figure 5). Liposomes consists of phospholipids that form a cell membrane as a single layer or a multilayer (Daraee, 2016). Phospholipids are composed of hydrophilic head and long hydrophobic tail parts and are found as two layers in nature. They form a spherical structure in water resulting from the tail parts escaping from the water and the head parts interacting with the water. The micelle is a monolayer structure, and the liposome is a bilayer. These unique properties of liposomes allow both hydrophobic and hydrophilic molecules to be protected from metabolic processes. As the hydrophobic drug molecules increase water solubility by being delivered in liposomes, they can be used in the design of a targeted drug delivery system. Their biocompatibility is unquestionable because they are formed entirely from natural molecules (cell membrane material). With liposomes, not only drug molecules but also gene carriers can be developed. Liposomes and other nano-carriers can be combined with different recognition elements to develop a targeted delivery system. For instance, liposomes are formed with cationic lipids to interact with negatively charged DNA in the gene carrier and to move towards the anionic cell membrane.

Composite Nanostructures

Nanostructures used in biomedical applications can be inorganic or polymeric as well as composite. Composite nanostructures have a multi-phase structure and improve the properties of the nanostructures they form. Ceramic, metallic, carbon-based and polymeric composite nanostructures may have extraordinary properties. The most frequently encountered nanostructures in multiphase nanostructures are the core-shell nanoparticles. These nanostructures have low toxicity, high biocompatibility, and high interaction with bioactive molecules and also high thermal and chemical stability. Core-shell nanoparticles are generally designed to bind drugs, receptors, and ligands by surface chemistry (Chatterjee, 2014). For instance, a hydrophobic drug can be

Figure 6. Top-down and bottom-up approaches

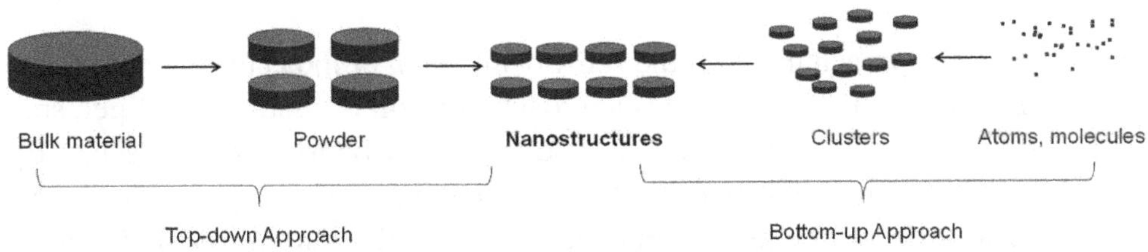

released from the biodegradable polymer layer on the biodegradable polymer, which is degraded by ionic strength, temperature, or pH change after the nanocarrier has been delivered. The core material is important for core-shell nanoparticles, which are used not only for treatment but also for diagnostic procedures. In general, the core material is responsible for the imaging property, whereas biocompatibility and targeting fall into the responsibility of the shell material.

FABRICATION OF NANOMATERIALS

There are two main approaches for the production of nanostructures: 1) the bottom-up approach and 2) the top-down approach (Figure 6). The bottom-up approach is based on the principle of self-organization of molecules and atoms. With this approach, highly complicated structures are obtained starting from molecules and atoms. Examples of this approach are the sol-gel method, spin coating, polymerization reactions, and precipitation reactions, self-assembly methods, and reduction of metallic oxides. In the top-down approach, microscopic structures are broken up and milled to produce nanostructures. This approach, which is based on the gradual reduction of the material until the desired nanostructure appears, can be thought of as a detailed sculpture from a large block of marble (Filipponi, 2013). The adaptation of a pattern produced on a larger scale to a nanoscale can be considered as a top-down approach. All lithographic techniques fall under this approach.

Two main conditions are important for both approaches. These are: production conditions (energy of the electron beam, etc.) and environmental conditions (dustiness of the environment, pollution, etc.). Since both conditions are significant for nanoscale production, nanomaterials are produced in vacuum clean chambers using special production tools.

Bottom-Up Approach

The bottom-up approach includes the self-organization of molecules or atoms. All self-assembly methods fall under this approach. Solvent evaporation, sol-gel, spin coating and polymerization reactions are also considered bottom-up approaches. By using the solvent evaporation method, thermal and ion-assisted evaporation 0D, 1D, 2D and 3D nanostructures can be obtained (Tiwari, 2012). In this method, atomic clusters around the cold-powder collecting surface are formed by homogeneous condensation of evaporated atoms or molecules as a result of the loss of energy through collisions with gas atoms or molecules. The resulting clusters must be removed from the deposition region to prevent aggregation or coalescence of the clusters.

The sol-gel method is a chemical process used mainly for synthesizing metal oxides, ceramic, glass materials and polymer nanoparticles (Arole, 2014). This method involves starting from a solution (or sol) that acts as the precursor for an integrated network (or gel). The advantages of the method are listed as follows; low processing temperature, the homogenous final product and the possibility of synthesizing complex composition materials.

One of the most common techniques used for the fabrication of 2D nanostructures is spin coating. This technique is based on the deposition of very thin uniform films to substrates. The fact that it is a quick and simple procedure, has a broad film thickness that ranges from a few nanometers to a few micrometers makes this technique attractive for the production of 2D nanostructures.

Polymerization processes, particularly radical polymerization processes, involve starting from a simple monomer, hence the name bottoms-up. Precipitation polymerization is a process in which monomers and initiators are completely soluble and initially begins with a homogeneous system in the continuous phase. At the end of the process insoluble polymer nanoparticles are formed and precipitated. Suspension polymerization is a heterogeneous radical polymerization process performed via mechanical agitation to have a homogenous mixture of monomers, organic phase, in a liquid phase, such as water. Followed by polymerization of monomers, nano-/micro-spheres of polymers are formed. Another similar process involves an emulsion of monomer and surfactant in the aqueous phase. Upon the formation of micelles, polymerization takes place, and polymer nano/microparticles are formed inside the micelles. These polymerization processes usually produce spherical nanoparticles unless they are applied on a surface.

Metallic nanoparticles can be fabricated via the reduction of metal complexes by using various precursors, reducing agents and polymeric stabilizers. The most common metallic nanoparticles such as gold, platinum and iron nanoparticles can be synthesized by reduction. It is also possible to produce composite nanoparticles with metallic core and polymer shell by using bottom-up approach.

Top-Down Approach

The top-down approach is based on breaking of bulk materials to produce nanostructures. This technique can be thought of as obtaining a detailed sculpture from a large block of marble. Lithographic techniques are the most common top-down fabrication techniques. The word *lithography*, which means printing from a stone, is a combination of two Greek words: *litho* meaning stone and *graphein* meaning writing. This printing technique, which was developed in the early 19th century, is defined as the transfer of a pattern from stone to paper and is based on the repulsion forces between oil and water molecules (Weaver, 1964). Today, nanostructure fabrication techniques that are based on the principle of transferring a certain pattern to a surface are called lithography. Lithography is a simple, inexpensive, effective, rapid, alternative way to fabricate periodic 2D and 3D nanostructure arrays. Over the past decade, nanostructure arrays have been successfully fabricated using the lithography approach (Xu, 2004). Photolithography, electron beam lithography, soft lithography and dip-pen nanolithography are examples of these techniques.

Photolithography, also called optical lithography or UV lithography, is a method used for creating well-defined features with high resolution (Jones, 2005). The photolithography process requires a photosensitive material (the photoresist), and a photomask. The process strategy is based on placing a mask between the radiation source and the photoresist, which is then irradiated. As light passes through the mask, a pattern is formed, which depending on the photoresist can form in two different ways: 1) by photodegradation of the exposed areas (positive pattern) and 2) by crosslinking (curing) them (negative pattern (Figure 7).

Figure 7. Schematic representation of the photolithography

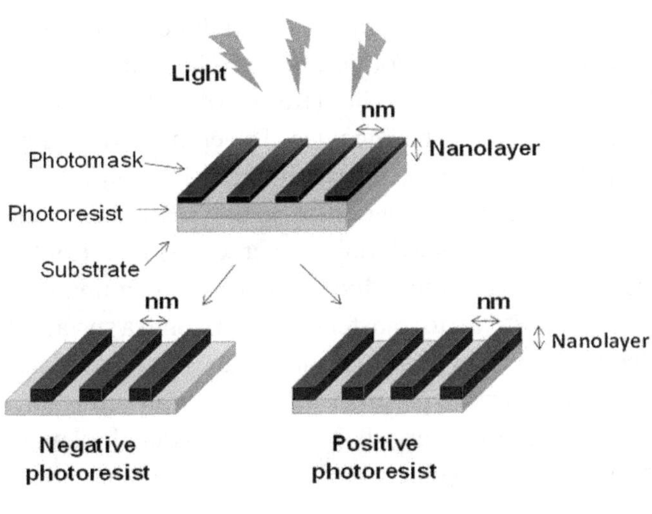

The development of nanoelectromechanical systems (NEMS), bio-microelectromechanical systems (Bio-MEMS), microfluidics, optics, photonics, multifunctional devices and the ability to create well-controlled nano/micro patterns provide alternative opportunities to design intelligent therapeutics (Tran, 2017). To give an example, biocompatible lithographically defined nanoparticles were patterned with different layers of metals like gold, iron, and nickel (Kim, 2010) (Fu, 2018). On the other hand, for patterning biomaterials like cells and proteins by photolithography, near-infrared (NIR) light should be preferred compared to UV light since it has less energy, thus it is less photodamaging (Lee, 2015). Huang et al. fabricated a voltammetric biosensor for albuterol by constructing lab-on-chip devices via photolithography (Huang, 2004) and developed acrylic MIP patterns with enhanced pattern resolution and recognition properties (Huang, 2007). In another study, microdot arrays with MIP nanofilaments were produced by photolithography (Linares, 2011).

Electron beam lithography can be defined as writing extremely fine patterns in thin films of photosensitive materials using a focused electron beam (Pease, 1981). Unlike photolithography, electron beam lithography does not require a mask, therefore the variety of patterns are much wider.

Additionally, soft lithography, another lithographic technique, which does not require an optical patterning, was developed by Whitesides et al. (Xia, 1998). The technique is based on using an elastomeric stamp, which is made of Polydimethylsiloxane (PDMS), to transfer the desired nanopattern to the substrate. Microcontact printing (μCP) and microtransfer molding (μTM) are the two main approaches used for many applications.

Microcontact printing can be used to pattern various materials, including proteins, colloidal crystals, DNA, polymeric nanocrystals, polyelectrolytes, thermoplastics, metals and semiconductor nanoparticles and dendrimers (Zhang, 2014) (Lange, 2004). PDMS stamps are used to generate multi-wells containing various nano- and micropatterns (Yliperttula, 2008). For instance, PEG hydrogel microwell array was fabricated with cultured embryoid bodies (Karp, 2007). Cell-based studies involve stem cells, osteogenic cells, and hepatocytes. The combination of nanotechnology and high-throughput screening systems can improve LOC systems.

Last but not least, "dip-pen" nanolithography (DPN) has been developed to fabricate tailored novel substrates at the nanometer scale (Piner, 1999) (Ginger, 2004). The technique is a direct-write tool which is based on scanning probe lithography that uses an ink-coated AFM tip to transfer the pattern onto a surface (Salaita, 2007). By using this technique, it is possible to print soft and hard materials from scanning probe tips onto a surface with high precision and sub-50-nm resolution. The first study of DPN was reported by Piner, who transferred alkanethiol molecules to a gold surface with 15 nm resolution (Piner, 1999). DPN based fabrication technique can be used to create bio-molecular micro/nanoarrays and tailored chemical surfaces for biological recognition. Nanoarrays can have more features compared to microarrays and the total area can be dramatically reduced, so that sample volumes and analysis times are decreased (Santra, 2015). For instance, antibody nanoarrays of the anti-p24 were fabricated to screen for HIV-1 virus (HIV-1) p24 antigen in serum samples (Lee, 2004). Another example of nanoarrays designed by DPN provides a platform to investigate the protein recognition (Lee, 2006). Lee constructed arrays of proteins with 100- to 350-nanometer features and used them to investigate cellular adhesion at the submicrometer scale (Lee, 2002). Apart from biomolecules, DPN provides the deposition of organic molecules (Zhang, 2003), polymers (Noy, 2002), and nanoparticles (Ben, 2002) onto a solid substrate.

The top-down approach allows researchers to develop functional surfaces that can be designed as lab-on-a-chip devices which are essential for point-of-care diagnostics. LOC is a microfluidic platform that can perform a number of chemical analyzes simultaneously and quickly with a little amount of sample (Manz, 1990) (Shi, 2018). Point-of-care diagnostics devices provide immediate results of medical tests close to the patients at home or hospitals. Additionally, such devices should be cheap, precise and easily accessible. For this purpose, nowadays researchers focus on the development of the LOC devices. One of the fabrication techniques is creating micro/nanoarrays that help to design multifunctional platforms. One example was reported by Brøgger et al. in 2012 (Brøgger, 2012). In this study, DNA probes were immobilized on PMMA microchannels and a microfluidic disc was developed for the detection of chromosomal translocations. In another study, multi-walled carbon nanotubes (MWCNT) were aligned vertically and an electrochemical biosensing platform was produced (Kim, 2013). MWCNT array electrode chip was fabricated by functionalization of MWCNT tips with ssDNA probes for bacteria analysis (Jiang, 2014). An alternative biosensor was developed by Ruecha et al. by using antibodies for the detection of proteins/antigens in body fluids and blood plasma (Ruecha, 2014).

Additionally, tissue microarrays (TMA) were developed for in situ tissue analyzes (Kononen, 1998) (Hutchins, 2018). TMAs are used for many biomedical applications such as predictive biomarker that predicts response to therapy (Egervari, 2007) and control tissue that establishes experimental protocols for diagnostic immunohistochemistry. They can also be used to determine the expression of proteins in healthy tissue (Richani, 2006). A special type of nanoarrays was designed with nanoscale voids on the surface of a metallic material (O'mahony, 2012). Having extraordinary optical transmission (EOT) and large electric field intensities make nanohole arrays suitable candidates for optofluidic platforms to perform label free testing and biomolecular sensing (Prasad, 2019).

3D Bioprinting

3D printing, also known as additive manufacturing (AM), layered manufacturing (LM), rapid prototyping (RP), is the process of printing a three-dimensional object in solid form which is designed virtually. The technique was first created by Hull in 1986 (Hull, 1986). Nowadays, 3D printing has been used for fabrication of not only industrial materials but also tissue, organ or biomedical tools. Biocompatible ink, used to produce artificial living tissue, is defined as bio-ink and 3D printing of bio-ink is described as 3D bioprinting (Sultan, 2017) (Mironov, 2005). Compared to conventional fabrication methods, more complex structures can be designed by 3D printing. Stereolithography, extrusion, laser-assisted, and inkjet are the four common 3D bioprinting techniques (Derakhshanfar, 2018). 3D bioprinting helps to fabricate complex native-like tissue architectures for regenerative medicine (Jessop, 2017), surgical devices, medical instruments, anatomical models for surgical planning and training (Liaw, 2017), organ-on-a-chip devices for drug testing, cancer research, tissue engineering (Vijayavenkataraman, 2018). In literature there are several tissue types produced by 3D printing such as liver (Billiet, 2014), nervous tissue (Hsieh, 2015), bone (Xu, 2014), cartilage (Mouser, 2017), skeletal muscle (Kim, 2016), skin (Vijayavenkataraman, 2016), cardiac tissue (Duan, 2017). The material, used for 3D printing should have good properties like printability, biocompatibility, biodegradability, structural and mechanical properties. Apart from biomolecules and cells, synthetic biodegradable polymers are used as bio-ink. For instance, poly(ethylene glycol) dimethacrylate (PEGDMA), polypropylene fumarate (PPF), trimethylene carbonate (TMC), ε-Caprolactone (CL) are used with photoinitiator (Arcaute, 2006). Graphene is also one of the favorite ink materials used for 3D bioprinting (Vlăsceanu, 2019). Cellulose nanocrystals, cellulose nanofibers are used in several biomedical applications such as cartilage tissue growth (Markstedt, 2015), auricular cartilage regeneration (Ávila, 2016) and wound dressing (Rees, 2015). Polyether-ether-ketone (PEEK) is also used for biomedical applications. (Singh, 2019). It is well known that PEEK has high mechanical properties, chemical, and biological stability and biocompatibility. Thanks to these properties, PEEK has been used in several biomedical applications, such as spine treatment, orthopedic tools, and products. PEEK and its composites with hydroxyapatite (HA) and/or chitosan help bone fixation and bone implant integration (Barton, 1996) (Yu, 2005). Recently, PEEK/HA composite scaffold with tailored pore size was produced by 3D printing (Vaezi, 2016). In this study, the adherent of human bone marrow stromal cells on the surface of the scaffold was successfully showed. 3D printing of PEEK is used to produce hip joints (Giannatsis, 2009), dental implants (Xu, 2017), drug delivery systems (Tan, 2018), biosensors and stents (Gittard, 2010).

BIOMEDICAL APPLICATIONS

Drug Delivery Systems

Drug delivery systems can be defined as the smart systems for the targeted delivery and controlled release of therapeutic agents (Figure 8). These systems provide promising results for many diseases, especially cancer. The delivery of the drug molecules to the target sides serve two purposes: 1) reducing the side effects of the drug molecule by not affecting the healthy tissues and 2) increasing the therapeutic effect of the drug molecule by activating locally. Thus, nanostructured drug delivery is a major focus of interest in many applications, particularly for the local chemotherapy of cancerous tumors, tissue, and organs. Nanocarriers bring the chemotherapeutic agents to the cancerous tissue and perform the controlled release of these agents so that the chemotherapeutic agents show high activity without damaging the healthy tissues. Nano drug delivery systems provide many other benefits, such as enhanced solubility of the drug molecule, increased oral bioavailability, increased rate of dissolution, increased surface area, decreased toxicity of the drug molecule, low dosage requirement (Bhatia, 2016). Nanosystems, which are called smart nanocarriers, are designed with stimuli-responsive polymers that respond to environmental conditions to ensure that the drug molecule is activated at the desired site. These smart nanosystems that are activated by environmental factors such as

Figure 8. Schematic representation of a multifunctional nanocarrier

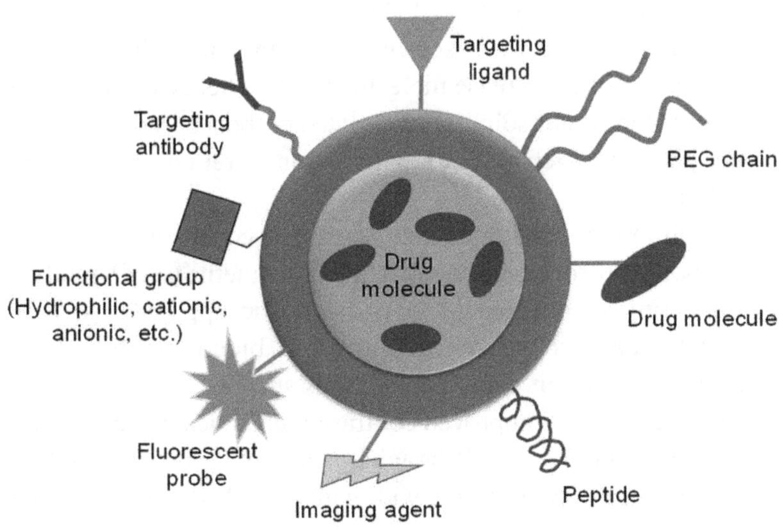

pH, temperature, ion concentration and external factors such as light, magnetic field, play an important role in many biomedical applications.

Targeting drug delivery can be designed by two different approaches: active targeting and passive targeting. The active targeting approach requires a binding ligand or a functional group that can interact with the desired site, whereas the passive targeting approach carries the drug molecule by benefiting from either external physiological changes or enhanced permeability and retention effect (EPR effect). EPR effect does not allow the drug molecules to enter into the healthy tissue. Instead, this effect allows the nano drug delivery system, which is loaded drug molecules, to penetrate only to the cancerous tissue and accumulate there. The damaged and porous structure of the cancerous tissue allows large nanostructures to enter into such tissues, whereas regular and healthy tissue does not allow nanostructures to penetrate and accumulate them. However, a commercial chemotherapy agent, mostly a small molecule, can also enter into healthy cells and affect them as well. The nanocarrier system, loaded with the drug molecule, is larger than the drug molecule itself, therefore it cannot enter into the healthy cell. Instead, it penetrates through the pores of the cancerous tissue. In addition to nanosystems designed with EPR effect, there are also nanosystems designed by utilizing the pH difference of cancerous and healthy tissues that can also be defined as passive targeting.

It is important to remember that targeted drug delivery systems not only serve for therapeutic purposes but also for diagnostic purposes. For example, a fluorescence-emitting molecule or quantum dot may be incorporated into the drug delivery system to enhance the imaging quality of the desired site. Yang et al. reported an example of a nano drug delivery system. In their work, they investigated in vivo behaviors of nanographene sheets (NGS) with polyethylene glycol (PEG) coated by a fluorescent label (Yang, 2010). PEG is a water-soluble biocompatible polymer which is used for drug delivery systems to increase molecular weight hence the size of the system and to make the system water soluble. PEGylated carbon-based nanocarrier shows efficient tumor passive targeting and low retention in reticuloendothelial systems due to the EPR effect.

Furthermore, iron oxide nanoparticles, can be used for diagnostic/therapeutic applications. Among the iron oxide nanoparticles, magnetite (Fe_3O_4) and maghemite (γ-Fe_2O_3) is used in in vitro and in vivo diagnostic applications. Due to their superparamagnetic properties, low toxicity and biocompatibility, iron oxide nanoparticles are preferred in many applications such as imaging, separation and treatment. For example, FDA approved contrast agents, dextran-coated Endorem® and Feridex®, are used for liver MR imaging (Laurent, 2008). In another example concerning the treatment of cancer, iron oxide nanoparticles were transported directly to the tumor by a magnetic force controlled externally. Iron oxide nanoparticles heat up and burn the tumor cells by increasing the magnetic field locally (Wang

L. a., 2006). The studies of magnetic nanoparticles have already been conducted in veterinary medicine and will be successfully applied to humans. Magnetic nanoparticles can be developed as a hyperthermic agent and drug carrier at the same time (Hervault, 2016). The existence of local heating effects in the vicinity of magnetic NPs leading to high temperatures at the magnetic NP surface, causing the release of drug molecule from the thermoresponsive polymer. Magnetic nanoparticles give promising results in magnetic hyperthermia treatments with or without the combination of thermoresponsive polymers (Figure 9).

In order to design drug delivery systems, 1D electrospun nanofibers can be used as well instead of nanoparticles. In literature, there are many examples of nanofibers which are employed in drug delivery applications (Chen, 2018). For instance, nanofibers were used to obtain biphasic release behavior that is described as an initial burst release followed by prolonged release (Han, 2013). The biphasic mechanism is based on both drug diffusion and polymer degradation. Additionally, stimuli-responsive nanofibers have been designed to increase the therapeutic efficiency of drug molecules, particularly chemotherapy agents. External stimulants can be temperature, ultrasound (Chen, 2014) (Yohe, 2013), light, magnetic field (Goodman, 2017), pH, ionic strength, enzyme concentration (Mura, 2013).

Figure 9. Magnetic hyperthermia therapy

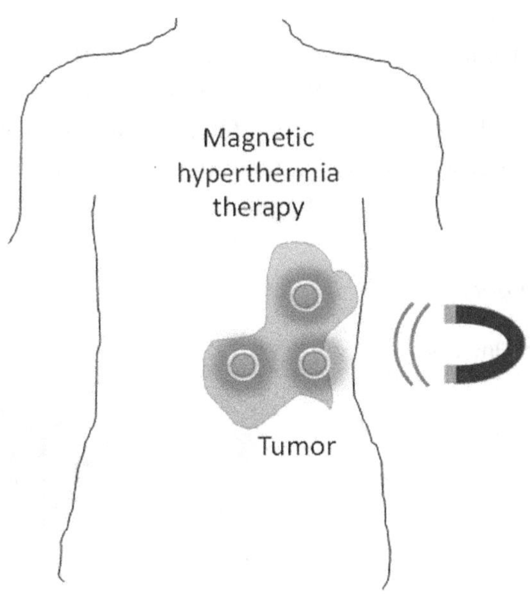

Bioimaging

Silica nanoparticles, which act as support materials for imaging agents such as fluorescent molecules, are used to detect biomolecules such as proteins and nucleic acids (Wang L. a., 2006). Silica nanoparticles are widely used in the polymer industry and biotechnology applications such as biological imaging. They are preferred in many applications due to their easy and cheap production, easy control of particle sizes, biocompatibility and highly active surfaces. The simple functionalization of the surfaces provides biomolecules and ligand affinity to silica nanoparticles and allows these nanoparticles to be used in many biomedical applications. Silica nanoparticles, which don't carry only imaging contrast agents as well as drug molecules, can easily be designed as drug delivery systems.

Quantum dots are very small semiconductor particles that are only a few nanometers in size. They are so small that their optical and electronic properties are very different from the larger particles that are composed of the same atoms. QDs are commonly used in imaging and bio-labeling processes in the field of biology, as they can emit light at different frequencies (in colors) when stimulated by electricity or light, and these frequencies can be controlled by particle size (Figure 10). QDs, also referred to as artificial atoms, may consist of single atoms such as selenium, or may consist of Group II-VI compounds such as CdSe, CdS, CdTe, ZnSe, ZnO, ZnS and Group III-V compounds such as GaN, GaP, InAs, and GaAs. The most commonly used compound is the CdSe QD with dimensions of 2 to 10 nm and different colors. When small dots are blue, the wavelength shifts towards red as the particle size of the dots grow (Chuto, 2010). An imaging example was reported by Yang, who in his study synthesized peptide-conjugated near-infrared QDs to oral squamous carcinoma cells by endocytosis for visual *in vivo* imaging (Yang K. C., 2010).

In addition to semiconductor QDs, there is a new class of carbon-based materials, namely graphene quantum dots (GQDs). GQDs have many advantages and extraordinary properties due to their nano sizes. They can be employed in many biomedical applications especially in imaging methods as they are photoluminescent,

Figure 10. Quantum dots

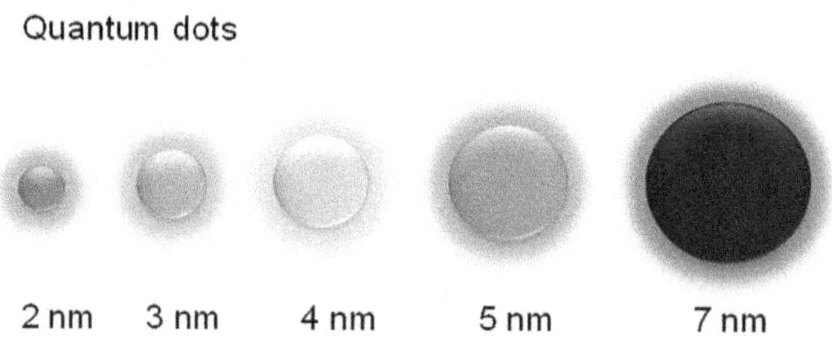

conductive and biocompatible. A successful study was carried out concerning the development of drug delivery and bioimaging systems for pancreatic cancer. In this study, hyaluronic acid was functionalized and green fluorescent graphene quantum dot (GQD)-labeled human serum albumin nanoparticles were prepared and applied for bioimaging and targeted delivery of gemcitabine to pancreatic cancer.

There are many examples in the literature regarding QD based imaging systems. However, it should be noted that all in vivo applications of QDs have been limited to animals.

Fluorescein and rhodamine molecules are organic dyes that have been used for fluorescence imaging for many years. The problem of photodegradation of these organic dyes, which are used in the labeling of biomolecules, has been overcome by inorganic QDs. QD imaging and labeling have begun to be used as an alternative to fluorescent molecules.

Silver and gold nanoparticles are good candidates as well for imaging applications. For instance, nano-hybrid carbon dots/polyethyleneimine/gold (C-dots/PEI/Au), and carbon dots/polyethyleneimine/silver (C-dots/PEI/Ag) were prepared to employ in diagnostic bioimaging applications (Emam, 2017).

Biosensor

Nanobiosensors can be described as analytical devices that combine a biologically active element with a suitable physical transducer to produce a signal that measures and quantifies the number of molecules in any sample on the nanoscale (Touhami, 2014). Nanobiosensors consist of two important parts, signal transduction, and biorecognition. The biorecognition elements can be enzymes, antibodies, nucleic acids, proteins, microorganisms or tissues, as well as synthetic biomimetic polymer-based organic and inorganic constructs. The main purpose of nanobiosensors is to detect any biochemical and biophysical signal associated with a particular disease at a single molecule or cell level. CNT-based nanobiosensors designed with gold/silver nanoparticles yield promising results. For example, CNTs aligned perpendicular to the surface (Wang J., 2005), nanowire coated DNA molecules, polypeptides and fibrin proteins play an important role in molecular recognition (Touhami, 2014). CNT based nanobiosensors are designed for DNA biomarkers, cell surface sugars, protein receptors, antibodies, and enzymes.

For the design of the highly sensitive devices, not only carbon nanotubes but also semiconductor materials, especially silicon nanotubes, are also used. For example, a very sensitive application of silicon nanowires was shown in a study in which high-affinity antibodies were attached to 1B nanowires, and the interaction of these antibodies with the virus was measured with high sensitivity due to the nanowire conductivity (Patolsky, 2004). The sensor designed in this study was able to detect only one single virus.

Lab-on-a-Chip (LOC)

Lab-on-a-chip (LOC) is defined as micro/nanochips (circuits) on which one or more laboratory processes are carried out. LOC devices formed by the combination of microfluidic technology with nanostructures are employed in many biomedical applications. The cost and process time of LOC devices, which require only a small sample volume, are significantly reduced due to the reaction speed (Niemeyer, 2004). In this regard, LOC nanostructures made way for point of care devices, a new area for diagnosis and rapid treatment applications.

Gold nanoparticles, which give different colors with different particle sizes, have been used in in biotechnology for a long time. Gold nanoparticles have numerous advantages such as chemical inertness, wide variety of surface treatment, easy synthesis, catalytic activity, high surface area/volume ratio, low toxicity, easy control of particle size. Thus, they are used in fields such as imaging, biosensors, drug delivery systems and cancer therapy. User-friendly strip tests like pregnancy tests are examples of gold nanoparticle usage (Figure 11). The fact that proteins and antibodies can be immobilized on gold nanoparticles without any change in their biological activity allows these gold-biocomposites to be frequently preferred in immunological test applications (Luo, 2007).

Bioseparation

In addition to imaging processes, iron oxide nanoparticles are used to separate biomolecules (proteins, antibodies, nucleic acids, etc.) via external magnetic force from

Figure 11. Pregnancy test

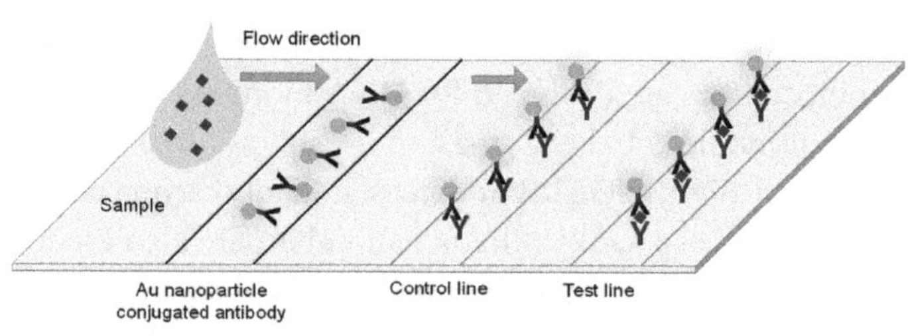

Figure 12. Magnetic separation

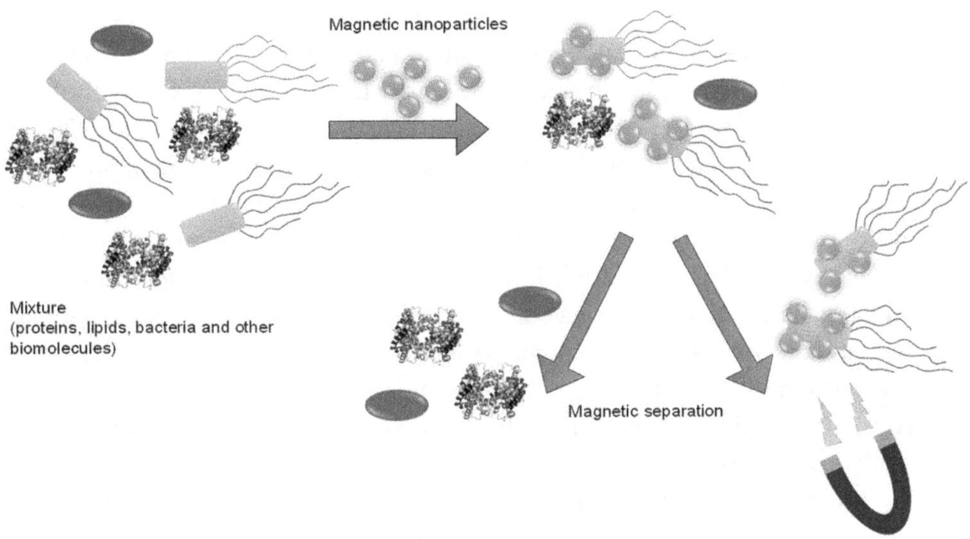

media simply and effectively way and can also be used successfully in the isolation of bacteria (HuiáShin, 2012) (Figure 12). The combination of superparamagnetic properties and molecularly imprinted biopolymers provide an eco-friendly and worth welting bio-sorbent. In a study conducted by Ostovan, this bio-compatible nano sorbent was applied to selective dispersive solid phase extraction (d-SPE) and the selective separation of baclofen from urine samples (Ostovan, 2018). In another study, it was shown that molecularly imprinted polymer nanotube membranes could be successfully used for bioseparation in a diverse field of biochemical species, such as ions, drug molecules, proteins and DNA (Wang H. J., 2006). A model system of this principle was applied for the affinity separation of β-estradiol. The researchers showed that MIP nanotubes with uniform pores could recognize and isolate a biomolecule from the mixture.

It is difficult to detect trace and ultra-trace the amount of drugs in plasma, blood, urine, and other metabolites. Adequate analytical methods should be used for the quantification of drugs at the trace levels. MIP carbon nanotubes are good candidates which can be employed for drug analyses in biological and environmental samples (Ansari, 2017).

Tissue Engineering

The emerging field of "tissue engineering" was created by Robert Langer from MIT (Langer, 2000). The principle is based on the ability to grow a network of cells, from either the patients themselves or donors, that will form functional tissues (Gazit, 2013). Nanostructures will play a more important role in tissue engineering applications in the future. Every day, the number of tissues engineering studies concerning the development of artificial tissues and scaffolds, and the investigation of cell adhesion character of nanomaterials have been increasing. For example, designing an artificial pancreas may provide a cure for both diabetes type I and cancer. Organ transplantation has associated problems with biocompatibility, thus nanostructures can be a solution to overcome the problem of biocompatibility. Nanomaterials can be used in orthopedic or dental implants. Their surface modifications or coatings can greatly enhance the biocompatibility by favoring the interaction of living cells with the biomaterial. Additionally, raw nanomaterials can also be used in drug encapsulation, bone replacements, prostheses, and implants as well (Bhatia, 2016). Hydrogels have also been used for many years in drug delivery systems and tissue scaffolds. Poly (N-isopropyl acrylamide) (PNIPAM) has been mostly preferred as the hydrogel exhibits a phase transition around 33°C, which is closed to body temperature. For the scaffold designs, biomolecules such as plant and animal viruses or bacteriophages and specific antibodies can be used as well. Biological assemblies can serve as a "smart scaffold" for the self-association of complex organic and inorganic nano-machines and nano-devices (Gazit, 2013).

Self-assembling peptides form hydrogels, by mimicking the extracellular matrix, can incorporate growth factors and have recently been designed to display cell-binding motifs and/or to incorporate protease sites for remodeling. Such multifunctional artificial matrices are promising materials for 3D cell culture and regenerative medicine in the near future (Collier, 2010).

Tissue regeneration requires essential molecules such as biomolecules, proteins and growth factors. It is important to deliver these multiple biomolecules precisely. To achieve this goal, delivery systems should be embedded into scaffolds. Biomolecules loaded nanoparticles and nanofibers are designed to have precise delivery (Samorezov, 2015). Lee et al. developed bioactive nanofiber scaffold for localized delivery of recombinant human bone morphogenetic protein-2 to the site of healing (Lee, 2015). Nanofibers can also be synthesized from natural polymers such as gelatin, chitosan, hyaluronic acid, and collagen, which have specific interaction size for cells, so these polymers support cell adhesion and proliferation (Zhang, 2015). Additionally, nanofibers can be developed as in vitro 3D tissue models, particularly tumor models for drug development studies (Hopkins, 2015).

Nano-Biomolecules

Biomedical nanotechnology includes the control of biomolecules at the nanoscale and as well as the use of synthetic nanostructures in the field of biology. In addition, bioengineers seek to design easy ways of synthesizing natural proteins by using nanomachines, and proteins with synthetic amino acids (Goodsell, 2004). One of the notable structures among nanobiopeptides is peptide nucleic acids. Peptide nucleic acids, composed of the components of the DNA molecule, contain a peptide bond instead of a sugar-phosphate bond, unlike the normal DNA chain. It has been shown in studies that these DNAs, which are partly artificial, are more stable than normal DNA. These changes made on nanoscale on proteins and nucleic acids have contributed to the advance of biomedical nanotechnology.

THE FUTURE OF BIOMEDICAL NANOTECHNOLOGY

The development of nanotechnology over the last 50 years showed that it is difficult to predict what will be developed in the next ten years. With advances in genetic science, DNA analysis will become easier, and perhaps it will become as simple as a pregnancy test. DNA mutations can be detected very quickly with a microfluidic LOC system that can be developed in a similar way to pregnancy test. The artificial organs produced from the cells of the patients will be a solution to the organ transplantation problems by virtually eliminating the problem of biocompatibility. With the intelligent nano scaffolding systems to be developed, stem cell treatments will be facilitated, and artificial organs can be produced. With the rapid development of carbon materials such as CNTs, graphenes, fullerenes and intelligent polymers, tissue engineering applications will be improved. Apart from these developments, nanorobots for diagnostic and therapeutic purposes will be developed to replace the microsurgery. Nanorobots will not only be used in surgical applications but will also play a leading role in the cell-level intervention of diseases such as cancer. Finally, we need to acknowledge that nanotechnology is a world full of unknowns, while it makes our lives easier it also involves significant risks.

ACKNOWLEDGMENT

Special thanks to Derya Uysal Ertan, Nazende Gunday Tureli and Neslihan Cetinkaya for their valuable and constructive suggestions and Arif Eren Cepni for his support in drawing creative carbon structures. This research received no specific grant from any funding agency in the public, commercial, or not-for-profit sectors.

REFERENCES

Ansari, S. (2017). Novel developments and trends of analytical methods for drug analysis in biological and environmental samples by molecularly imprinted polymers. *TrAC Trends in Analytical Chemistry*, *89*, 146–162.

Arcaute, K., Mann, B. K., & Wicker, R. B. (2006). Stereolithography of three-dimensional bioactive poly (ethylene glycol) constructs with encapsulated cells. *Annals of Biomedical Engineering*, *34*(9), 1429–1441.

Arole, V. M. (2014). Fabrication of nanomaterials by top-down and bottom-up approaches-an overview. JAAST:Material Science, 89-93.

Ávila, H. M., Schwarz, S., Rotter, N., & Gatenholm, P. (2016). 3D bioprinting of human chondrocyte-laden nanocellulose hydrogels for patient-specific auricular cartilage regeneration. *Bioprinting*, *1*, 22–35.

Barton, A. J., Sagers, R. D., & Pitt, W. G. (1996). Bacterial adhesion to orthopedic implant polymers. *Journal of Biomedical Materials Research: An Official Journal of The Society for Biomaterials and The Japanese Society for Biomaterials*, *30*(3), 403–410.

Ben Ali, M., Ondarcuhu, T., Brust, M., & Joachim, C. (2002). Atomic force microscope tip nanoprinting of gold nanoclusters. *Langmuir*, *18*(3), 872–876.

Bhatia, S. (2016). Nanoparticles types, classification, characterization, fabrication methods and drug delivery applications. In *Natural polymer drug delivery systems* (pp. 33–93). Cham: Springer.

Billiet, T., Gevaert, E., De Schryver, T., Cornelissen, M., & Dubruel, P. (2014). The 3D printing of gelatin methacrylamide cell-laden tissue-engineered constructs with high cell viability. *Biomaterials*, *35*(1), 49–62.

Brøgger, A. L., Kwasny, D., Bosco, F. G., Silahtaroglu, A., Tümer, Z., Boisen, A., & Svendsen, W. E. (2012). Centrifugally driven microfluidic disc for detection of chromosomal translocations. *Lab on a Chip*, *12*(22), 4628–4634.

Chatterjee, K. S. (2014). Core/shell nanoparticles in biomedical applications. *Advances in Colloid and Interface Science*, *209*, 8–39.

Chen, M., Li, Y. F., & Besenbacher, F. (2014). Electrospun Nanofibers-Mediated On-Demand Drug Release. *Advanced Healthcare Materials*, *3*(11), 1721–1732.

Chen, S., Li, R., Li, X., & Xie, J. (2018). Electrospinning: An enabling nanotechnology platform for drug delivery and regenerative medicine. *Advanced Drug Delivery Reviews, 132*, 188–213.

Chuto, G. R. (2010). Les nanoparticules. *Médecine Nucléaire (Paris)*, ▪▪▪, 370–376.

Collier, J. H. (2010). Multi-component extracellular matrices based on peptide self-assembly. *Chemical Society Reviews, 39*(9), 3413–342.

Çakir, P. C. (2013). Protein-Size Molecularly Imprinted Polymer Nanogels as Synthetic Antibodies, by Localized Polymerization with Multi-initiators. *Advanced Materials, 25*(7), 1048–1051.

Daraee, H. E. (2016). Application of liposomes in medicine and drug delivery. *Artificial Cells, Nanomedicine, and Biotechnology, 44*(1), 381–391.

Derakhshanfar, S., Mbeleck, R., Xu, K., Zhang, X., Zhong, W., & Xing, M. (2018). 3D bioprinting for biomedical devices and tissue engineering: A review of recent trends and advances. Bioactive materials, 3(2), 144-156.

Duan, B. (2017). State-of-the-art review of 3D bioprinting for cardiovascular tissue engineering. *Annals of Biomedical Engineering, 45*(1), 195–209.

Eglash, R. (2011). Nanotechnology and Traditional Knowledge Systems. In Nanotechnology and Global Sustainability (pp. 74-97). CRC Press.

Egervari, K., Szollosi, Z., & Nemes, Z. (2007). Tissue microarray technology in breast cancer HER2 diagnostics. *Pathology, Research and Practice, 203*(3), 169–177.

Eigler, D. M. (1990). Positioning single atoms with a scanning tunnelling microscope. *Nature, 344*(6266), 524–526.

Emam, A. N., Loutfy, S. A., Mostafa, A. A., Awad, H., & Mohamed, M. B. (2017). Cyto-toxicity, biocompatibility and cellular response of carbon dots–plasmonic based nano-hybrids for bioimaging. *RSC Advances, 7*(38), 23502–23514.

Fakhrullin, R. (2014). *Cell surface engineering: fabrication of functional nanoshells*. Royal Society of Chemistry.

Feynman, R. P. (1960). There's plenty of room at the bottom. *Engineering and Science, 23*(5), 22–36.

Filipponi, L. (2013). *Nanotechnologies: principles, applications, implications and hands-on activities*. Luxembourg: Publications Office of the European Union.

Fu, X., Cai, J., Zhang, X., Li, W. D., Ge, H., & Hu, Y. (2018). Top-down fabrication of shape-controlled, monodisperse nanoparticles for biomedical applications. *Advanced Drug Delivery Reviews.*

Gazit, E. (2013). *Plenty of room for biology at the bottom: An introduction to bionanotechnology*. World Scientific.

Giannatsis, J., & Dedoussis, V. (2009). Additive fabrication technologies applied to medicine and health care: A review. *International Journal of Advanced Manufacturing Technology*, *40*(1-2), 116–127.

Ginger, D. S., Zhang, H., & Mirkin, C. A. (2004). The evolution of dip-pen nanolithography. *Angewandte Chemie International Edition*, *43*(1), 30–45.

Gittard, S. D., & Narayan, R. J. (2010). Laser direct writing of micro-and nano-scale medical devices. *Expert Review of Medical Devices*, *7*(3), 343–356.

Goodman, A. M., Neumann, O., Nørregaard, K., Henderson, L., Choi, M. R., Clare, S. E., & Halas, N. J. (2017). Near-infrared remotely triggered drug-release strategies for cancer treatment. *Proceedings of the National Academy of Sciences of the United States of America*, *114*(47), 12419–12424.

Goodsell, D. S. (2004). *Bionanotechnology: lessons from nature*. John Wiley & Sons.

Han, F., Jia, X., Dai, D., Yang, X., Zhao, J., Zhao, Y., & Yuan, X. (2013). Performance of a multilayered small-diameter vascular scaffold dual-loaded with VEGF and PDGF. *Biomaterials*, *34*(30), 7302–7313.

Hervault, A. D. (2016). Doxorubicin loaded dual pH-and thermo-responsive magnetic nanocarrier for combined magnetic hyperthermia and targeted controlled drug delivery applications. *Nanoscale*, *8*(24), 12152–12161.

Hopkins, A. M., DeSimone, E., Chwalek, K., & Kaplan, D. L. (2015). 3D in vitro modeling of the central nervous system. *Progress in Neurobiology*, *125*, 1–25.

Hsieh, F. Y., & Hsu, S. H. (2015). 3D bioprinting: A new insight into the therapeutic strategy of neural tissue regeneration. *Organogenesis*, *11*(4), 153–158.

Huang, H. C., Lin, C. I., Joseph, A. K., & Der Lee, Y. (2004). Photo-lithographically impregnated and molecularly imprinted polymer thin film for biosensor applications. *Journal of Chromatography. A*, *1027*(1-2), 263–268.

Huang, H. C., Huang, S. Y., Lin, C. I., & Lee, Y. D. (2007). A multi-array sensor via the integration of acrylic molecularly imprinted photoresists and ultramicroelectrodes on a glass chip. *Analytica Chimica Acta*, *582*(1), 137–146.

HuiáShin, H. a. (2012). A facile and sensitive detection of pathogenic bacteria using magnetic nanoparticles and optical nanocrystal probes. *Analyst (London)*, *137*(16), 3609–3612.

Hull, C. W. (1986). U.S. Patent No. 4,575,330. Washington, DC: U.S. Patent and Trademark Office.

Hutchins, G., & Grabsch, H. I. (2018). How to make tissue microarrays. *Diagnostic Histopathology*, *24*(4), 127–135.

Jessop, Z. M., Al-Sabah, A., Gardiner, M. D., Combellack, E., Hawkins, K., & Whitaker, I. S. (2017). 3D bioprinting for reconstructive surgery: Principles, applications and challenges. *Journal of Plastic, Reconstructive & Aesthetic Surgery; JPRAS*, *70*(9), 1155–1170.

Jiang, X., Shao, N., Jing, W., Tao, S., Liu, S., & Sui, G. (2014). Microfluidic chip integrating high throughput continuous-flow PCR and DNA hybridization for bacteria analysis. *Talanta*, *122*, 246–250.

Jones, S. W. (2005). Introduction to integrated circuit technology. IC Knowlegde LLC, Georgetown, MA Revision, Nov.

Kim, D. H., Rozhkova, E. A., Ulasov, I. V., Bader, S. D., Rajh, T., Lesniak, M. S., & Novosad, V. (2010). Biofunctionalized magnetic-vortex microdiscs for targeted cancer-cell destruction. *Nature Materials*, *9*(2), 165.

Karp, J. M., Yeh, J., Eng, G., Fukuda, J., Blumling, J., Suh, K. Y., ... Khademhosseini, A. (2007). Controlling size, shape and homogeneity of embryoid bodies using poly (ethylene glycol) microwells. *Lab on a Chip*, *7*(6), 786–794.

Kim, J., Elsnab, J., Gehrke, C., Li, J., & Gale, B. K. (2013). Microfluidic integrated multi-walled carbon nanotube (MWCNT) sensor for electrochemical nucleic acid concentration measurement. *Sensors and Actuators. B, Chemical*, *185*, 370–376.

Kim, J., Ko, I., Seol, Y., Atala, A., Yoo, J. J., & Lee, S. (2016, December). 3D Bioprinting of Functional Skeletal Muscle Tissue for Volumetric Muscle Tissue Loss. In Tissue Engineering Part A, (Vol. 22, pp. S5-S5). 140 HUGUENOT STREET, 3RD FL, NEW ROCHELLE, NY 10801 USA: MARY ANN LIEBERT, INC.

Kononen, J., Bubendorf, L., Kallionimeni, A., Bärlund, M., Schraml, P., Leighton, S., & Kallionimeni, O. P. (1998). Tissue microarrays for high-throughput molecular profiling of tumor specimens. *Nature Medicine*, *4*(7), 844.

Lange, S. A., Benes, V., Kern, D. P., Hörber, J. H., & Bernard, A. (2004). Microcontact printing of DNA molecules. *Analytical Chemistry*, *76*(6), 1641–1647.

Langer, R. (2000). Biomaterials in drug delivery and tissue engineering: One laboratory's experience. *Accounts of Chemical Research*, *33*, 94–101.

Laurent, S. F. (2008). Magnetic iron oxide nanoparticles: Synthesis, stabilization, vectorization, physicochemical characterizations, and biological applications. *Chemical Reviews*, *108*(6), 2064–2110.

Lee, K. B., Park, S. J., Mirkin, C. A., Smith, J. C., & Mrksich, M. (2002). Protein nanoarrays generated by dip-pen nanolithography. *Science*, *295*(5560), 1702–1705.

Lee, K. B., Kim, E. Y., Mirkin, C. A., & Wolinsky, S. M. (2004). The use of nanoarrays for highly sensitive and selective detection of human immunodeficiency virus type 1 in plasma. *Nano Letters*, *4*(10), 1869–1872.

Lee, M., Kang, D. K., Yang, H. K., Park, K. H., Choe, S. Y., Kang, C., & Kang, I. C. (2006). Protein nanoarray on Prolinker™ surface constructed by atomic force microscopy dip-pen nanolithography for analysis of protein interaction. *Proteomics*, *6*(4), 1094–1103.

Lee, S. S., Hsu, E. L., Mendoza, M., Ghodasra, J., Nickoli, M. S., Ashtekar, A., & Nelson, D. (2015). Gel scaffolds of BMP-2-binding peptide amphiphile nanofibers for spinal arthrodesis. *Advanced Healthcare Materials*, *4*(1), 131–141.

Lee, T. T., García, J. R., Paez, J. I., Singh, A., Phelps, E. A., Weis, S., & García, A. J. (2015). Light-triggered in vivo activation of adhesive peptides regulates cell adhesion, inflammation and vascularization of biomaterials. *Nature Materials*, *14*(3), 352.

Liaw, C. Y., & Guvendiren, M. (2017). Current and emerging applications of 3D printing in medicine. *Biofabrication*, *9*(2), 024102.

Linares, A. V., Falcimaigne-Cordin, A., Gheber, L. A., & Haupt, K. (2011). Patterning nanostructured, synthetic, polymeric receptors by simultaneous projection photolithography, nanomolding, and molecular imprinting. *Small*, *7*(16), 2318–2325.

Luo, L. Z. (2007). Development of a gold nanoparticles based chemiluminescence imaging assay and its application. *Analytica Chimica Acta*, ▪▪▪, 106–111.

Manz, A., Graber, N., & Widmer, H. Á. (1990). Miniaturized total chemical analysis systems: A novel concept for chemical sensing. *Sensors and Actuators. B, Chemical*, *1*(1-6), 244–248.

Markstedt, K., Mantas, A., Tournier, I., Martínez Ávila, H., Hägg, D., & Gatenholm, P. (2015). 3D bioprinting human chondrocytes with nanocellulose–alginate bioink for cartilage tissue engineering applications. *Biomacromolecules*, *16*(5), 1489–1496.

Mironov, V. (2005). The second international workshop on bioprinting, biopatterning and bioassembly. *Expert Opinion on Biological Therapy*, *5*(8), 1111–1115.

Mouser, V. H., Levato, R., Bonassar, L. J., D'Lima, D. D., Grande, D. A., Klein, T. J., & Malda, J. (2017). Three-dimensional bioprinting and its potential in the field of articular cartilage regeneration. *Cartilage*, *8*(4), 327–340.

Mura, S., Nicolas, J., & Couvreur, P. (2013). Stimuli-responsive nanocarriers for drug delivery. *Nature Materials*, *12*(11), 991.

Niemeyer, C. M. (2004). *Nanobiotechnology: concepts, applications and perspectives*. John Wiley & Sons.

Noy, A., Miller, A. E., Klare, J. E., Weeks, B. L., Woods, B. W., & DeYoreo, J. J. (2002). Fabrication of luminescent nanostructures and polymer nanowires using dip-pen nanolithography. *Nano Letters*, *2*(2), 109–112.

O'mahony, J. (2012). U.S. Patent Application No. 13/503,902.

Ostovan, A. G. (2018). Fabrication of water-compatible superparamagnetic molecularly imprinted biopolymer for clean separation of baclofen from bio-fluid samples: A mild and green approach. *Talanta*, *179*, 760–768.

Patolsky, F. Z. (2004). Electrical detection of single viruses. *Proceedings of the National Academy of Sciences of the United States of America*, *101*(39), 14017–14022.

Pease, R. F. (1981). Electron beam lithography. *Contemporary Physics*, *22*(3), 265–290.

Pérez-Madrigal, M. M. (2015). Insulating and semiconducting polymeric free-standing nanomembranes with biomedical applications. *Journal of Materials Chemistry. B, Materials for Biology and Medicine*, *3*(29), 5904–5932.

Piner, R. D., Zhu, J., Xu, F., Hong, S., & Mirkin, C. A. (1999). " Dip-pen" nanolithography. science, 283(5402), 661-663.

Pokropivny, V. V. (2007). Classification of nanostructures by dimensionality and concept of surface forms engineering in nanomaterial science. *Materials Science and Engineering C*, *27*(5-8), 990–993.

Prasad, A., Choi, J., Jia, Z., Park, S., & Gartia, M. R. (2019). Nanohole array plasmonic biosensors: Emerging point-of-care applications. *Biosensors & Bioelectronics*.

Rees, A., Powell, L. C., Chinga-Carrasco, G., Gethin, D. T., Syverud, K., Hill, K. E., & Thomas, D. W. (2015). 3D bioprinting of carboxymethylated-periodate oxidized nanocellulose constructs for wound dressing applications. *BioMed Research International.*

Reisner, D. E. (2008). *Bionanotechnology: global prospects.* CRC Press.

Salaita, K., Wang, Y., & Mirkin, C. A. (2007). Applications of dip-pen nanolithography. *Nature Nanotechnology*, *2*(3), 145.

Richani, K., Romero, R., Kim, Y. M., Cushenberry, E., Soto, E., Han, Y. M., & Kim, C. J. (2006). Tissue microarray: An effective high-throughput method to study the placenta for clinical and research purposes. *The Journal of Maternal-Fetal & Neonatal Medicine*, *19*(8), 509–515.

Ruecha, N., Rangkupan, R., Rodthongkum, N., & Chailapakul, O. (2014). Novel paper-based cholesterol biosensor using graphene/polyvinylpyrrolidone/polyaniline nanocomposite. *Biosensors & Bioelectronics*, *52*, 13–19.

Samorezov, J. E., & Alsberg, E. (2015). Spatial regulation of controlled bioactive factor delivery for bone tissue engineering. *Advanced Drug Delivery Reviews*, *84*, 45–67.

Santra, S., De Luca, A., Bhaumik, S., Ali, S. Z., Udrea, F., Gardner, J. W., ... Guha, P. K. (2015). Dip pen nanolithography-deposited zinc oxide nanorods on a CMOS MEMS platform for ethanol sensing. *RSC Advances*, *5*(59), 47609–47616.

Singh, S., Prakash, C., & Ramakrishna, S. (2019). 3D Printing of Polyether-ether-ketone for Biomedical Applications. *European Polymer Journal*, *114*, 234–248.

Shi, H., Nie, K., Dong, B., Long, M., Xu, H., & Liu, Z. (2018). Recent progress of microfluidic reactors for biomedical applications. *Chemical Engineering Journal*, *361*, 635–650.

Soenen, S. J. (2015). (Intra) cellular stability of inorganic nanoparticles: Effects on cytotoxicity, particle functionality, and biomedical applications. *Chemical Reviews*, ▪▪▪, 2109–2135.

Srinivasan, S. (1997). Wootz steel: an advanced material of the ancient world.

Sultan, S., Siqueira, G., Zimmermann, T., & Mathew, A. P. (2017). 3D printing of nano-cellulosic biomaterials for medical applications. *Current Opinion in Biomedical Engineering*, *2*, 29–34.

Tan, D., Maniruzzaman, M., & Nokhodchi, A. (2018). Advanced pharmaceutical applications of Hot-Melt Extrusion coupled with Fused Deposition Modelling (FDM) 3D printing for personalised drug delivery. *Pharmaceutics*, *10*(4), 203.

Tiwari, J. N. (2012). Zero-dimensional, one-dimensional, two-dimensional and three-dimensional nanostructured materials for advanced electrochemical energy devices. *Progress in Materials Science*, *57*(4), 724–803.

Touhami, A. (2014). Biosensors and Nanobiosensors: Design and Applications. *Nanomedicine (London)*, ▪▪▪, 374–400.

Tran, K. T., & Nguyen, T. D. (2017). Lithography-based methods to manufacture biomaterials at small scales. *Journal of Science: Advanced Materials and Devices*, *2*(1), 1–14.

Vaezi, M., Black, C., Gibbs, D., Oreffo, R., Brady, M., Moshrefi-Torbati, M., & Yang, S. (2016). Characterization of new PEEK/HA composites with 3D HA network fabricated by extrusion freeforming. *Molecules (Basel, Switzerland)*, *21*(6), 687.

Vijayavenkataraman, S., Yan, W. C., Lu, W. F., Wang, C. H., & Fuh, J. Y. H. (2018). 3D bioprinting of tissues and organs for regenerative medicine. *Advanced Drug Delivery Reviews*, *132*, 296–332.

Vijayavenkataraman, S., Lu, W. F., & Fuh, J. Y. H. (2016). 3D bioprinting of skin: A state-of-the-art review on modelling, materials, and processes. *Biofabrication*, *8*(3), 032001.

Vlăsceanu, G. M., Iovu, H., & Ioniţă, M. (2019). Graphene inks for the 3D printing of cell culture scaffolds and related molecular arrays. *Composites. Part B, Engineering*.

Wang, H. J. (2006). Template synthesized molecularly imprinted polymer nanotube membranes for chemical separations. *Journal of the American Chemical Society*, *128*(50), 15954–15955.

Wang, J. (2005). Carbon-nanotube based electrochemical biosensors: A review. *Electroanalysis*, *17*(1), 7–14.

Wang, L. a. (2006). Multicolor FRET silica nanoparticles by single wavelength excitation. *Nano Letters*, ▪▪▪, 84–88.

Ward, M. A. (2011). Thermoresponsive polymers for biomedical applications. *Polymers*, *3*(3), 1215–1242.

Weaver, P. (1964). *The technique of lithography*. London: BT Batsford.

Williams, L. D. (2006). *Nanotechnology demystified*. McGraw Hill Professional.

Xia, Y. a. (1998). Soft lithography. *Annual Review of Materials Science*, *28*(1), 153–184.

Xie, J. L. (2008). Putting electrospun nanofibers to work for biomedical research. *Macromolecular Rapid Communications*, *29*(22), 1775–1792.

Xu, N., Ye, X., Wei, D., Zhong, J., Chen, Y., Xu, G., & He, D. (2014). 3D artificial bones for bone repair prepared by computed tomography-guided fused deposition modeling for bone repair. *ACS Applied Materials & Interfaces*, *6*(17), 14952–14963.

Xu, Q. T. (2004). Fabrication of free-standing metallic pyramidal shells. *Nano Letters*, *4*(12), 2509–2511.

Xu, X., He, L., Zhu, B., Li, J., & Li, J. (2017). Advances in polymeric materials for dental applications. *Polymer Chemistry*, *8*(5), 807–823.

Yadugiri, V. T. (2010). 'Plenty of room'-fifty years after the Feynman lecture. Current Science, (00113891), 99(7).

Yang, K. C. (2010). Quantum dot-based visual in vivo imaging for oral squamous cell carcinoma in mice. *Oral Oncology*, *46*(12), 864–868.

Yang, K. Z. (2010). Graphene in mice: Ultrahigh in vivo tumor uptake and efficient photothermal therapy. *Nano Letters*, *10*(9), 3318–3323.

Yliperttula, M., Chung, B. G., Navaladi, A., Manbachi, A., & Urtti, A. (2008). High-throughput screening of cell responses to biomaterials. european journal of pharmaceutical sciences, 35(3), 151-160.

Yohe, S. T., Kopechek, J. A., Porter, T. M., Colson, Y. L., & Grinstaff, M. W. (2013). Triggered Drug Release from Superhydrophobic Meshes using High-Intensity Focused Ultrasound. *Advanced Healthcare Materials*, *2*(9), 1204–1208.

Yu, S., Hariram, K. P., Kumar, R., Cheang, P., & Aik, K. K. (2005). In vitro apatite formation and its growth kinetics on hydroxyapatite/polyetheretherketone biocomposites. *Biomaterials*, *26*(15), 2343–2352.

Zarschler, K. R. (2016). Ultrasmall inorganic nanoparticles: State-of-the-art and perspectives for biomedical applications. *Nanomedicine; Nanotechnology, Biology, and Medicine*, 1663–1701.

Zhang, D., Ni, N., Chen, J., Yao, Q., Shen, B., Zhang, Y., & Mo, X. (2015). Electrospun SF/PLCL nanofibrous membrane: A potential scaffold for retinal progenitor cell proliferation and differentiation. *Scientific Reports*, *5*, 14326.

Zhang, H., Chung, S. W., & Mirkin, C. A. (2003). Fabrication of sub-50-nm solid-state nanostructures on the basis of dip-pen nanolithography. *Nano Letters*, *3*(1), 43–45.

Zhang, P., Xia, J., Wang, Z., & Guan, J. (2014). Gold nanoparticle-packed microdisks for multiplex Raman labelling of cells. *Nanoscale*, *6*(15), 8762–8768.

KEY TERMS AND DEFINITIONS

Bottom-Up Approach: The method of constructing a complex system atom by atom and molecule by molecule from the bottom.

Core-Shell Nanostructures: Nanostructures composed of an inner core and an outer shell made of at least two different materials.

Lab-on-a-Chip: Micro/nanochips on which one or more laboratory processes are performed simultaneously.

Liposome: A spherical vesicle consisting of at least one lipid bilayer.

Nanobiosensor: Nanostructured devices that measure a biological event using optical, electronic and magnetic technology.

Nanotechnology: Manipulation of matter at nanoscale.

Polymer: Long chain molecules formed by the addition of relatively small molecules called monomers to each other.

Quantum Dots: They are small semiconductor particles of a few nanometers in size with different optical and electronic properties than large materials.

Top-Down Approach: The method for fabrication of micro- or nanostructures in which large particles are broken up or milled

Chapter 4
Measuring Consciousness in the Clinic

Nithin Nagaraj
Consciousness Studies Programme, National Institute of Advanced Studies, Bengaluru, India

ABSTRACT

We don't doubt for a moment that we are conscious, but what is 'Consciousness'? Understanding consciousness, its nature, and characteristics has remained a hard problem for several centuries. While philosophers, neuroscientists, physicists, psychologists, and psychiatrists grapple with this hard problem, clinicians are in need of a practical way to 'measure' consciousness (or its surrogate). Determining whether a patient is conscious or not, and measuring the degree of consciousness, could be critical and potentially life-saving in a clinical scenario. In this chapter, we will review recent scientific approaches for modelling and measuring consciousness, and their clinical applications with an emphasis on a host of issues (theoretical, philosophical, methodological, technological, & clinical) and challenges that need to be satisfactorily and convincingly addressed going forward.

INTRODUCTION

'Consciousness' or conscious experience is the subjective qualitative feeling of 'what it is like to be?' (Nagel, 1974). Even as you read these words, you experience visual perceptions of words on a white background. At the same time, you may have an inner experience of a rich set of thoughts, feelings and bodily sensations (such as the tingling sensation in your toe) – these together with the sensory perceptions constitute your mind, body and world.

DOI: 10.4018/978-1-7998-0326-3.ch004

The central puzzle in gaining an understanding of 'Mind' which all theories of mind have to address is the nature and properties of 'Consciousness'. Not surprisingly, there is no universally agreed upon theory or even a singular definition of consciousness, but its central importance in understanding of mind is more or less universally accepted. The very existence of consciousness, its nature and relationship with other nonconscious aspects of reality ('Matter') remains heavily disputed till date with the entire spectrum of philosophical positions possible, namely – the non-existence of consciousness (only matter or only mind ever exists); as a derived existence or emergent property (of matter, or mind which are taken as more fundamental); as a dualistic existence (consciousness and non-conscious entities both fundamentally exist but are distinct and different), and finally as a non-dualistic fundamental element of reality (consciousness alone exists – matter and mind being emergent manifestations). There are also in-between positions which do not fall in any of the positions described above.

The exact nature of relationships between Consciousness-Mind-Matter is far from being philosophically settled. However, clinicians are more interested in knowing whether this conscious experience can in fact be measured in the clinic (under an appropriately chosen definition of consciousness). Recently, it has been fiercely debated by philosophers, scientists and medical practitioners whether conscious experience could at all be reduced to some kind of neural activity in brain networks. If indeed one can measure consciousness via measuring activity in the brain, then it can be readily used in the clinic to determine whether an incommunicative patient is conscious or not. Furthermore, measuring the level of consciousness (or its surrogate) could well be critical and potentially life-saving in a clinical scenario.

While there are differing viewpoints on this topic of measuring consciousness without any consensual agreement, there have been several attempts to study consciousness scientifically in the past couple of decades. The recent emphasis on developing a 'Science of Consciousness' is evident in the number of scientific measures of consciousness that have been proposed in the literature (Seth et al., 2008; Nagaraj & Virmani, 2017; Virmani & Nagaraj, 2019 and references there in). We shall delve into these, but first we take an overview of the approaches to understanding consciousness from different disciplines.

The Problem of Consciousness: Debate Across Disciplines

As previously alluded, the puzzle of consciousness – its definition, properties and relationship with 'mind' and 'matter' is a rich debate spanning several disciplines. Here, we provide a brief overview of this debate (by no means exhaustive).

The history of the deliberation on what constitutes consciousness probably goes back to the history of humans itself. Spiritual beliefs in preliterate cultures indicate an early reflection about the nature of conscious awareness. In ancient India, there were several philosophical schools which had rich ideas on consciousness and its relationship with the world and the individual being. Biological approaches have mostly linked consciousness and conscious awareness to mental phenomena, having endowed non-human animals and humans or other cognitive systems with consciousness in a variety of different senses (sentience, wakefulness, self-consciousness, subject of consciousness etc. (Van Gulick, 2018)). Thomas Nagel's 'what it is like?' criterion (hinted at the beginning of this chapter) is a subjective notion of being a conscious organism (like being a bat or being a human) that became quite famous (Nagel, 1974). From a purely subjective notion of being a conscious organism, one can never truly understand *what it is to be like* another conscious entity ('I' can never truly know what it is to be like 'you' – though admitting that 'I' and 'You' are both conscious entities). This gap between an account of first-person experience and third person observation of conscious processes is very difficult to bridge. This has been the real challenge of a scientific exploration of consciousness (Josephson, 1996).

It is well known that there are fundamental limits to knowing in science (Heisenberg's uncertainty principle) and mathematics (Gödel's incompleteness theorem). Joseph Levine (1983) suggested the existence of an *explanatory gap* in our understanding of consciousness, especially the relationship between consciousness and a nonconscious (physical) substrate. This gap is because of either a *practical* limit owing to the state of our current theories and models which could hopefully be resolved in the future (with improved theories, models and technological advancements); or there could be a fundamental *cognitive limit* in our human capacities that will prevent us from filling this gap forever.

Dualist theories place consciousness (or some aspect of it) in a realm outside the physical. However, dualism itself comes in several flavours depending on whether non-physical entities (minds) exist separately from physical substances (substance dualism) or if both physical and non-physical properties are instantiated by the very same thing (property dualism or dual-aspect theory).

There are a number of theories which associate consciousness with a distinct cognitive architecture or with special pattern of activity - such as Global Workspace theory (Baars, 2005), Attended and Intermediate Representation (Prinz, 2012). Neural theories of consciousness appeal to various neural processes or properties to explain consciousness. Last, but not the least, Quantum theories of consciousness place the locus of consciousness to the micro-physical level of quantum phenomena. A popular theory in this category is the Orchestrated Objective Reduction (Orch-OR) proposed by Roger Penrose and Stuart Hameroff (1998) which posits that consciousness is an arising owing to quantum effects that occur within subcellular structures in microtubules which are internal to neurons.

Having briefly surveyed the different approaches to consciousness, we shall now shift our focus to scientific theories and further narrow down to the ones that can be measured in the clinic.

Towards a Science of Consciousness (Narrowing the Focus)

The two fundamental pillars of science are 'theory' and 'experiments'. In order to develop a coherent scientific theory of consciousness, it is imperative that the phenomenon under study is amenable to experimental investigation. Experimental investigation would always imply performing a 'measurement' of some kind, which is subsequently subject to analysis and interpretation. Thus, we are inevitably faced with the problem of 'measuring' consciousness if we are serious in our effort to develop a science of consciousness. But, to measure consciousness, we would also need a sound theoretical framework to guide our experiments in order to measure, analyze and interpret the experimental observations. Thus, 'Theory' and 'Experiment' mutually feed to each other in almost every scientific endeavour.

While reductionist theories are very successful in explaining, predicting and controlling physical/biological/natural phenomena (that does not involve the observer), the same is not true when it is applied to consciousness (which is very much pertaining to a conscious observer). By the very nature of its definition, all conscious experiences are first person's perspective and reductionist approaches are valid only for third person's account or observations. There is a disconnect between first person's perspective and third person's account in several conscious experiences such as deep sleep, coma, anaesthetic and drug induced states. It is also not clear how a neurobiological account of activity in the brain can convincingly explain my inner experience of 'redness' when I perceive a red rose, or my feeling of a headache. These experiences, by their very nature, seem to defy reductionist approaches at modelling and understanding.

In 1995, David Chalmers laid the foundation for a nonreductive theory of consciousness in his now much celebrated paper (Chalmers, 1995). Chalmers proposed 'psychophysical laws' – principles which connects physical processes with consciousness (Chalmers, 1995; Chalmers, 1996). The first of these is the coherence principle which connects consciousness to awareness, or global availability. The second is the principle of structural coherence that connects the structure of awareness to the structure of consciousness. The third is the law of organizational invariance which states that two systems (for eg., one made up of neurons and the other made up silicon chips) with exactly the same fine-grained functional organization will have qualitatively identical experiences. Chalmers also proposed a basic fundamental principle in the form of 'double-aspect information' which attempts to link phenomenal experiential states with physical states (for eg., brain states). However, despite being philosophically very well grounded, Chalmers' double-aspect information is not clinically feasible. In fact, it is not even clear how one would go about measuring double-aspect information in order to quantify or measure consciousness.

In a series of papers, Giulio Tononi (with others) has proposed a neuroscientific theory of consciousness based on ideas from information theory (Tononi et al., 1994; Tononi, 2004; Oizumi et al., 2014). Tononi claims that consciousness can be mathematically defined (and hence measured) as the inherent capacity of a system to integrate intrinsic information. As per Tononi, consciousness seems to be generated by certain parts of the brain (thalmocortical networks) than others (cerebellum) though the later may even boast of significantly greater number of neuronal connections. This can be explained, as per Tononi, by the fact that thalmocortical networks integrate a larger amount of intrinsic information. Though Tononi's theory has been subject to intense debate and criticism by several neuroscientists and philosophers, it has several good features, one of them being the possibility of a clinical assessment. Perturbational Complexity Index or PCI (Casali et al., 2013) is one such clinically applicable measure which claims theoretical links with Tononi's integrated information theory of consciousness.

There have been a plethora of measures of consciousness (please refer to Nagaraj & Virmani, 2017; Virmani & Nagaraj, 2019, and references therein). Table 1 gives a non-exhaustive list of measures of consciousness which have been recently proposed. Very few of these measures are practically feasible in the clinic owing to various challenges, issues and limitations which we will discuss in the next section.

MEASURING CONSCIOUSNESS IN THE CLINIC: ISSUES AND CHALLENGES

Why is it hard to measure consciousness in the clinic? There are a number of issues and challenges which we describe in this section.

Theoretical and Philosophical Issues

It has largely been a philosophical exercise to determine an acceptable definition of consciousness and conscious experience. However, there seems to be no universally acceptable definition of consciousness, one that would be equally agreeable to philosophers, scientists and researchers. Since we are interested in 'measuring' consciousness in the clinic, any definition that is reasonable and quantitative is desirable.

Table 1. Measures of consciousness and their clinical viability

Sl. No.	Consciousness Measure	What Does It Measure?	Clinical Viability	Remarks
1	Chalmer's Double-Aspect Information (Chalmers, 1995; 1996)	Doesn't measure, but proposes a bridge between the physical and phenomenal aspects of reality/experience	No	Philosophically well grounded but not practically viable
2	Neural Complexity (Tononi, Sporns, & Edelman, 1994)	Brain complexity	Low	Based on information theory
3	Causal Density (Seth, 2005)	Causal interactions in brain networks as a measure of consciousness	Medium	Granger causality measure is used
4	IIT 1.0 (Tononi, 2004)	Information integration	Low	Effective information defined using Mutual-Information
5	IIT 2.0 (Tononi, 2008)	Information integration	Low	Probabilistic model, requires perturbation analysis
6	IIT 3.0 (Oizumi, Albantakis, & Tononi, 2014)	Information integration	Low	Probabilistic model, cause-effect space, requires perturbation analysis
7	PCI (Casali et al., 2013)	Information integration in thalamocortical networks	Very High	Clinically measurable using TMS-EEG, claims link with integration theory

The role of a scientific theory in defining a measure of consciousness can't be undermined. For example, in order to measure temperature, a statistical theory of thermodynamics is needed. Without such a foundational theory, defining and measuring temperature has no real meaning. Similarly, in order to measure consciousness in the clinic, a theoretical framework needs to be in place first.

Broadly speaking, there are two classes of measures – behavioural measures and brain based measures (Seth et al., 2008). Behavioural measures of consciousness rely on the person's ability to respond or choose a behaviour which then becomes an index of his/her conscious level. The issue with this approach is that it can't be applied to patients who are in deep sleep or coma or anaesthetic state. Even for infants and animals, such a measure would not be applicable. Even when behavioural measure is applicable, it is difficult to measure graded conscious levels (i.e. a scale of conscious levels being low for deep-sleep, coma and vegetative states and high for waking with dream being intermediate level).

Brain based scientific measures of consciousness are increasingly becoming popular, and a large class of them fall under 'Complexity Theories of Consciousness' (Seth et al., 2008). As per integration theories, conscious contents are available widely to several cognitive/neural processes. Neuroscience theories have given rise to several putative measures of consciousness which quantify the simultaneous differentiation and integration of neural dynamics in brain networks. These theories argue that every conscious experience is also simultaneously differentiated and integrated (Seth et al., 2006). The fundamental issue with these approaches is whether these measures really capture level of consciousness as they claim, or they are merely indicative of conscious level at a gross approximation. In other words, could there be states or levels of consciousness which are beyond the ability of these measures to capture.

Methodological Issues

As noted earlier, one of the biggest issues with studying and measuring conscious experience is the fact that by its very nature is a first person's perspective or account of what he/she is experiencing. It seems that methods of science can't be directly applied to this case. To illustrate with an example, consider the scenario of the experience of anaesthesia. As a first person's account, my experience of anaesthetic state is very different from the third person's perspective (the doctor). Typically, such an experience is felt as timeless or instantaneous for myself as the subject of experience, i.e., it feels like the moment of losing waking consciousness and regaining it is instantaneous without any elapsed duration. Whereas, the doctor, who is not the subject of this experience, indicates that around 45 minutes of duration has indeed elapsed as per the external clock. This mismatch of the perception of time between the inner experience (myself, the subject of experience) and the external evidence (doctor's clock) leads to a methodological problem of measuring consciousness while in the anaesthetic state. When should we take the first person's report as useful evidence of conscious level and quality, and when can it be ignored as a mere illusion? There are no clear answers to this dilemma.

If we restrict ourselves to brain-based measures of consciousness, then first person's account is completely ignored. At this point, there are no frameworks to handle this methodological issue of taking into account first person's report along with brain-based measurements to arrive at a comprehensive measure of conscious level. This is indeed a work for the future.

Technological Challenges

Even if we grant that measuring neural activity (or capacity) of brain networks can be a good proxy or surrogate for determining the level of consciousness, there are technological challenges to achieve a robust, reliable and clinically applicable measure.

In order to record brain activity, there are several technologies available —including non-invasive techniques such as electroencephalography (EEG), magnetoencephalography (MEG), functional magnetic resonance imaging (fMRI) as well as invasive single-unit recordings which allow for single-neuron recordings. Single-unit recordings are very precise, but they are invasive and hence can't be applied widely, and definitely not to subjects who are normal. On the other hand, EEG, MEG and fMRI are non-invasive tools to study the central nervous system but do not provide very high spatial and temporal resolution. In order to map brain activity to behaviour, researchers need to create neuronal maps describing the flow of information through the brain. Stimulating different responses is a powerful technique to visualize which portion of the brain is activated and this can be used to explore networks pertaining to cognition, memory, perception, language, emotions and motor control. For measuring consciousness via complexity theories of consciousness (brain based complexity measures), it is required to determine which brain networks perform high amounts of information integration and differentiation.

Obtaining measurements of brain activity is only the first step. Sophisticated algorithmic techniques based on sound mathematical principles needs to be developed to glean out a measure of consciousness from these measurements. The challenges faced by these techniques/algorithms are the high amount of noise, interference, nonlinear feedback leading to cascading of errors, nonstationarity, missing data and non-gaussianity inherent in the measurements. Sources of noise could be several and the method needs to be robust, reliable and coherent. Repeatability and reproducibility is a must. The cost of these measurements and the development of software tools are quite high as of now to prevent large scale application and deployment. Further progress in hardware and software technologies can overcome these obstacles.

Clinical Challenges

Last but not the least, to bring all these under one roof, in a clinic, on real patients/subjects, is a very big challenge. Clinical applications have further challenges beyond the aforementioned theoretical & philosophical issues, methodological and technological challenges. These are in terms of ethical issues of what can be used and what can't be used on a patient or subject in the clinic. Even if a measure could be used in the clinic, what kind of medical decisions can actually be taken based on these measures? We are not at a stage yet where these measures could be used to take a potential life-saving/threatening decision. However, the hope is that such measures can eventually aid the clinician/surgeon to give further evidence to aid diagnosis/decision making on the operation table.

In Table 2, the issues and challenges described are highlighted, along with their severity, whether it will be resolved in the near future, and how important it is for a clinically viable solution for measuring consciousness. It is unlikely that philosophical issues will ever be resolved satisfactorily, though its importance to clinical application is rather low. Resolution of theoretical issues is possible in the near future given the

Table 2. A matrix of issues and challenges for developing a clinically viable measure of consciousness, along with severity, whether it will be resolved in the near future, and how important it is.

No.	Type of Issue/ Challenge	Severity	Whether It Will Be Resolved Soon	Importance for Clinical Applications
1	Philosophical	High	Unlikely	Low
2	Theoretical	Medium	Possible	Medium
3	Methodological	High	Probably soon	High
4	Technological	Medium	Yes	High
5	Clinical (Ethical)	High	No	High

rapid progress in integration theories and their critical analysis and refinements. Methodological issues are more severe, but also potentially resolvable in the near future by a hybrid approach of including first person's account along with brain based measures in a suitable and reasonable manner. Technological issues can be resolved owing to rapid advances in electronics, software, networking, communication and information processing systems. Ethical and other clinical challenges are unlikely to be resolved soon. This is because of the rise of artificial intelligence, machine learning and deep learning solutions, it is not clear what will be the nature of these problems when our society will allow robots to perform complex neuro-surgeries in place of humans. Also, whether we can ever come to use the output of these measures to determine and decide the life/death of an individual is a very controversial topic of debate, unlikely to be resolved anytime soon. But we will have to grapple with these issues and challenges going forward.

PERTURBATIONAL COMPLEXITY INDEX

In this section, we describe a recently proposed measure of consciousness – Perturbational Complexity Index (PCI) which has been applied in the clinic. We shall evaluate the pros and cons of such an approach.

Perturbational Complexity Index or PCI (Casali et al., 2013) is a clinical measure of consciousness which claims to be theoretically based on integrated information theory. PCI measures the information content of the response of thalamocortical networks in the brain by a measure of complexity known as Lempel-Ziv complexity (Lempel & Ziv, 1976), when the brain is excited by a magnetic pulse (Casali et al., 2013). PCI takes into account the theoretical considerations which indicate that consciousness is contingent on the complex activity resulting in the brain. This complex activity in brain networks is simultaneously information-rich (differentiated in space and time) and integrated (shared by interacting cortical areas). PCI as an objective clinical measure for the computation of consciousness, exhibits promising results when the values of PCI are compared across 3 kinds of subjects: (i) healthy subjects in wakefulness, non-rapid eye movement (NREM) sleep and dreaming states, (ii) subjects induced with sedation by anaesthetic agents: midazolam, xenon & propofol, and (iii) patients emerged from coma (vegetative state, minimally conscious state, and locked-in syndrome). PCI has the advantage of being non-invasive, and the assessment of consciousness is unaffected by the integrity of specific sensory pathways or motor efferent systems. PCI results are also invariant to the placement of TMS pulse across several cortical sites.

Though PCI has been measured in the clinic, there are issues that need to be addressed. It is not clear whether PCI does indeed measure consciousness as it claims since it does not directly measure the capacity of brain networks to integrate intrinsic information, as required by integrated information theory. Further, PCI values don't explicitly demonstrate how higher values in wakefulness correspond to higher integration and information-richness (differentiation) in cortical areas and inversely for lower values of PCI. As per integrated information theory, the quantitative value of consciousness as indicated by information integration can be computed only by perturbing the elements (in this case neurons or a group of neurons) by all possible inputs. Since PCI makes use of a single TMS pulse, it is not clear whether this is sufficient to indeed capture information integration of thalamocortical network.

CONCLUSION: THE WAY FORWARD

Consciousness continues to remain a challenging puzzle and arguably in many ways the final frontier of all research. Scientific theories of consciousness have witnessed significant progress in recent decades. However, there are several issues and challenges to be addressed for measuring consciousness in the clinic and these will require the coming together of researchers, cognitive scientists, mathematicians, computer scientists, philosophers and clinicians. The way forward to measuring consciousness depends on how we collectively address the issues raised in this chapter, and other unforeseen problems that will present to us in the future. One thing we can all agree is the immediacy of the need for building a science of consciousness and a robust, reliable and interpretable measure of consciousness in the clinic. There are exciting times ahead of us.

ACKNOWLEDGEMENTS

The author gratefully acknowledges the financial support of Science and Technology for Yoga and Meditation (SATYAM-DST) Grant no. DST/SATYAM/2017/45(G) and Tata Trusts towards this work.

REFERENCES

Baars, B. J. (2005). Global workspace theory of consciousness: Toward a cognitive neuroscience of human experience. *Progress in Brain Research, 150*, 45–53. doi:10.1016/S0079-6123(05)50004-9 PMID:16186014

Casali, A. G., Gosseries, O., Rosanova, M., Boly, M., Sarasso, S., Casali, K. R. ... Massimini, M. (2013). A theoretically based index of consciousness independent of sensory processing and behavior. *Science translational medicine, 5*(198).

Chalmers, D. J. (1995). Facing up to the problem of consciousness. *Journal of Consciousness Studies, 2*(3), 200–219.

Chalmers, D. J. (1996). The conscious mind: In search of a fundamental theory. Oxford, UK: Oxford University Press.

Josephson, B. D. (1996). First-Person Experience and the Scientific Exploration of Consciousness. In Biomedical and Life Physics (pp. 383-389). Vieweg+ Teubner Verlag. doi:10.1007/978-3-322-85017-1_38

Lempel, A., & Ziv, J. (1976). On the complexity of finite sequences. *IEEE Transactions on Information Theory, 22*(1), 75–81. doi:10.1109/TIT.1976.1055501

Levine, J. (1983). Materialism and qualia: The explanatory gap. *Pacific philosophical quarterly, 64*(4), 354-361.

Nagaraj, N., & Virmani, M. (2017). Is 'Information' Fundamental for a Scientific Theory of Consciousness? In *Self, Culture and Consciousness* (pp. 357–378). Singapore: Springer. doi:10.1007/978-981-10-5777-9_21

Nagel, T. (1974). What is it like to be a bat? *The Philosophical Review, 83*(4), 435–450. doi:10.2307/2183914

Oizumi, M., Albantakis, L., & Tononi, G. (2014). From the phenomenology to the mechanisms of consciousness: Integrated information theory 3.0. *PLoS Computational Biology, 10*(5). doi:10.1371/journal.pcbi.1003588 PMID:24811198

Penrose, R., & Hameroff, S. (1998). The PenroseHameroff 'Orch OR'Model of Consciousness. *Philosophical Transactions of the Royal Society of London. Series A, Mathematical and Physical Sciences, 356*, 1869–1896.

Prinz, J. (2012). The conscious brain. Oxford, UK: Oxford University Press. doi:10.1093/acprof:oso/9780195314595.001.0001

Seth, A. K. (2005). Causal connectivity of evolved neural networks during behavior. *Network (Bristol, England), 16*(1), 35–54. doi:10.1080/09548980500238756 PMID:16350433

Seth, A. K., Dienes, Z., Cleeremans, A., Overgaard, M., & Pessoa, L. (2008). Measuring consciousness: Relating behavioural and neurophysiological approaches. *Trends in Cognitive Sciences, 12*(8), 314–321. doi:10.1016/j.tics.2008.04.008 PMID:18606562

Seth, A. K., Izhikevich, E., Reeke, G. N., & Edelman, G. M. (2006). Theories and measures of consciousness: An extended framework. *Proceedings of the National Academy of Sciences of the United States of America, 103*(28), 10799–10804. doi:10.1073/pnas.0604347103 PMID:16818879

Tononi, G. (2004). An information integration theory of consciousness. *BMC Neuroscience, 5*(1), 42. doi:10.1186/1471-2202-5-42 PMID:15522121

Tononi, G. (2008). Consciousness as integrated information: A provisional manifesto. *The Biological Bulletin, 215*(3), 216–242. doi:10.2307/25470707 PMID:19098144

Tononi, G., Sporns, O., & Edelman, G. M. (1994). A measure for brain complexity: Relating functional segregation and integration in the nervous system. *Proceedings of the National Academy of Sciences of the United States of America, 91*(11), 5033–5037. doi:10.1073/pnas.91.11.5033 PMID:8197179

Van Gulick, R. (2018). "Consciousness". *The Stanford Encyclopedia of Philosophy* (Spring 2018 Edition), Edward N. Zalta (Ed.). Retrieved from https://plato.stanford.edu/archives/spr2018/entries/consciousness/

Virmani, M., & Nagaraj, N. (2019). A novel perturbation based compression complexity measure for networks. *Heliyon (London), 5*(2). doi:10.1016/j.heliyon.2019.e01181 PMID:30828654

Chapter 5
A Decision Tree on Data Mining Framework for Recognition of Chronic Kidney Disease

Ravindra B. V.
SOIS, Manipal Academy of Higher Education, Manipal, India

Sriraam N.
https://orcid.org/0000-0003-3790-3900
Centre for Medical Electronics and Computing, M. S. Ramaiah Institute of Technology, India

Geetha M.
Department of CSE, MIT, Manipal Academy of Higher Education, Manipal, India

ABSTRACT

The term chronic kidney disease (CKD) refers to the malfunction of the kidney and its failure to remove toxins and other waste products from blood. Typical symptoms of CKD include color change in urine, swelling due to fluids staying in tissue, itching, flank pain, and fatigue. Timely intervention is essential for early recognition of CKD as it affects more than 10 million people in India. This chapter suggests a decision tree-based data mining framework to recognize CKD from Non chronic kidney disease (NCKD). Data sets derived from open source UCI repository was considered. Unlike earlier reported work, this chapter applies the decision rules based on the clustered data through k-means clustering process. Four cluster groups were identified and j48 pruned decision tree-based automated rules were formatted.

DOI: 10.4018/978-1-7998-0326-3.ch005

The performance of the proposed framework was evaluated in terms of sensitivity, specificity, precision, and recall. A new quantitative measure, relative performance, and MCC were introduced which confirms the suitability of the proposed framework for recognition of CKD from NCKD.

INTRODUCTION

Kidney is the primary part of the excretory system which removes the excessive body fluids and wastes. The required chemical homeostasis is thereby maintained and thus it prevents any damage to the internal organ. There are situations where kidneys fail to function towards removing toxins and waste product from the blood. Such condition leads to chronic kidney disease (CKD). (Matovinović, 2009; Collister et al., 2016; Levey et al., 2005; Jojoa et al., 2017) Chronic kidney disease (CKD) refers to failure to generate functional aspects of kidney where one has to go for renal dialysis if it is for chronic renal failure. The acute renal failure leads to occurrence of end-stage renal disease (ESRD). The process of dialysis helps in removing the toxins and waste and helps the kidney to function through an artificial mode. The complex renal failure leads to chronic condition where one has to undergo kidney transplantation.

According to a survey 10 – 15% of adult population are being affected by CKD in India can be noted that CKD has been found to be potential indicator for increased cardiovascular disease and death. Studies reveals that CKD has a huge impact on causing hypertension, diabetes, obesity etc. One can refer to the work reported on pathophysiology and kidney disease classification for future understanding (Matovinovic, 2009).The decrease in GFR causes accumulation of Urea, Creatinine and other in blood. Thus affects the regular function of kidney. According to the kidney disease improving global outcomes declaration, Potential indication of CKD can be recognized by GFR of less than 60 ml / minute / 1.73m^2 (Levy et al., 2005). A detailed review in progression in CKD has been reported (Collister et al., 2016).

Developing country like India needs special attention as the number of people affected crossed 10 million according to a survey reported recently (Matovinovic, 2009). The decline of excretory, metabolic and endocrine functionalities merely indicates the stage of CKD occurrence. The biomarker that identifies the presence of the CKD includes presence of the presence of sediments in the urine, increased level of albumin excretion rate (AER) and albumin creatinine ratio (ACR); structural deformation reflected through the two-dimensional imaging procedure. The occurrence of CKD can be prevented through early intervention mechanism where computer aided intelligent decision system helps in recognizing the condition of CKD and non-chronic kidney disease (NCKD) of an individual.

This study suggests the application of data mining framework for recognition of CKD and NCKD patterns. Kidney dialysis parameters collected from Indian population available in the open source UCI repository was considered for the study which includes both healthy controls and kidney failure patients. Unlike earlier work reported earlier in the literature. The proposed study makes use of k-means clustering and four groups have been identified. Pattern classification was then performed by analyzing the rules that has been framed using J48 pruned decision tree data mining. Figure 1 shows the proposed data mining framework.

The performance of the proposed framework was evaluated using qualitative metrics such as precision, recall, kappa statistics, MCC, F-SCORE. The ROC characteristics through AUC confirm the suitability of the proposed framework.

Related Work

Data mining has played a crucial role towards pattern classification of medical data (Kusiak et al., 2003; Mai Shouman et al., Shah et al., 2006; Sephri et al., 2011; Sriraam et al., 2006). Kusiak et al., (2001, 2003) have reported data mining algorithms for kidney dialysis patients. Sriraam et al., (2006) have applied decision tree mining for survival prediction of kidney failure patients. For chronic kidney disease classification, several works have been reported in the literature. A specific report made by Nahas et al., (2005) highlighted the challenges involved towards CKD recognition and diagnosis. Rubini & Eswaran (2015) have reported a study on prediction of CKD. Three models, radial basis function neural network multilayer perception neural network and linear logistic regression model was employed for the study. Though the results were reported, no detailed information on neural network model configuration was reported. Ravindra et al., have made a special study towards clustering phenomena for kidney dialysis data (Ravindra et al., 2015) Neural network and SVM based classification procedure was reported recently (Ravindra et al., 2018; Ravindra et al., 2019).

Figure 1. Proposed data mining framework

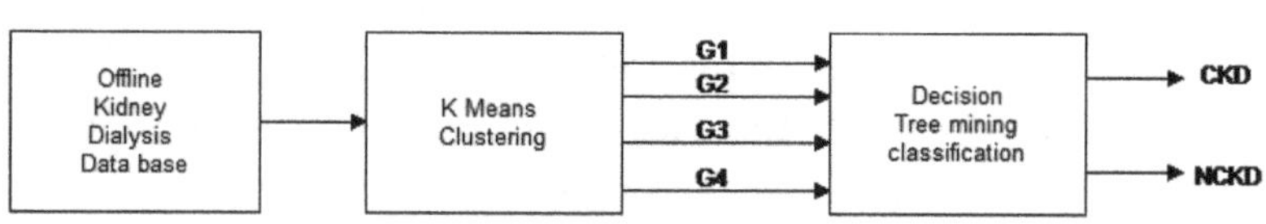

Table 1. Attributes and their properties in patient dataset

No	Attribute	Type	Units or Values
1	Age	Numerical	Years
2	Blood Pressure	Numerical	mm/Hg
3	Specific Gravity	Nominal	(1.005,1.010,1.015,1.020,1.025)
4	Albumin	Nominal	(0,1,2,3,4,5)
5	Sugar	Nominal	(0,1,2,3,4,5)
6	Red Blood Cells	Nominal	(normal, abnormal)
7	Pus Cell	Nominal	(normal, abnormal)
8	Pus Cell clumps	Nominal	(present, not present)
9	Bacteria	Nominal	(present, not present)
10	Blood Glucose Random	Numerical	mgs/dl
11	Blood Urea	Numerical	mgs/dl
12	Serum Creatinine	Numerical	mgs/dl
13	Sodium	Numerical	mEq/L
14	Potassium	Numerical	mEq/L
15	Hemoglobin	Numerical	gms
16	Packed Cell Volume	Numerical	
17	White Blood Cell Count	Numerical	cells/cumm
18	Red Blood Cell Count	Numerical	millions/cmm
19	Hypertension	Nominal	(yes, no)
20	Diabetes Mellitus	Nominal	(yes, no)
21	Coronary Artery Disease	Nominal	(yes, no)
22	Appetite	Nominal	(good, poor)
23	Pedal Edema	Nominal	(yes, no)
24	Anemia	Nominal	(yes, no)
25	Class	Nominal	(ckd, not ckd)

Study Database

The dataset contained 400 patient records, which were reported to be obtained from India, and was posted with the University of California Irvine Machine Learning Repository (Dua & Graff, 2019; Rubini & Eswaran, 2015). Description of 25 attributes in the dataset is presented in Table 1.Table 2 shows the baseline characteristics (Dua & Graff, 2019).

Table 2. Baseline characteristics of the study population (n=150 NCKD) and (N-250 CKD)

Variable	NCKD Mean ± Standard Deviation	CKD Mean ± Standard Deviation
Age	46.517 ± 15.631	54.21 ± 17.389
Blood Pressure	71.351 ± 8.543	79.625 ± 15.234
Specific Gravity	1.022 ± 0.003	1.014 ± 0.005
Albumin	0 ± 0	1.722 ± 1.373
Sugar	0 ± 0	0.767 ± 1.349
Blood Glucose Random	107.722 ± 18.565	175.42 ± 92.082
Blood Urea	32.79 ± 11.45	72.389 ± 58.587
Serum Creatinine	0.869 ± 0.255	4.415 ± 6.95
Sodium	141.731 ± 4.818	133.902 ± 12.403
Potassium	4.388 ± 0.587	4.878 ± 4.322
Hemoglobin	15.188 ± 1.278	10.648 ± 2.186
Packed Cell Volume	46.336 ± 4.134	32.94 ± 7.029
White Blood Cell Count	7705.05 ± 1839.771	9069.536 ± 3580.521
Red Blood Cell Count	5.379 ± 0.596	3.945 ± 0.865

K-means clustering procedure as reported in our earlier work (Ravindra et al., 2017, Ravindra et al., 2018) was applied to cluster closely related attributes. For the proposed study, four cluster groups G1, G2, G3, G4 were considered and Table 3 shows the group for classification & understanding groups are referred to as CASEA, B, C and D respectively.

Table 3. Parameters considered in each group

CASE A	CASE B	CASE C	CASE D
Blood Pressure	Albumin	Packed Cell Volume	Albumin
Specific Gravity	Sugar	White Blood Cell Count	Sugar
Serum Creatinine	Blood Glucose Random	Red Blood Cell Count	Blood Glucose Random
	Hemoglobin		Blood Urea
			Serum Creatinine
			Sodium
			Potassium

Decision Tree Data Mining

A decision tree referred to as integrated structure that comprises of root node, branches and leaf nodes (Danham & Sridhar, 2006; Witten et al., 1999; Breslow & Aha., 1997). Any given attribute is tested by the internal node with the branch shows the outcome of the test and the class label is represented by the leaf. Root node refers to the topmost node in the tree. A decision tree is pruned to obtain a tree that confirms the generalization of the given training dataset. A best way of pruning a decision tree is to impose a minimum on the number of the training attributes of the given dataset.

In the proposed study, an univariate approach referred as J48 decision tree algorithm is proposed. J48 classifier derived from simple C4.5 decision tree performs the binary tree operation for classifying the given dataset. A decision tree is pruned to obtain a tree that confirms the generalization of the training dataset (Rokach & Maimon, 2005). A best way of pruning a decision tree is to impose minimum on the number of training attributes of the given dataset (Mohamed et al., 2012). For the proposed study J48 decision tree considers minimum default functions as 2 to generate number of leaves and trees. For better understanding and brevity, the structure of J48 decision tree algorithm is given below: (Danham & Sridhar, 2006)

```
INPUT
        I         // Training data
OUTPUT
•        // Decision tree
DTBUILD (*I)
{
        O = ψ;
        O = Initiate rot node and label with spitting
attribute;
        O = ADD arc to root node for each split predicate and
label;
For each arc perform
        I = Dataset created by applying splitting predicate to
I;
If stopping node reached for this path, then
                O' = Create leaf node and label with
appropriate class;
Else
                O' = DTBUILD (I);
```

Table 4. Confusion Matrix

CKD/NCKD	Classified as CKD	Classified as NCKD
NCKD	T_P	F_N
CKD	F_P	T_N

Where $T_{P:}$ True positive
$T_{N:}$ True negative
$F_{P:}$ False positive
$F_{N:}$ False negative

```
O = add O' to arc;
}
```

Evaluation

The following parameters were included to evaluate the performance of decision tree classifier:

$$\text{Specificity} = T_P / (T_P+T_N) * 100\% \quad (1)$$

$$\text{Sensitivity} = T_N / (F_P+T_N) * 100\% \quad (2)$$

$$\text{Accuracy} = (T_P+T_N) / (T_P+F_P+T_N+F_N) * 100\% \quad (3)$$

$$\text{Recall} = T_P / (T_P+T_N) \quad (4)$$

$$\text{Precision} = T_P / (T_P+F_N) \quad (5)$$

$$\text{Fscore} = ((2* T_P)/(2* T_P + F_P + T_N)) \quad (6)$$

$$\text{MCC} = (((T_P * T_N)-(F_P * F_N)) / (\text{SQRT} ((T_P + T_N)*(T_N + F_P)*(T_P + F_P)*(F_N * T_N)))) \quad (7)$$

Figure 2. Set of rules obtained by J48 algorithm for CASE A

```
sc <= 1.2
|   sg <= 1.015: ckd (39.66/1.0)
|   sg > 1.015: notckd (158.77/12.29)
sc > 1.2: ckd (201.57/2.52)
```

Kappa test = (Observed agreement - Expected agreement) / (100 - Expected agreement) (8)

Where observed agreement is overall accuracy and

Expected agreement is = $\{((TP + F_P)*(FN + T_P)) + ((T_N + F_N)*(F_P + T_N))$ (9)

Table 4 shows the confusion matrix for the proposed classification.

For each clustered group, J48 decision tree mining algorithm was applied and decision rules were generated in terms of CKD and NCKD for each case. The combination of different kidney dialysis attributes with data mining framework resulted in recognition of CKD from NCKD. The set of rules generated by the decision tree algorithms and its corresponding tree structure for CASE A, B,C and D were shown in Figures 2,3,4 and 5 respectively. Tables 5,6,7 and 8 shows the decision generated as CKD,NCKD based on the decision tree rules.


```
sc <= 1.2
|   sg <= 1.015: ckd (39.66/1.0)
|   sg > 1.015: notckd (158.77/12.29)
sc > 1.2: ckd (201.57/2.52)
```


Table 5. Decision Tree Rules generated for CASE A for CKD-NCKD recognitions

Rules Generated	CASE A	CKD/NCKD
Rule1	sc<=1.2 & sg <=1.015	CKD
Rule2	sc<=1.2 & sg > 1.015	NCKD
Rule3	sc > 1.2	CKD

Figure 3. Set of rules obtained by J48 algorithm for CASE B

```
hemo <= 12.9: ckd (205.75/3.09)
hemo > 12.9
|   al <= 0
|   |   bgr <= 141: notckd (156.43/10.59)
|   |   bgr > 141: ckd (10.18/0.37)
|   al > 0: ckd (27.64/0.71
```

Table 6. Decision Tree Rules generated for CASE B for CKD-NCKD recognitions

Rules Generated	CASE B	CKD/NCKD
Rule1	Hemo <= 12.9	CKD
Rule2	(Hemo > 12.9) & (al <= 0 & bgr <= 141)	NCKD
Rule3	(Hemo > 12.9) & (al <= 0 & bgr > 141)	CKD
Rule4	(Hemo > 12.9) & (al > 0)	CKD


```
hemo <= 12.9: ckd (205.75/3.09)
hemo > 12.9
|   al <= 0
|   |   bgr <= 141: notckd (156.43/10.59)
|   |   bgr > 141: ckd (10.18/0.37)
|   al > 0: ckd (27.64/0.71
```


Figure 4. Set of rules obtained by J48 algorithm for CASE C

```
pcv <= 39: ckd (183.59/1.84)
pcv > 39
|   pcv <= 44
|   |   rbcc <= 4.4: ckd (6.22/0.23)
|   |   rbcc > 4.4: notckd (95.9/36.11)
|   pcv > 44: notckd (114.29/26.14)
```

Table 7. Decision Tree Rules generated for CASE C for CKD-NCKD recognitions

Rules Generated	CASE C	CKD/NCKD
Rule1	Pcv <=39	CKD
Rule2	Pcv > 39 & Pcv <= 44 &rbcc <= 4.4	CKD
Rule3	Pcv > 39 & Pcv <= 44 &rbcc > 4.4	NCKD
Rule4	Pcv > 39 & Pcv > 44	NCKD

```
pcv <= 39: ckd (183.59/1.84)
pcv > 39
|   pcv <= 44
|   |   rbcc <= 4.4: ckd (6.22/0.23)
|   |   rbcc > 4.4: notckd (95.9/36.11)
|   pcv > 44: notckd (114.29/26.14)
```

```
sc <= 1.2
|   bgr <= 144
|   |   al <= 0: notckd (148.0/10.0)
|   |   al > 0
```

Figure 5. Set of rules obtained by J48 algorithm for CASE D

```
sc <= 1.2
|  bgr <= 144
|  |  al <= 0: notckd (148.0/10.0)
|  |  al > 0
|  |  |  su <= 0: ckd (11.0)
|  |  |  su > 0: notckd (5.0)
|  bgr > 144
|  |  pot <= 4.7: ckd (23.0)
|  |  pot > 4.7: notckd (3.0/1.0)
sc > 1.2: ckd (210.0/5.0)
```

Table 8. Decision Tree Rules generated for CASE D for CKD-NCKD recognitions

Rules Generated	CASE D	CKD/NCKD
Rule1	sc > 1.2	CKD
Rule2	sc<=1.2 & bgr > 144 & pot<= 4.7	CKD
Rule3	sc<=1.2 & bgr > 144 & pot > 4.7	NCKD
Rule4	sc<=1.2 & bgr <= 144 & al <= 0	NCKD
Rule5	sc<=1.2 & bgr <= 144 & al > 0 & su <= 0	CKD
Rule6	sc<=1.2 & bgr <= 144 & al > 0 & su > 0	NCKD

```
|   |   |   su <= 0: ckd (11.0)
|   |   |   su > 0: notckd (5.0)
|   bgr > 144
|   |   pot <= 4.7: ckd (23.0)
|   |   pot > 4.7: notckd (3.0/1.0)
sc > 1.2: ckd (210.0/5.0)
```

The performance of the proposed data mining framework for classification of CKD and NCKD was evaluated in terms of Precision, Recall, F Measures. Table 9 shows the confusion matrix obtained using the decision tree classifier.

The quantitative performance metrics as depicted in Figure 6 confirms the suitability of the proposed data mining framework for recognition of CKD. The precision and F-measure metrics almost indicate >98.5% attainment. Almost the four groups except group B other groups perform well. Figure 7a shows the

Table 9. Confusion Matrix for Decision Tree Classifier

		Classified as CKD	Classified as NCKD
CASE A	CKD	239	11
	NCKD	5	145
CASE B	CKD	246	4
	NCKD	6	144
CASE C	CKD	223	27
	NCKD	22	128
CASE D	CKD	237	13
	NCKD	8	142

Figure 6. Decision tree classifier performance

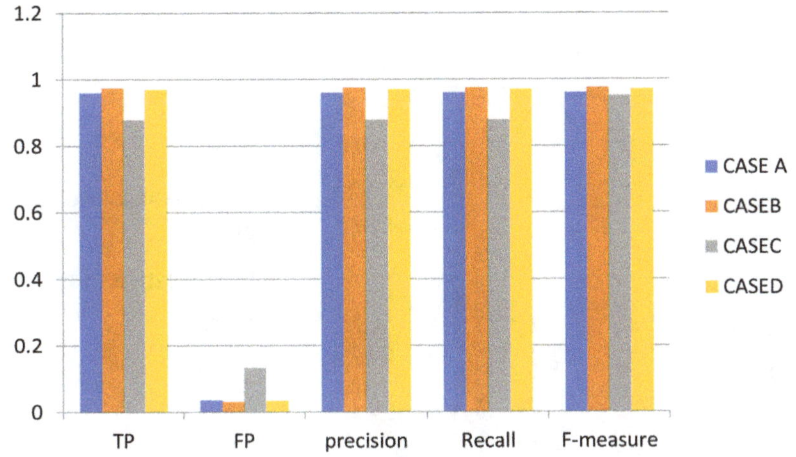

performance of the proposed classifier in terms of MSE, and kappa statistics, and Figure 7b shows the relative error.

The result confirm cluster group A and D found to be a potential candidate for necessary clinical diagnosis. The overall performance was finally evaluated in terms of relative performance of the decision tree classifier which is defined as:

Relative performance = Precision/computational time (10)

Figure 7a. Error status and Kappa statistics

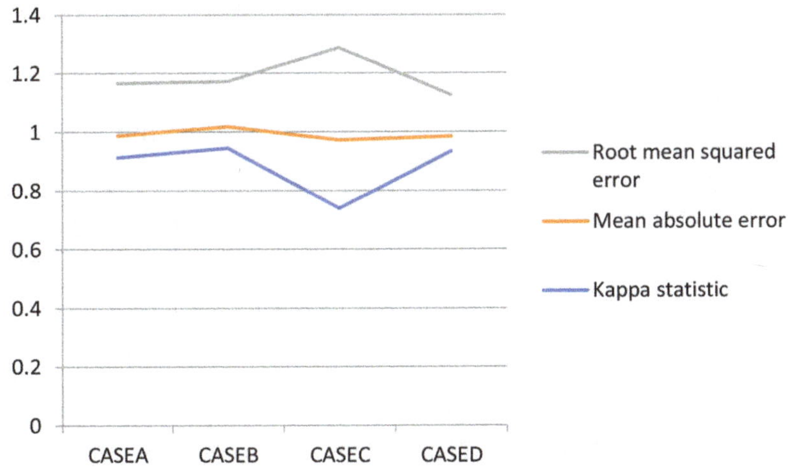

Figure 7b. Relative absolute and root relative squared error

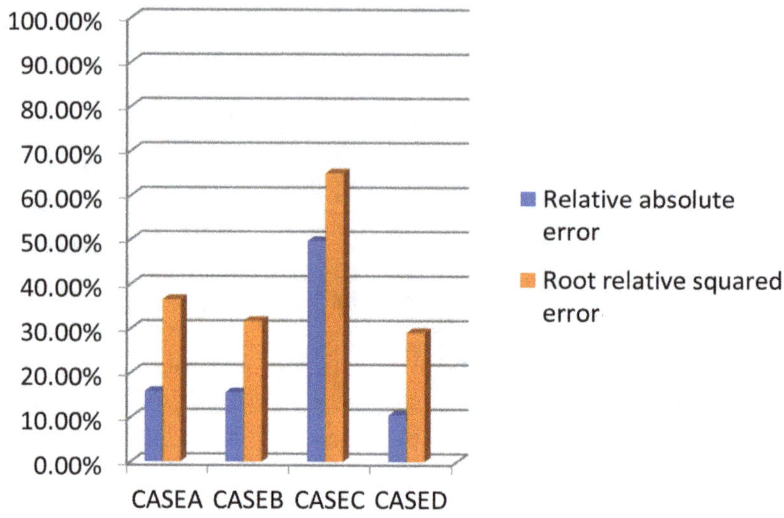

Figure 8. Shows the results which indicates CASE A and CASE D could be a potential cluster parameter for early recognition of CKD.

DISCUSSION

It is very important to identify the key priority parameters that contributes significantly towards the recognition of CKD FROM patient's dialysis attributes, unlike earlier

Figure 8. Relative performance

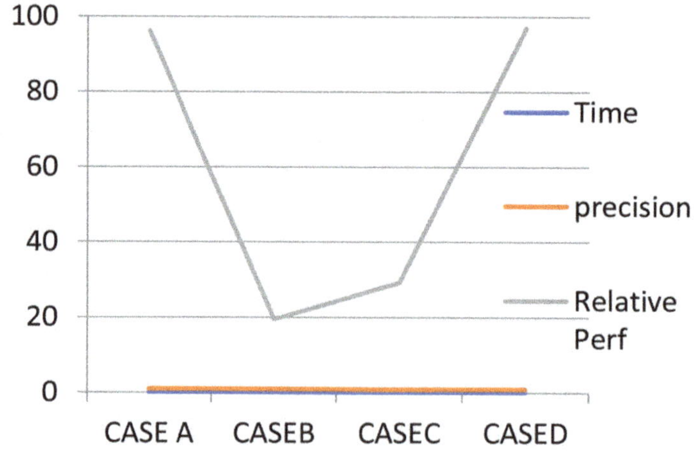

Table 10. Optimal decision tree classifier performance

	No of Leaves	Size of Tree	AUC
CASE A	3	5	96.8
CASE B	4	7	97.5
CASE C	4	7	95
CASE D	6	11	94.75

reported study. The proposed data mining framework considered closely correlated kidney dialysis attributes for recognition of CKD. Four cases/groups have been framed by means of clustering. Among the four cases CASE B yields better specificity and less sensitivity following were inferred from the proposed study.

Serum Creatinine was dominant towards the recognition of CKD among these attributes for CASE A.

Hemoglobin and Albumin were equally contributed towards CKD for CASE B

Packed cell volume and red blood cell count contributed significantly towards recognition of CKD for CASE C.

For CASE D, among the seven attributes four attributes were dominated (Serum Creatinine, Blood Glucose Random, albumin and potassium).

It can be further noted the level of Serum Creatinine could be a potential biomarker for recognition of CKD from NCKD.

The efficiency of the decision tree data mining framework lies on the attributes, no of leaves and size of the tree. The optimal decision tree classifier performance based on the above attributes is shown in the Table 10.

From Table 10, the area under the ROC curve (AUC) of the decision tree classifier confirms again the efficiency of the proposed framework for CKD-NCKD classification. It can be further noted that the relative performance shows the importance of close correlation between the kidney dialysis parameters for recognition of CKD and NCKD group

REFERENCES

Breslow, L. A., & Aha, D. W. (1997). *Simplifying Decision Trees: A Survey*. Washington, DC: Navy Center for Applied Research in Artificial Intelligence, Naval Research Laboratory.

Collister, D., Ferguson, T., Komenda, P., & Tangri, N. (2016). The Patterns, Risk Factors, and Prediction of Progression in Chronic Kidney Disease: A Narrative Review. *Seminars in Nephrology*, *36*(4), 273–282. doi:10.1016/j.semnephrol.2016.05.004 PMID:27475658

Dua, D. & Graff, C. (2019). UCI Machine Learning Repository. Retrieved from http://archive.ics.uci.edu/ml. Irvine, CA: University of California, School of Information and Computer Science.

Dunham, M. H. (2006). *Data Mining: Introductory and Advanced Topics. Pearson Education India* (p. 315). Pearson Education India. Retrieved from http://www.amazon.com/Data-Mining-Introductory-Advanced-Topics/dp/0130888923

El Nahas, M. (2005). The global challenge of chronic kidney disease. *Kidney International*, *68*(6), 2918–2929. Retrieved from http://www.ncbi.nlm.nih.gov/pubmed/21212690. doi:10.1111/j.1523-1755.2005.00774.x PMID:16316385

Kumar, M. (2016). Prediction of Chronic Kidney Disease Using Random Forest Machine Learning Algorithm. *Journal of Computer Science and Mobile Computing*, *5*(2), 24–33.

Kusiak, A. (2001). Feature transformation methods in data mining. *IEEE Transactions on Electronics Packaging Manufacturing*, *24*(3), 214–221. doi:10.1109/6104.956807

Kusiak, A. (2003). Data mining based decision-making approach for predicting survival of kidney dialysis patients. In IFAC Proceedings Volumes (IFAC-Papers Online)(Vol. 36, pp. 35–39). IFAC Secretariat. 10.1016/S1474-6670(17)33468-7

Lasisi, T. J., Raji, Y. R., & Salako, B. L. (2016). Salivary creatinine and urea analysis in patients with chronic kidney disease: A case control study. *BMC Nephrology*, *17*(1), 10. doi:10.118612882-016-0222-x PMID:26775026

Levey, A. S., Eckardt, K. U., Tsukamoto, Y., Levin, A., Coresh, J., Rossert, J., ... Eknoyan, G. (2005). Definition and classification of chronic kidney disease: A position statement from Kidney Disease: Improving Global Outcomes (KDIGO). *Kidney International*, *67*(6), 2089–2100. doi:10.1111/j.1523-1755.2005.00365.x PMID:15882252

Lichman, M. (2013). *UCI Machine Learning Repository. Retrieved from* http://archive.ics.uci.edu/ml. Irvine, CA: University of California, School of Information and Computer Science.

Matovinović, M. S. (2009). 1. Pathophysiology and Classification of Kidney Diseases. *EJIFCC, 20*(1), 2–11. Retrieved from http://www.ncbi.nlm.nih.gov/pubmed/27683321. PMID:27683321

Mohamed, W. N. H. W., Salleh, M. N. M., & Omar, A. H. O. (2012). A comparative study of Reduced Error Pruning method in decision tree algorithms. In *Proceedings - 2012 IEEE International Conference on Control System, Computing and Engineering, ICCSCE.* (pp. 392–397). 10.1109/ICCSCE.2012.6487177

Jojoa, J. A., Rivera, C. E., Delgado, E. M., Casas, H. M., Rosas, G. M., Rosero, C. Y., & Montenegro, F. A. (2017). (2017). New ABC Chronic Kidney Disease Classification. *Int J Nephrol Kidney Failure, 3*(2). doi:10.16966/2380-5498.144

Nisha, R., Srinivasa, K. S. R., Thanga, M. K., & Jagatha, P. (2017). Biochemical evaluation of creatinine and urea in patients with renal failure undergoing hemodialysis. *Journal of Clinical Pathology and Laboratory Medicine, 1*(2), 1–5.

Potharaju, S. P., & Sreedevi, M. (2016). An improved prediction of kidney disease using SMOTE. *Indian Journal of Science and Technology, 9*(31). doi:10.17485/ijst/2016/v9i31/95634

Ravindra, B. V., Sriraam, N., & Geetha, M. (2018). Chronic kidney disease detection using back propagation neural network classifier. In *Proceedings of the 2018 International Conference on Communication, Computing and Internet of Things, IC3IoT 2018* (pp. 65–68). Piscataway, NJ: IEEE. 10.1109/IC3IoT.2018.8668110

Ravindra, B. V., Sriraam, N., & Geetha, M. (2017). Classification of non-chronic and chronic kidney disease using SVM neural networks. *International Journal of Engineering & Technology, 7*(1.3), 191. doi:10.14419/ijet.v7i1.3.10669

Rokach, L., & Maimon, O. (2005). Top-Down Induction of Decision Trees Classifiers – A Survey. *IEEE Transactions on Systems, Man and Cybernetics. Part C, Applications and Reviews, 35*(4), 476–487. doi:10.1109/TSMCC.2004.843247

Rubini, L., & Eswaran, P. (2015). Generating comparative analysis of early stage prediction of Chronic Kidney Disease. *International Journal Of Modern Engineering Research, 5*(49), 49–55.

Sriraam, N., Natasha, V., & Kaur, H. (2011). Data Mining Techniques and Medical Decision Making for Urological Dysfunction. In Data Warehousing and Mining (pp. 2506–2516). Hershey, PA: IGI Global. doi:10.4018/978-1-59904-951-9.ch153

Subas, A., Alickovic, E., & Kevric, J. (2017). Diagnosis of chronic kidney disease by using random forest. In IFMBE proceedings, 62, pp. 589–594. Germany: Springer Verlag. doi:10.1007/978-981-10-4166-2_89

Udhayarasu, M., Ramakrishnan, K., & Periasamy, S. (2017). Assessment of chronic kidney disease using skin texture as a key parameter: For South Indian population. *Healthcare Technology Letters*, *4*(6), 223–227. doi:10.1049/htl.2016.0098 PMID:29383256

Witten, H., Frank, E., Trigg, L., Hall, M., Holmes, G., & Cunningham, S. J. (1999). Weka: Practical Machine Learning Tools and Techniques with Java Implementations.

APPENDIX

Glossary

Al: Albumin. Patients with ESRD Hypoalbuminemia is common it affected by a blend of increased degradation of albumin and reduced synthesis.

Ba: Bacteria. End-stage renal disease (ESRD) patients and persons who are a healthy analysis of Microbial DNA exposed that raise in the comparative profusion for 190 (OTUs)operational taxonomic units which they belong to the ESRD group. Whereas healthy group OTUs belong to other good health groups.

Bgr: Blood glucose random. Diabetes is challenging to manage in patients who have end-stagerenal disease (ESRD), as both uremia and dialysis can complicate glycemic control by affecting the secretion, clearance, and peripheral tissue sensitivity of insulin. Insulin doses should be lowered in those with low glomerular filtration rates.

Bp: Blood pressure. Hypertension is a Major cause for the decline in GFR which results in a strong independent factor for ESRD. Both systolic (SBP) and diastolic (DBP) are the major causes for CKD.

Bu: Blood urea. BUN level increases when kidneys unable to eliminate urea from blood hence there is a direct link between CKD & blood urea.

Hemo: Hemoglobin. Hemoglobin in patients' blood is used to evaluate anemia's early stage followed by the progression of chronic kidney disease.

Pc: Pus cell. Pus cells are nothing but white blood cells they indicate infection indication.

Pcc: Pus cell clumps. Pus cell clumps are nothing but white blood cells they indicate infection indication.

Pcv: Packed cell volume. Packed cell volume in the patients is a predictive factor for Anemia and intern anemia stage indicate the early renal disease.

Rbc: Red blood cells. Enough EPO cannot be made by the damaged kidneys which cause bone marrow makes fewer red blood cells initiating anemia.

Rc: Red blood cell count. Enough EPO cannot be made by the damaged kidneys which cause bone marrow makes fewer red blood cells initiating anemia.

Sc: Serum creatinine. The damage of the kidney advancement is noticeable by two important chemicals in the blood one among them is creatinine evaluation in serum assists to measure Glomerular Filtration Rate (GFR) followed by renal function.

Sg: Specific gravity. When the kidney is functioning normal, urine specific gravity will be in the range 1.002 and 1.030 otherwise it is one of the critical parameters for CKD.

Su: Sugar. It is vital in the treatment of ESRD diabetic patients to prevent additional harm to other organs (eyes, kidneys, and heart) it is suggested that blood sugar control need to be taken care.

Wc: White blood cell count. The WBC (white blood cell count) and absolute neutrophil count are directly associated with impermanence risk in ESRD.

Chapter 6
Classification of EMG Signals Using Eigenvalue Decomposition-Based Time-Frequency Representation

Rishi Raj Sharma
Defence Institute of Advanced Technology, Pune, India

Mohit Kumar
Vel Tech Rangarajan Dr. Sagunthala R & D Institute of Science and Technology, Chennai, India

Ram Bilas Pachori
Indian Institute of Technology, Indore, India

ABSTRACT

Electromyogram (EMG) signals are commonly used by doctors to diagnose abnormality of muscles. Manual analysis of EMG signals is a time-consuming and cumbersome task. Hence, this chapter aims to develop an automated method to detect abnormal EMG signals. First, authors have applied the improved eigenvalue decomposition of Hankel matrix and Hilbert transform (IEVDHM-HT) method to obtain the time-frequency (TF) representation of motor unit action potentials (MUAPs) extracted from EMG signals. Then, the obtained TF matrices are used for features extraction. TF matrix has been sliced into several parts and fractional energy in each slice is computed. A percentile-based slicing is applied to obtain discriminating features. Finally, the features are used as an input to the classifiers such as random forest, least-squares support vector machine, and multilayer perceptron to classify the EMG signals namely, normal and ALS, normal and myopathy, and ALS and myopathy, and achieved accuracy of 83%, 80.8%, and 96.7%, respectively.

DOI: 10.4018/978-1-7998-0326-3.ch006

INTRODUCTION

The muscular system is responsible to generate the force for the movement of the body and providing the shape to the body. Nerve impulses are responsible for the movement of the muscles. These impulses originated in the brain and travel through the peripheral nervous system to a specific location in the body. Neuromuscular disorder (NMD) is a disorder which interrupts the communication path between the nervous system and the muscles (Kandel et al., 2000; Anthea et al., 1993). Motor neuron diseases, disorders of neuromuscular transmission, neuropathy, amyotrophic lateral sclerosis (ALS), and myopathy come under the category of NMD (Karpati et al., 1970). Myopathy is a disease which affects the skeletal muscle tissue directly. It affects the functioning of the muscles. However, neuropathy is related to the disease that causes damage to the nerves which is involved in the muscular control (Yousefi et al., 2014). The ALS is also a type of NMD which can also be responsible for the death of the patient (Mishra, et al., 2016, February). The commonly found symptoms of ALS are respiratory failure, atrophy, and weakness. It may have serious impact on the functioning of motor neurons. With the time, it may result in the paralysis. Hence, in time diagnosis and proper treatment are of prime importance. Electromyogram (EMG) is a common tool utilized by the clinician for the diagnosis of the NMD.

In general, neurophysiologists utilized the properties of motor unit action potentials (MUAPs) to assess the NMDs (Nikolic & Krarup, 2011). Hence, MUAPs have an important role in the diagnosis of the NMDs. The MUAPs consist a complex structure which makes the manual assessment, a difficult task. Moreover, the accurate manual detection of the abnormalities present in the characteristics of MUAPs requires a lot of skills and experience. Hence, the detection accuracy of these abnormalities may not be sufficient to take the further step. Therefore, it is required to perform computer aided analysis of MUAPs using signal processing techniques.

Several computer aided methods are available in the literature for the analysis of normal and NMD EMG signals. In (Pattichis & Elia, 1999), the time domain measures, cepstral coefficients, autoregressive (AR) coefficients, and AR spectral measures are computed from the MUAPs for the analysis of normal and diseased EMG signals. In (Fattah et al., 2012), time and frequency domain-based features such as zero crossing rate, autocorrelation, and Fourier transform are suggested for the detection of the ALS patients. The interference pattern analysis is found useful in studying the muscle activity (Fuglsang-Frederiksen, 2000). A method for ALS detection based on short time Fourier transform (STFT) is proposed in (Doulah et al., 2012, May). In (Pfeiffer, 1999), a sequential Baysen algorithm-based approach is used to analyze the EMG signals. An AR method and wavelet neural network-based approach is utilized for the discrimination of different classes of EMG signals (Subasi et al., 2006). The principal component analysis (PCA) based method is proposed to analyze the EMG signals in (Shaw & Bagha, 2012). In (Doulah & Fattah, 2014, April), the mel-frequency cepstral coefficients are computed from the MUAPs and fed to the K-nearest neighbour (K-NN) classifier. This method is found effective for the detection of the ALS.

In (Güler & Koçer, 2005), a fast Fourier transform (FFT) and PCA based algorithm is applied to discriminate the normal, neuropathy, and myopathy EMG signals. In (Katsis et al., 2007), a clustering-based approach is followed for the analysis of normal, neuropathy, and myopathy EMG signals. The continuous wavelet transform is applied to the EMG signals for the classification of MUAPs (Gazzoni et al., 2004). In (Kouchaki, 2012, May), Kolmogorov complexity (KC) is used as a feature for the discrimination of the different types of EMG signals. The KC feature is obtained from the intrinsic mode functions (IMFs) extracted using the empirical mode decomposition (EMD). EMD based features are also utilized for the classification of normal and ALS EMG signals in (Mishra et al., 2017). In (Christodoulou & Pattichis, 1999), two different techniques based on pattern recognition are proposed for the classification of EMG signals. One method is based on artificial neural network (ANN) algorithm, and a statistical pattern recognition based technique is used in the second approach. A time-frequency (TF) based approach is proposed for the analysis of normal and diseased EMG signals in (Sharma et al., 2019a), and correntropy and cross information potential are used as a feature to discriminate the various types of EMG signals. In (Joshi et al., 2017, February), tunable-Q wavelet transform (TQWT) method is used to decompose the EMG signals into sub-bands. The authors have computed various linear and non-linear features from these sub-bands for detecting the abnormal EMG signals.

In this work, we have aimed to propose a method for classifying the normal, ALS, and myopathy EMG signals. Initially MUAPs are extracted from EMG signals of each class and thereafter TF matrix is obtained for each MUAP. The TF matrix is obtained using improved eigenvalue decomposition of Hankel matrix and Hilbert transform (IEVDHM-HT) method (Sharma & Pachori, 2017a; Sharma & Pachori, 2017b, February). The IEVDHM-HT method decomposes a multi-component non-stationary signal into mono-component signals and compute their instantaneous amplitudes and frequencies in order to represent signal in TF domain. This method has provided better TF representation (TFR) as compared to Hilbert-Huang transform (HHT) (Huang, et al., 1998, March) as HHT suffers from mode-mixing phenomena while the IEVDHM-HT method is free from mode-mixing. The IEVDHM-HT method is also used for complex data analysis in (Sharma & Pachori, 2018a), in which a complex signal is represented in TF plane in entire positive and negative frequency range. A methodology for cross-terms elimination in Wigner-Ville distribution using eigenvalue decomposition method is proposed in (Sharma & Pachori, 2018b). The baseline wander and power line interference removal from electrocardiogram (ECG) signal using eigenvalue decomposition method is presented in (Sharma & Pachori, 2018c). The performance of the extracted features is evaluated using least squares support vector machine (LS-SVM) (Suykens & Vandewalle, 1999) and random forest classifiers (Breiman, 2001) to find the most suitable combination of the features. Flow chart of the proposed work can be seen in Figure 1.

This chapter is organized in the following way: In the second section, information of the dataset, TFR, various TF based features and classification method is provided. The results of the work are presented in the third section and discussed in the fourth section. The work is concluded in the fifth section.

METHODOLOGY

Dataset Used in the Proposed Work

In this work, we have used the publicly available data set of EMG signals from the EMGLABs database (McGill et al., 2005). A concentric needle electrode is availed for the recording of the EMG signals. In order to monitor the signal, a slight and constant contraction was made in muscle. The concentric needle electrodes of the area of 0.07 mm2 are used for the recording (Nikolic, 2001). The recorded ECG signal was amplified by a factor of 4000 and subject to a band-pass filter of cut-off frequency of 2 Hz and 10 kHz. The sampling frequency of the recorded signals were 23437.5 Hz (McGill et al., 2005). The dataset contains three groups of subjects. There are two groups of patients namely, myopathy and ALS. The group of myopathy patients has 7 subjects of the age group of 19-63 years. There are 8 patients in the

Figure 1. The block diagram representing the steps involved in the proposed method

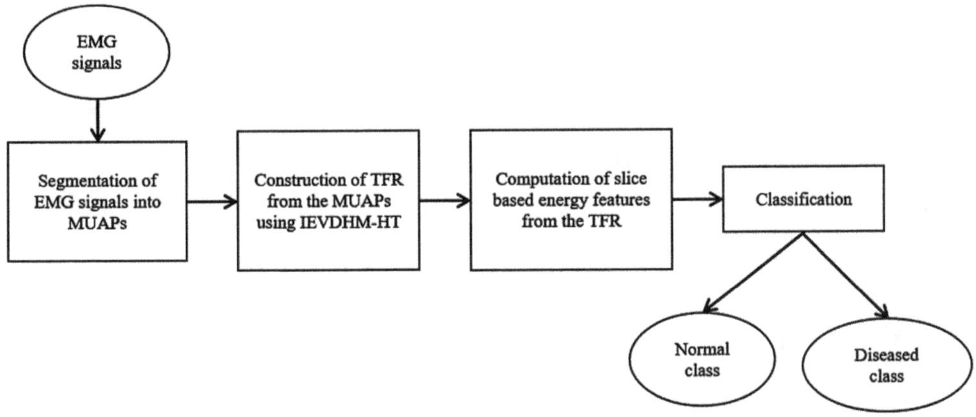

ALS group of the age group of 35-67 years. The third group contains 10 subjects, who do not have any neuromuscular disease. The age of the healthy group varies between 21-37 years. The typical plots of the EMG signals of normal, ALS, and myopathy are depicted in Figure 2.

Extraction of MUAPs

MUAPs have been obtained from the EMG signals in the following way: First, a window of 5.6 ms is applied to the EMG signal to divide them into the timeframes having the MUAPs (Nikolic & Krarup, 2011). The timeframes which have one MUAP are known as segments. The time-frames which have superimposed MUAPs are termed as compound segments. The portions of EMG signal which do not have MUAP are called baseline. The timeframe is considered as MUAP, if the variance of the portion of the timeframe within the window is greater than the threshold value. It may be a single MUAP or may have many superimposed MUAPs (Nikolic & Krarup, 2011). In order to estimate the threshold, an amplitude density function is used which is computed from the normalized variance signal. Thereafter, we formed a group by keeping the similar looking segments together. It may consist of multiple segments. If a group has five or more segments then it is named as potential class (PCL). Then, each of the PCL is represented by the template corresponding to the active MUAP of the EMG signal (Nikolic & Krarup, 2011).

TFR Using IEVDHM-HT

The TFR of each MUAP is obtained using IEVDHM-HT method. For the database given in (McGill, 2005), each MUAP contains 625 samples and can be represented as m[p], where p is varying from 1 to 625. Therefore a Hankel matrix, HM of size P×P is formed, where P = 313 samples. The matrix HM can be mathematically expressed as follows (Sharma et al., 2019c):

$$\begin{bmatrix} m[1] & m[2] & . & . & m[313] \\ m[2] & m[3] & & . & . & . \\ . & . & & . & . & . \\ . & . & & . & . & . \\ m[313] & m[314] & . & . & m[625] \end{bmatrix} \quad (1)$$

Figure 2a. Typical plots of different classes of EMG signals: Normal class

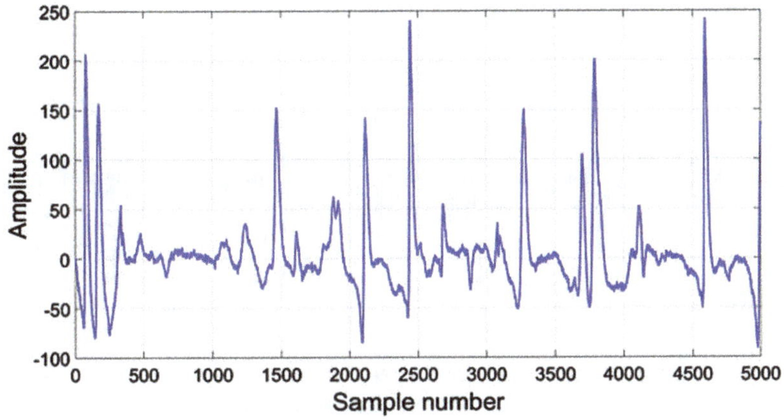

The eigenvalue decomposition of matrix HM is performed to compute eigenvalue matrix E_{val} and eigenvector matrix E_{vec} and can be mathematically expressed as follows (Sharma et al., 2019d):

$$HM = E_{vec} E_{val} E'_{vec} \tag{2}$$

Further, we have utilized the modified significant threshold point (MSTP) method to recognize the useful eigenvalues to decompose the signal into its components. The MSTP stated that if the sum of magnitude of larger eigenvalues is higher than the 95% of sum of magnitude of all the eigenvalues, consider them as useful

Figure 2b. Typical plots of different classes of EMG signals: ALS class

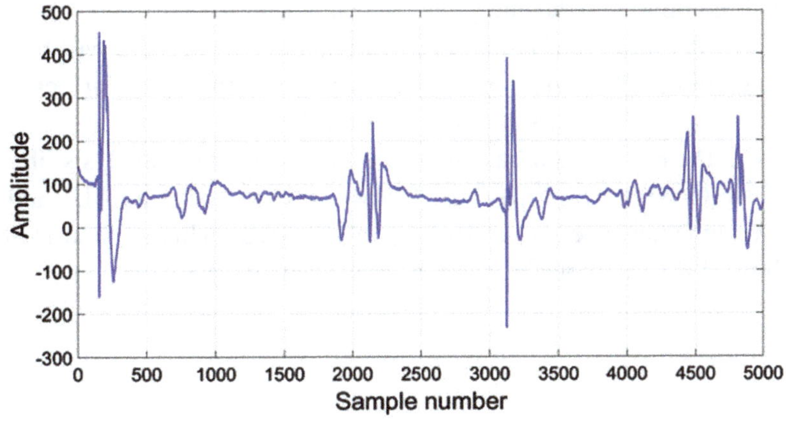

Figure 2c. Typical plots of different classes of EMG signals: Myopathy class

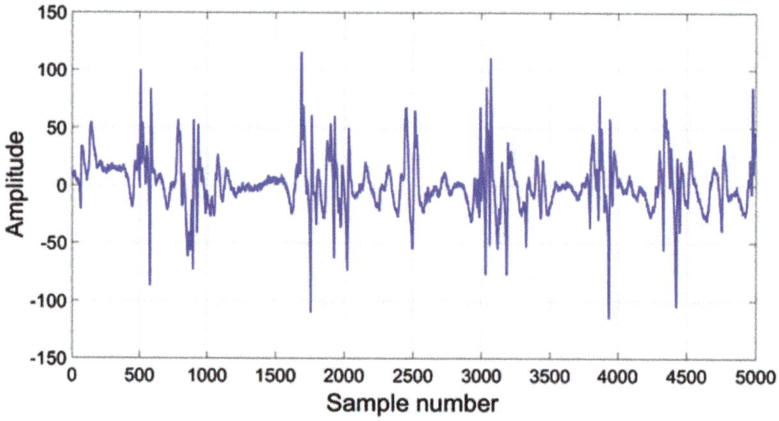

eigenvalues (Sharma & Pachori, 2017a). All the useful eigenvalues are considered for obtaining decomposed components. The mathematical expressions for obtaining the decomposed component are derived in (Sharma & Pachori, 2017a). The obtained decomposed components are examined to satisfy the modified mono-component signal criteria (MMSC) explained in (Sharma & Pachori, 2017a). The MMSC contains two conditions which can be stated as follows (Sharma & Pachori, 2017a, Huang et al., 1998, March):

Condition 1: The local extrema counts and total number of zero-crossings should be differ by maximum one.
Condition 2: The average value of upper envelope and lower envelope should be zero.

All the MMSC unsatisfying components are required to follow the above discussed process. Further, the sum of the energy of the components (E_{nsc}) which do not satisfy the MMSC is compared to the energy of the original signal m[p]. If we find that the E_{nsc} is greater than the 5% of the original signal then the process will be repeated from the beginning. Otherwise, the process will be terminated. Further details of this method are provided in (Sharma & Pachori, 2017a).

The IEVDHM-HT method has been recently used for the analysis of coronary artery disease (CAD) in (Sharma et al., 2019c) and for analyzing ALS and normal EMG signals in (Sharma et al., 2019a, Chandra, 2018). This method is also used for providing TFR of complex signals in (Sharma & Pachori, 2018a).

Table 1. Parameters obtained in different sliced TF plane

Iteration Number	Slice Range	Parameter
1	$\left(0, \frac{e_{\max}}{10}\right)$	$\rho_1(n,k)$
2	$\left(\frac{e_{\max}}{10}, \frac{e_{\max}}{5}\right)$	$\rho_2(n,k)$
3	$\left(\frac{e_{\max}}{5}, \frac{3e_{\max}}{10}\right)$	$\rho_3(n,k)$
4	$\left(\frac{3e_{\max}}{10}, \frac{2e_{\max}}{5}\right)$	$\rho_4(n,k)$
5	$\left(\frac{2e_{\max}}{5}, \frac{e_{\max}}{2}\right)$	$\rho_5(n,k)$
6	$\left(\frac{e_{\max}}{2}, \frac{3e_{\max}}{5}\right)$	$\rho_6(n,k)$
7	$\left(\frac{3e_{\max}}{5}, \frac{7e_{\max}}{10}\right)$	$\rho_7(n,k)$
8	$\left(\frac{7e_{\max}}{10}, \frac{4e_{\max}}{5}\right)$	$\rho_8(n,k)$
9	$\left(\frac{4e_{\max}}{5}, \frac{9e_{\max}}{10}\right)$	$\rho_9(n,k)$
10	$\left(\frac{9e_{\max}}{10}, e_{\max}\right)$	$\rho_{10}(n,k)$

Time-Frequency Based Features

The energy of each TF matrix of each MUAP is sliced in segments. The slicing is performed vertically in TF plane with respect to maximum energy of TF plane in a way that each slice contains equal energy band. Recently, TF average based new parameters are proposed and applied for CAD identification (Sharma et al., 2019d). In this work, 10 slices are considered. Let us consider a TF matrix which possesses maximum instantaneous energy e_{max}. The energy of TF plane is segmented into 10 slices and each slice contains energy band of $e_{max}/10$. Therefore, the band of energy range of each slice will be $(0, e_{max}/10)$, $(e_{max}/10, e_{max}/5)$, $(e_{max}/5, 3e_{max}/10)$, $(3e_{max}/10, 2e_{max}/5)$, $(2e_{max}/5, e_{max}/2)$, $(e_{max}/2, 3e_{max}/5)$, $(3e_{max}/5, 7e_{max}/10)$, $(7e_{max}/10, 4e_{max}/5)$, $(4e_{max}/5, 9e_{max}/10)$, and $(9e_{max}/10, e_{max})$. The band of each slice of TF matrix is represented in Table 1. The parameter, $Slice_{en}$ given in (3) is computed which is correlated with the energy of each slice where $\rho(n; k)$ is the energy density at time n and frequency k.

$$Slice_{en} = \sum_{n=1}^{P}\sum_{k=1}^{Q}\rho\left(n,k\right) \tag{3}$$

CLASSIFICATION

We have used random forest [30] and LS-SVM classifiers for evaluating the effectiveness of the proposed features. Random forest classifier constructs a set of decision trees from randomly selected data set. Final decision of the class is based on the average of the votes from different decision trees. The decision of the class is based on the margin function (MG). It is defined for a training set that is drawn randomly from the distribution of random vector *B, A* as (Breiman, 2001):

$$MG\left(A,B\right) = avg_t\left[H_t\left(A\right) = B\right] - \max_{i \neq Bavg_t} F\left[H_t\left(A\right) = i\right] \tag{4}$$

Where, $H_t(A) = H(y, \gamma_t)$, $F(.)$ represents an indicator function, and the operator avg_t refers to the average value. The γ_t is representing the random vector, assigned to the tth tree. The $H(y, \gamma_t)$ denotes the tree classifier, which is the result of the growth of a random tree based on the input vector *y* and the γ_t. If the margin is attained higher value then it refers to the high confidence in the classification. The

Waikato environment for knowledge analysis (WEKA) toolbox (Hall et al., 2009) has been employed to implement the random forest classifier. It is explored for the detection of atrial fibrillation in (Kumar et al., 2018) and for the analysis of myocardial infarction ECG signals in (Kumar et al., 2017a).

In LS-SVM classification method, kernel functions are used to map the input vectors into higher dimensional space. Finally, for separating the different classes of data, a hyperplane is constructed in this space (Suykens & Vandewalle, 1999). It's mathematical equation is given as follows (Suykens & Vandewalle, 1999):

$$T = sign\left[\sum_{a=1}^{z} \propto_a w_a E\left(v, v_a\right) + b\right] \tag{5}$$

where, α_a represents the Lagrangian multiplier, $E(v,v_a)$ denotes a kernel function, v_a is used for representing the ath input vector of D-dimension, w_a is indicating the target vector, and b refers to the bias term.

The polynomial of order 2 (Poly2), order 3 (Poly3), and radial basis function (RBF) are availed as the kernels of LS-SVM. The polynomial kernel is represented as follows (Suykens & Vandewalle, 1999):

$$E\left(v, v_a\right) = \left(v_a^T + 1\right)^r \tag{6}$$

Where, r denotes the order of the kernel. The representation of RBF kernel is as follows (Khandoker et al., 2007):

$$E\left(v, v_a\right) = e^{\frac{-v - v_a^2}{2\sigma^2}} \tag{7}$$

Where, σ controls the width of RBF kernel. The performance of the classifiers is measured in terms of specificity (Sp), accuracy (Ac), and sensitivity (Se) (Azar, & El-Said, 2014). The LS-SVM classifier is employed for various biomedical signal classification problems in the literature such as, detection of diabetic heart rate variability (HRV) signals (Pachori et al., 2016), analysis of heart diseases (Patidar et al., 2015; Patidar & Pachori, 2014; Kumar et al., 2016; Sharma et al. 2019b).

The multilayer perceptron (MLP), a neural network-based classifier (Lippmann, 1987, Madyastha, Aazhang, 1994), is also employed in this work to test the classification performance of the features. It consists of a multilayer feed-forward neural network. It has one input layer, one output layer, and may have one or more

Figure 3. A plot of normal MAUP and its TFR

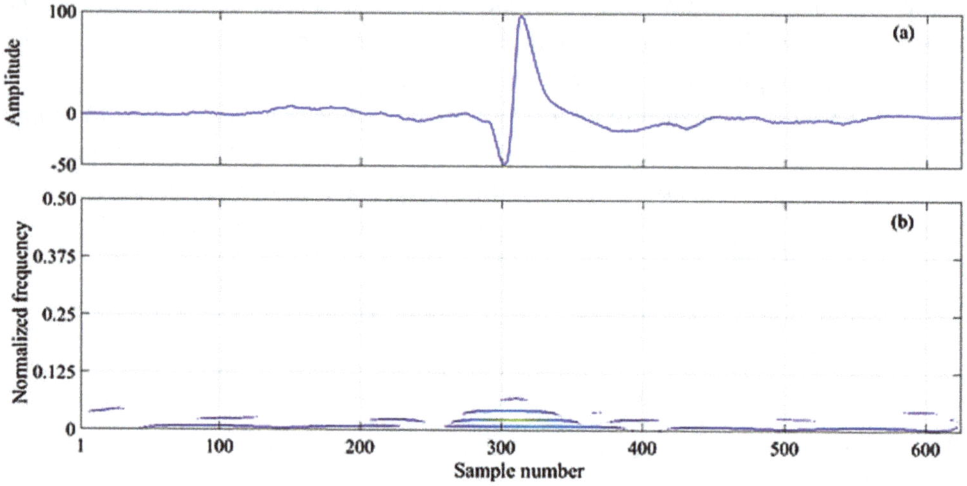

hidden layers. There is a weighted network which connects one node to the other nodes. For weight optimization, the backpropagation algorithm (Lippmann, 1987) is a widely used algorithm. MLP classifier is implemented for the classification of sleep stages in (Sharma et al., 2017).

RESULTS AND DISCUSSION

In the proposed work, first the EMG signals are segmented into MUAPs. The MUAPs are subjected to the IEVDHM-HT method to construct the TFR. The plots of MAUPs of each class and corresponding TFR are depicted in Figures 3-5. From these TFR, we have computed the TF based features. The ranges of these features are provided in Table 2. From this table, we can observe that the features computed from the ALS MAUPs have obtained highest values among the three classes. However, features computed from the myopathy MUAPs have shown lowest values among three classes.

The discrimination ability of the features are also examined using Kruskal-Wallis (KW) test [50]. The p-values obtained using KW test are arranged in the Table 3. The p-values lesser than 0.05 are considered significant in several applications of biomedical signal analysis (Pachori et al., 2015; Sood et al., 2016; Kumar et al., 2017; Pachori, 2008). From Table 3, it can be observed that all the features have shown good discrimination ability as all the features have lesser p-values ($p < 0.05$).

Moreover, we have also utilized random forest and LS-SVM classifier with 10-fold cross-validation (TFCV) method (Kohavi, 1995) to compute the effectiveness

Figure 4. The plot of MAUP taken from ALS class and corresponding TFR

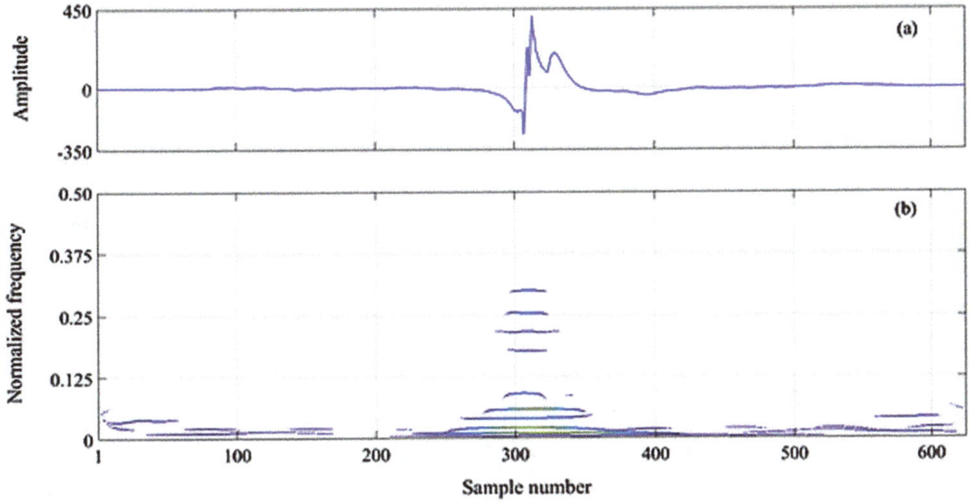

of the proposed features. In TFCV method, dataset is divided into 10 parts. From these 10 parts 9 parts are used for training and one part is used for testing, and the process is repeated for the 10 iterations. Finally, the average of the obtained accuracies for each fold is considered as the final result. The accuracy computed using these classifiers are shown in Table 4. From the Table 4, it can be seen that for normal and ALS classes, the features have shown 75.43% accuracy with random forest classier. We can see an improvement in the accuracy, when these features are applied to the LS-SVM classifier. LS-SVM have provided 76.76% accuracy when RBF is availed as the kernel function. The maximum accuracy observed in TFVC process for an iteration is 83% for this class.

For the normal and myopathy classes, these features have obtained 73.85% accuracy of classification with random forest classifier. When these features are subjected to the LS-SVM classifier, the accuracy is improved up to 74.45%. For TFCV method, the highest obtained accuracy for one fold is 78.6%. We have also examined the performance of the features for the ALS and myopathy classes. We have observed that these features have performed best for this category of EMG signals. We can see from Table 4, the random forest classifier has provided 83.83% classification accuracy for the proposed features. The proposed features have obtained 84.72% accuracy of classification for LS-SVM classifier. We have observed maximum accuracy of 88.71% for a fold of TFCV for ALS and myopathy classes. The accuracy of each fold for the TFCV method is depicted in Figures 6-8.

In some cases, while energy of TF plane is segmented into 10 slices corresponding to e_{max}, many values of $Slice_{en}$ becomes zero. It reduces the accuracy for the

Figure 5. A plot representing the myopathy MAUP and corresponding TFR

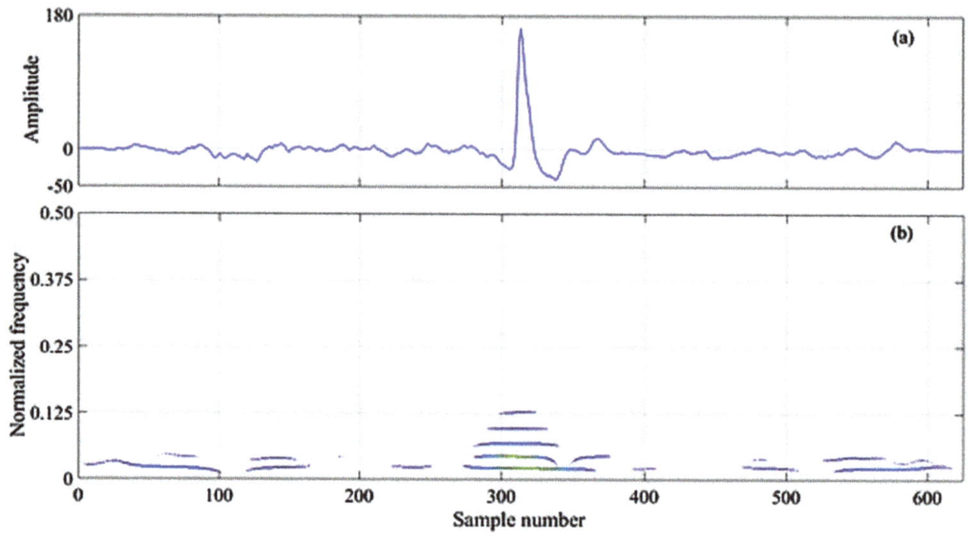

considered dataset. Therefore, another methodology of slicing is also presented which is based on percentile of maximum instantaneous energy of each TF plane. On slicing the TF plane into three slices of 33 percentile (33ptl), the range of slice becomes (0, 33.33ptl of e_{max}), (33ptl of e_{max}, 66.67ptl of e_{max}), (66.67ptl of e_{max}, e_{max}). The $Slice_{en}$ parameter for the above said slices have been computed for all three cases. In Tables 5 and 6, the classification performance of various classifiers are presented for features computed by slicing for three levels as given in Table 1 and

Figure 6. A plot showing the accuracy of each fold for the normal and ALS classes

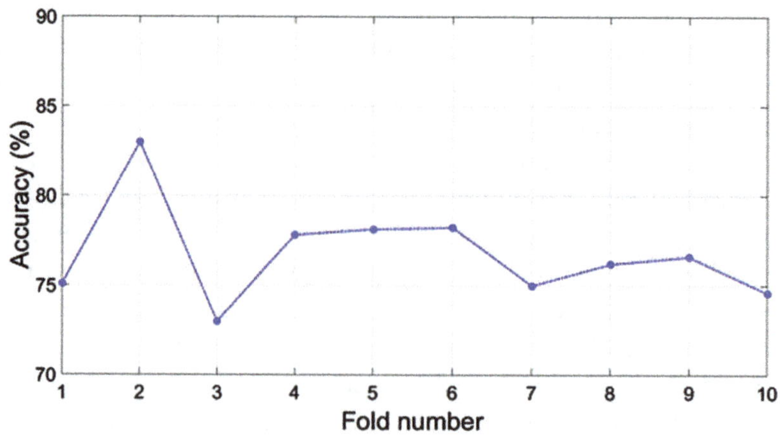

Table 2. Ranges of the features obtained from the different classes of EMG signals (The Std. refers to the standard deviation.)

Features		Normal	ALS	Myopathy
1	Mean	181889.9	1606951	90189.46
	Std.	229008.5	5570843	330897.64
2	Mean	85036.74	764212.3	35688.94
	Std.	129674.1	3060959	120749.57
3	Mean	56215.12	563901.3	22801.6
	Std.	72894.03	2975410	80764.81
4	Mean	44478.25	477029.9	17602.02
	Std.	59637.06	2549718	50211.11
5	Mean	37012.97	387354	15443.15
	Std.	45417.92	1769080	47614.77
6	Mean	35069.41	371203.9	14375.9
	Std.	45454.67	1691374	58125.41
7	Mean	34056.33	569359.1	14410.42
	Std.	41551.18	6300222	63766
8	Mean	35897.35	661774.9	16544.61
	Std.	46475.25	9144943	111988.04
9	Mean	42315.65	519653.3	16157.43
	Std.	56388.46	2383715	58310.82
10	Mean	91109.52	1207296	35983.49
	Std.	133129.1	5650886	127692.53

percentile based features respectively. From Tables 5 and 6, it can be observed that the percentile based features have shown better performance as compared to the simple slicing based features. The classification performance has been tested using three classifiers namely, random forest, SVM, and multilayer perceptron (MLP). From Table 6, it can be seen that the random forest classifier provided the highest classification accuracy of 83% for normal and ALS classes. The SVM and MLP classifiers achieved the classification accuracy of 79.9% and 81.1% for normal and ALS classes, respectively. The obtained highest accuracy for normal and myopathy classes is 80.8% using MLP classifier. For this case, the proposed algorithm also achieved 79.7% and 77.9% accuracy with random forest and SVM classifiers. The proposed methodology performed best to distinguish the ALS and myopathy classes. For the ALS and myopathy classes, the random forest, SVM, and MLP classifiers

Table 3.

Features	Normal and ALS Classes	Normal and Myopathy Classes
1	4.96E-92	3.45E-149
2	2.80E-74	1.38E-146
3	2.09E-78	2.22E-138
4	3.20E-86	3.33E-136
5	9.94E-94	2.28E-138
6	3.03E-99	5.48E-149
7	5.06E-108	9.69E-143
8	3.27E-113	8.68E-144
9	4.96E-121	1.89E-152
10	1.93E-130	3.58E-146

obtained classification accuracies of 96.7%, 87.7%, and 97.7%, respectively. The other classification parameters can be observed in Table 6.

In a recently proposed method (Joshi et. Al. 2017), classification accuracy for ALS and normal class is 89.16% using more than 14 different parameters while

Table 4. Classification performance of the proposed features for various classes

Classes	Classifier	Kernel Function	Parameters	Ac (%)	Sp (%)	Se (%)
Normal and ALS	Random forest		No. of trees = 100	75.43	87.8	58.6
	LS-SVM	Polynomial	r = 2	73.78	95.73	43.96
		Polynomial	r = 3	73.58	91.46	49.29
		RBF	$\sigma = 0.1$	76.76	86.77	63.17
Normal and Myopathy	Random forest		No. of trees = 100	73.85	77	70.7
	LS-SVM	Polynomial	r = 2	71.51	59.52	83.49
		Polynomial	r = 3	72.84	66.31	79.36
		RBF	$\sigma = 0.5$	74.45	75.42	73.48
ALS and Myopathy	Random forest		No. of trees = 100	83.83	79.1	87.3
	SVM	Polynomial	r = 2	75.48	45.58	97.48
		Polynomial	r = 3	78.31	54.14	96.08
		RBF	$\sigma = 0.1$	84.72	80.49	87.82

Figure 7. The plot of the accuracies of the fold of TFCV method for the normal and myo classes

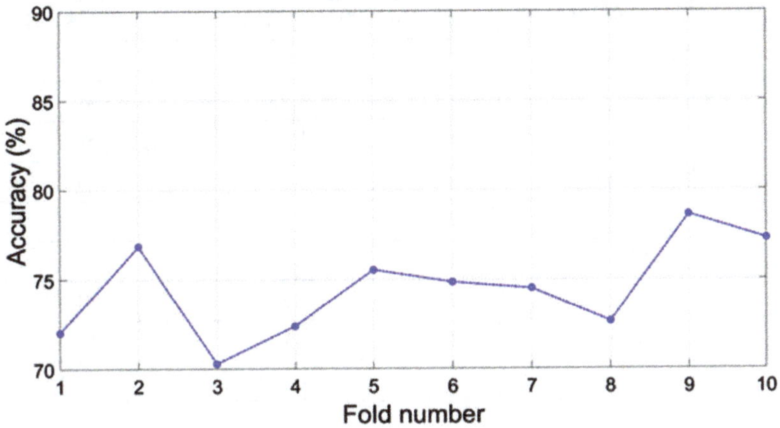

the proposed method achieves 83% using only one parameter. For normal versus myopathy class, (Joshi et al. 2017) achieves 82.41% accuracy and proposed method achieves 80.8%. In case of ALS versus myopathy, the proposed method obtained 96.7% accuracy in comparison with 94.42% accuracy obtained using (Joshi et al. 2017) method. The proposed method used only one parameter which is based on slices of TF plane and total three features are computed. In (Joshi et al., 2017), several time domain-based, entropy-based parameters are using simultaneously for classification. Therefore, it can be concluded that the TF plane-based slicing is better

Figure 8. A plot of the accuracy of each fold for the ALS and myo classes

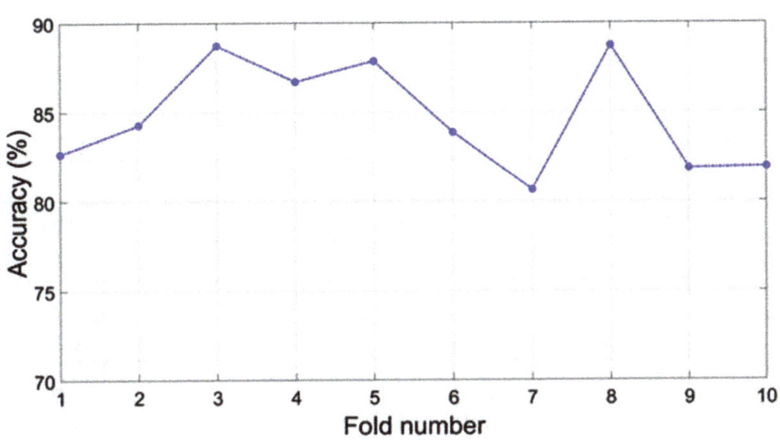

Table 5. Classification performance of the simple slicing based three features for various classes

Classes	Classifier	Accuracy (%)	Sensitivity (%)	Specificity (%)
Normal and ALS	Random forest	66.7	72	59.6
	SVM	60.1	95	40.5
	MLP	74.4	92.6	50.3
Normal and Myopathy	Random forest	61.4	61	61.9
	SVM	55.7	94.1	17.4
	MLP	70.4	72.4	68.5
ALS and Myopathy	Random forest	75.1	77.9	71.6
	SVM	60.3	100	06.5
	MLP	81.2	91.5	67.1

than the time domain based and entropy-based parameters. The percentile-based slicing has provided better accuracy as compared to the normal slicing method.

CONCLUSION

In this work, a novel methodology for EMG signal analysis and classification is proposed. The normal, ALS, and myopathy signals are segmented into MUAPs. Thereafter, TFRs of all the MUAPs are obtained. The TF based features are computed. The energy contained in TF matrix is sliced into ten segments with equal energy

Table 6. Classification performance of the percentile based three features for various classes

Classes	Classifier	Ac (%)	Sen (%)	Spe (%)
Normal and ALS	Random forest	83	85.9	79.2
	SVM	79.9	97.8	55.8
	MLP	81.1	94.1	63.5
Normal and Myopathy	Random forest	79.7	80	79.6
	SVM	77.9	90.2	65.6
	MLP	80.8	87.2	74.4
ALS and Myopathy	Random forest	96.7	97.1	96.3
	LS-SVM	87.7	99.2	72.2
	MLP	91.7	95	87

levels. We have studied the energy contained in each slice for all the MUAPs of each class. Finally, 76.76% accuracy is achieved for normal and ALS classes and 74.45% accuracy is achieved for normal and myopathy classes with LS-SVM classifier. For ALS and myopathy classes, we achieved 84.72% accuracy using LS-SVM classifier. We have also computed the percentile-based features to distinguish the different classes of EMG signals. The percentile-based features performed better than the other computed features. For percentile-based features, we have obtained 83% accuracy for normal and ALS, 80.8% accuracy for normal and Myopathy classes, 96.7% accuracy for ALS and myopathy classes. In future, the proposed TF slice-based parameters can also be studied for other muscle abnormalities. The proposed framework in this chapter can be studied for the automated classification of other physiological signals corresponding to normal and abnormal categories.

REFERENCES

Anthea, M., Hopkins, J., McLaughlin, C. W., Johnson, S., Warner, M. Q., LaHart, D., & Wright, J. D. (1993). *Human biology and health. 1993*. Englewood Cliffs, NJ: Prentice Hall.

Azar, A. T., & El-Said, S. A. (2014). Performance analysis of support vector machines classifiers in breast cancer mammography recognition. *Neural Computing & Applications*, *24*(5), 1163–1177. doi:10.100700521-012-1324-4

Breiman, L. (2001). Random forests. *Machine Learning*, *45*(1), 5–32. doi:10.1023/A:1010933404324

Chandra, P. (2018) *Eigenvalue decomposition based analysis and classification of electromyogram signals.* (Master's thesis), Indian Institute of Technology, Indore, India.

Christodoulou, C. I., & Pattichis, C. S. (1999). Unsupervised pattern recognition for the classification of EMG signals. *IEEE Transactions on Biomedical Engineering*, *46*(2), 169–178. doi:10.1109/10.740879 PMID:9932338

Doulah, A. B. M. S. U. & Fattah, S. A. (2014, April). Neuromuscular disease classification based on mel-frequency cepstrum of motor unit action potential. In *2014 International Conference on Electrical Engineering and Information & Communication Technology (ICEEICT),* (pp. 1-4). 10.1109/ICEEICT.2014.6919167

Doulah, A. B. M. S. U. & Jumana, M. A. (2012, May). ALS disease detection in EMG using time-frequency method. In *2012 International Conference on Informatics, Electronics & Vision (ICIEV),* (pp. 648-651).

Fattah, S. A., Iqbal, M. A., Jumana, M. A., & Doulah, A. S. U. (2012). Identifying the motor neuron disease in EMG signal using time and frequency domain features with comparison. *Signal and Image Processing: an International Journal, 3*(2), 99–114. doi:10.5121ipij.2012.3207

Fuglsang-Frederiksen, A. (2000). The utility of interference pattern analysis. *Muscle & Nerve: Official Journal of the American Association of Electrodiagnostic Medicine, 23*(1), 18–36. doi:10.1002/(SICI)1097-4598(200001)23:1<18::AID-MUS4>3.0.CO;2-B PMID:10590403

Gazzoni, M., Farina, D., & Merletti, R. (2004). A new method for the extraction and classification of single motor unit action potentials from surface EMG signals. *Journal of Neuroscience Methods, 136*(2), 165–177. doi:10.1016/j.jneumeth.2004.01.002 PMID:15183268

Güler, N. F., & Koçer, S. (2005). Classification of EMG signals using PCA and FFT. *Journal of Medical Systems, 29*(3), 241–250. doi:10.100710916-005-5184-7 PMID:16050079

Hall, M., Frank, E., Holmes, G., Pfahringer, B., Reutemann, P., & Witten, I. H. (2009). The WEKA data mining software: an update. *ACM SIGKDD explorations newsletter, 11*(1), 10-18.

Huang, N. E., Shen, Z., Long, S. R., Wu, M. C., Shih, H. H., Zheng, Q. . . . Liu, H. H. (1998, March). The empirical mode decomposition and the Hilbert spectrum for nonlinear and non-stationary time series analysis. In *Proceedings of the Royal Society of London A: mathematical, physical and engineering sciences* (Vol. 454, No. 1971, pp. 903-995). 10.1098/rspa.1998.0193

Joshi, D., Tripathi, A., Sharma, R., & Pachori, R. B. (2017, February). Computer aided detection of abnormal EMG signals based on tunable-Q wavelet transform. In *2017 4th International Conference on Signal Processing and Integrated Networks (SPIN),* (pp. 544-549). 10.1109/SPIN.2017.8050010

Kandel, E. R., Schwartz, J. H., Jessell, T. M., Jessell, M. B. T., Siegelbaum, S., & Hudspeth, A. (2000). Principles of neural science, 4. New York, NY: McGraw-Hill.

Karpati, G., Carpenter, S., & Nelson, R. F. (1970). Type I muscle fibre atrophy and central nuclei: A rare familial neuromuscular disease. *Journal of the Neurological Sciences, 10*(5), 489–500. doi:10.1016/0022-510X(70)90027-4 PMID:4910660

Katsis, C. D., Exarchos, T. P., Papaloukas, C., Goletsis, Y., Fotiadis, D. I., & Sarmas, I. (2007). A two-stage method for MUAP classification based on EMG decomposition. *Computers in Biology and Medicine*, *37*(9), 1232–1240. doi:10.1016/j.compbiomed.2006.11.010 PMID:17208215

Khandoker, A. H., Lai, D. T., Begg, R. K., & Palaniswami, M. (2007). Wavelet-based feature extraction for support vector machines for screening balance impairments in the elderly. *IEEE Transactions on Neural Systems and Rehabilitation Engineering*, *15*(4), 587–597. doi:10.1109/TNSRE.2007.906961 PMID:18198717

Kohavi, R. (1995) A study of cross-validation and bootstrap for accuracy estimation and model selection. *In proceedings of the 14th International Joint Conference on Artificial Intelligence*, Morgan Kaufmann Publishers, San Francisco, CA, pp. 1137-1143.

Kouchaki, S., Boostani, R., & Parsaei, H. (2012, May). A new feature selection method for classification of EMG signals. In *2012 16th CSI International Symposium on Artificial Intelligence and Signal Processing (AISP),* (pp. 585-590). 10.1109/AISP.2012.6313814

Kumar, M., Pachori, R. B., & Acharya, U. R. (2016). An efficient automated technique for CAD diagnosis using flexible analytic wavelet transform and entropy features extracted from HRV signals. *Expert Systems with Applications*, *63*, 165–172. doi:10.1016/j.eswa.2016.06.038

Kumar, M., Pachori, R. B., & Acharya, U. R. (2017). Characterization of coronary artery disease using flexible analytic wavelet transform applied on ECG signals. *Biomedical Signal Processing and Control*, *31*, 301–308. doi:10.1016/j.bspc.2016.08.018

Kumar, M., Pachori, R. B., & Acharya, U. R. (2017a). Automated diagnosis of myocardial infarction ECG signals using sample entropy in flexible analytic wavelet transform framework. *Entropy (Basel, Switzerland)*, *19*(9), 488. doi:10.3390/e19090488

Kumar, M., Pachori, R. B., & Acharya, U. R. (2018). Automated diagnosis of atrial fibrillation ECG signals using entropy features extracted from flexible analytic wavelet transform. *Biocybernetics and Biomedical Engineering*, *38*(3), 564–573. doi:10.1016/j.bbe.2018.04.004

Lippmann, R. (1987). An introduction to computing with neuralnets. *IEEE ASSP Magazine*, *4*(2), 4–22. doi:10.1109/MASSP.1987.1165576

Madyastha, R. K., & Aazhang, B. (1994). An algorithm for training multilayer perceptrons for data classification and function interpolation. *IEEE Transactions on Circuits and Systems. I, Fundamental Theory and Applications*, *41*(12), 866–875. doi:10.1109/81.340848

McGill, K. C., Lateva, Z. C., & Marateb, H. R. (2005). EMGLAB: An interactive EMG decomposition program. *Journal of Neuroscience Methods*, *149*(2), 121–133. doi:10.1016/j.jneumeth.2005.05.015 PMID:16026846

McKight, P. E. & Najab, J. (2010). Kruskal-Wallis Test. *The corsini encyclopedia of psychology*, 1-1.

Mishra, V. K., Bajaj, V., & Kumar, A. (2016, February). Classification of normal, ALS, and myopathy EMG signals using ELM classifier. In *2016 2nd International Conference on Advances in Electrical, Electronics, Information, Communication and Bio-Informatics (AEEICB),* (pp. 455-459).

Mishra, V. K., Bajaj, V., Kumar, A., Sharma, D., & Singh, G. K. (2017). An efficient method for analysis of EMG signals using improved empirical mode decomposition. *AEÜ. International Journal of Electronics and Communications*, *72*, 200–209. doi:10.1016/j.aeue.2016.12.008

Nikolic, M. (2001). *Detailed analysis of clinical electromyography signals: EMG decomposition, findings and firing pattern analysis in controls and patients with myopathy and amyotrophic lateral sclerosis* (Doctoral dissertation).

Nikolic, M., & Krarup, C. (2011). EMGTools, an adaptive and versatile tool for detailed EMG analysis. *IEEE Transactions on Biomedical Engineering*, *58*(10), 2707–2718. doi:10.1109/TBME.2010.2064773 PMID:20699205

Pachori, R. B. (2008). Discrimination between ictal and seizure-free EEG signals using empirical mode decomposition. *Research Letters in Signal Processing*, *2008*, 14. doi:10.1155/2008/293056

Pachori, R. B., Avinash, P., Shashank, K., Sharma, R., & Acharya, U. R. (2015). Application of empirical mode decomposition for analysis of normal and diabetic RR-interval signals. *Expert Systems with Applications*, *42*(9), 4567–4581. doi:10.1016/j.eswa.2015.01.051

Pachori, R. B., Kumar, M., Avinash, P., Shashank, K., & Acharya, U. R. (2016). An improved online paradigm for screening of diabetic patients using RR-interval signals. *Journal of Mechanics in Medicine and Biology*, *16*(01). doi:10.1142/S0219519416400030

Patidar, S., & Pachori, R. B. (2014). Classification of cardiac sound signals using constrained tunable-Q wavelet transform. *Expert Systems with Applications*, *41*(16), 7161–7170. doi:10.1016/j.eswa.2014.05.052

Patidar, S., Pachori, R. B., & Acharya, U. R. (2015). Automated diagnosis of coronary artery disease using tunable-Q wavelet transform applied on heart rate signals. *Knowledge-Based Systems*, *82*, 1–10. doi:10.1016/j.knosys.2015.02.011

Pattichis, C. S., & Elia, A. G. (1999). Autoregressive and cepstral analyses of motor unit action potentials. *Medical Engineering & Physics*, *21*(6-7), 405–419. doi:10.1016/S1350-4533(99)00072-7 PMID:10624737

Pfeiffer, G. (1999). The diagnostic power of motor unit potential analysis: An objective Bayesian approach. *Muscle & Nerve: Official Journal of the American Association of Electrodiagnostic Medicine*, *22*(5), 584–591. doi:10.1002/(SICI)1097-4598(199905)22:5<584::AID-MUS6>3.0.CO;2-0 PMID:10331357

Sharma, R., Pachori, R. B., & Upadhyay, A. (2017). Automatic sleep stages classification based on iterative filtering of electroencephalogram signals. *Neural Computing & Applications*, *28*(10), 2959–2978. doi:10.100700521-017-2919-6

Sharma, R. R., Chandra, P., & Pachori, R. B. (2019a). Electromyogram signal analysis using eigenvalue decomposition of the Hankel matrix. In Machine Intelligence and Signal Analysis (pp. 671-682). doi:10.1007/978-981-13-0923-6_57

Sharma, R. R., Kumar, A., Pachori, R. B., & Acharya, U. R. (2019b). Accurate automated detection of congestive heart failure using eigenvalue decomposition based features extracted from HRV signals. *Biocybernetics and Biomedical Engineering*, *39*(2), 312–327. doi:10.1016/j.bbe.2018.10.001

Sharma, R. R., Kumar, M., & Pachori, R. B. (2019c). Automated CAD identification system using time–frequency representation based on eigenvalue decomposition of ECG signals. In Machine Intelligence and Signal Analysis (pp. 597-608). doi:10.1007/978-981-13-0923-6_51

Sharma, R. R., Kumar, M., & Pachori, R. B. (2019d). Joint time-frequency domain based CAD disease sensing system using ECG signals. *IEEE Sensors Journal*, *19*(10), 3912–3920. doi:10.1109/JSEN.2019.2894706

Sharma, R. R., & Pachori, R. B. (2017a). Time–frequency representation using IEVDHM–HT with application to classification of epileptic EEG signals. *IET Science, Measurement & Technology*, *12*(1), 72–82. doi:10.1049/iet-smt.2017.0058

Sharma, R. R. & Pachori, R. B. (2017b, February). A new method for non-stationary signal analysis using eigenvalue decomposition of the Hankel matrix and Hilbert transform. In *2017 4th International Conference on Signal Processing and Integrated Networks (SPIN),* (pp. 484-488). 10.1109/SPIN.2017.8049998

Sharma, R. R., & Pachori, R. B. (2018a). Eigenvalue decomposition of Hankel matrix-based time-frequency representation for complex signals. *Circuits, Systems, and Signal Processing*, 1–17.

Sharma, R. R., & Pachori, R. B. (2018b). Improved eigenvalue decomposition-based approach for reducing cross-terms in Wigner–Ville distribution. *Circuits, Systems, and Signal Processing*, 1–21.

Sharma, R. R., & Pachori, R. B. (2018c). Baseline wander and power line interference removal from ECG signals using eigenvalue decomposition. *Biomedical Signal Processing and Control, 45*, 33–49. doi:10.1016/j.bspc.2018.05.002

Shaw, L., & Bagha, S. (2012). Online EMG signal analysis for diagnosis of neuromuscular diseases by using PCA and PNN. *International Journal of Engineering Science and Technology, 4*(10), 4453–4459.

Sood, S., Kumar, M., Pachori, R. B., & Acharya, U. R. (2016). Application of empirical mode decomposition–based features for analysis of normal and CAD heart rate signals. *Journal of Mechanics in Medicine and Biology, 16*(01). doi:10.1142/S0219519416400029

Subasi, A., Yilmaz, M., & Ozcalik, H. R. (2006). Classification of EMG signals using wavelet neural network. *Journal of Neuroscience Methods, 156*(1-2), 360–367. doi:10.1016/j.jneumeth.2006.03.004 PMID:16621003

Suykens, J. A., & Vandewalle, J. (1999). Least squares support vector machine classifiers. *Neural Processing Letters, 9*(3), 293–300. doi:10.1023/A:1018628609742

Yousefi, J., & Hamilton-Wright, A. (2014). Characterizing EMG data using machine-learning tools. *Computers in Biology and Medicine, 51*, 1–13. doi:10.1016/j.compbiomed.2014.04.018 PMID:24857941

Chapter 7
Identification of High Risk and Low Risk Preterm Neonates in NICU:
Pattern Recognition Approach

S. Tejaswini
M. S. Ramaiah Institute of Technology, India

N. Sriraam
https://orcid.org/0000-0003-3790-3900
Ramaiah Institute of Technology, India

Pradeep G. C. M.
M. S. Ramaiah Medical College and Hospital, India

ABSTRACT

Infant cries are referred as the biological indicator where infant distress is expressed without any external stimulus. One can assess the physiological changes through cry characteristics that help in improving clinical decision. In a typical Neonatal Intensive Care Unit (NICU), recognizing high-risk and low-risk admitted preterm neonates is quite challenging and complex in nature. This chapter attempts to develop pattern recognition-based approach to identify high-risk and low-risk preterm neonates in NICU. Four clinical conditions were considered: two Low Risk (LR) and two High Risk (HR), LR1- Appropriate Gestational Age (AGA), LR2- Intrauterine Growth Restriction (IUGR), HR1-Respiratory Distress Syndrome (RDS), and HR2- Premature Rupture of Membranes (PROM). An overall cry unit of 800 (n=20 per condition) was used for the proposed study. After appropriate pre-processing, Bark Frequency Cepstral Coefficient (BFCC) was estimated using three methods. Schroeder, Zwicker

DOI: 10.4018/978-1-7998-0326-3.ch007

and Terhardt; and Transmiller; and a non-linear Support Vector Machine (SVM) Classifier were employed to discriminate low-risk and high-risk groups. From the simulation results, it was observed that sensitivity specificity and accuracy of 91.47%, 91.42%, and 92.9% respectively were obtained using the BFCC estimated for classifying high risk and low risk with SVM classification.

INTRODUCTION

Recognition of low risk and high-risk neonates of preterm condition in a typical neonatal Intensive Care Unit (NICU) is quite challenging for clinical community. Factors such as low birth weights, under weights or over weight for gestation age, Apgar score (low/ minute score), mothers with complicated pregnancy have generally categorise as high risk infant. Preterm neonates are often refined as high risk as their birth happens before 37 completed weeks of pregnancy. Most preterm neonates are born between 32 and 37 weeks of gestation and needs special clinical attention (Ronald S Illingworth, 1972). For neonates born before 28 weeks gestation intensive care is essential to monitor closely the condition of the neonate in terms of its survival. Further preterm neonates with less than 2000 gm weight will considered as high risk with symptoms such as respiratory distress syndrome, apnoea, hyperglycaemia, congenital heart disease, hypoxia- ischemic encephalopathy (Abou-Abbas et al., 2017)

Preterm neonates admitted to NICU need to be monitored continuously understand the level of complication and to provide necessary clinical care. At any instant of time, clinician and the staff nurse need to know the level of risk of an individual neonate and the manual routine that is adopted in the current clinical practice is found to be cumbersome procedure (Kamińska et al., 2013) (Da Motta et al., 2015). Neonatal cry, the fundamental biological means of communication conveys valuable information to the mother, caretaker as well as the neonatologist in the typical NICU environment (Liu, Li, & Kuo, 2018) (Lubis & Gondawijaya, 2019). The condition of the cry such as wet diaper, hunger, burp, pain further can be exploited to evaluate the level of risk of neonates, high level/ low- level risk at NICU.

The fundamental acoustical properties of the neonatal cry and its corresponding cepstral analysis can be well investigated to distinguish the low-risk and high-risk preterm neonates and to improve the wellbeing of newborns. This specific study suggests an automated mechanism to recognize the low-risk and high-risk preterm neonates in NICU by considering the variants of cry patterns. Four selected clinical conditions Appropriate Gestation Age (AGA), Intrauterine Growth Restriction

(IUGR), Respiratory Distress Syndrome (RDS) and Premature Rupture of Membranes (PROM) were considered for the study, where AGA and IUGR were termed as Low-risk conditions and RDS and PROM were considered as high-risk conditions. Artificial intelligence-based pattern recognition phenomenon plays a crucial role towards object/ pattern recognition or classification with establishment of robust decision tool for clinical applications. In this research study, the cry recordings were collected from the NICU of Ramaiah Medical College and Hospitals, Bangalore, India and were pre-processed. Bark frequency Cepstral Coefficients (BFCC) were extracted from the cry acoustical recording by making use of Schroeder, Zwicker and Terhardt and Transmiller methods. The non-parametric statistical method confirms the suitability of BFCC features for distinguishing low risk and high risk preterm neonates. An automated supporter vector machine (SVM) pattern classifier was employed to identify and to perform binary classification.

Related Literature

Wrapped frequency space-based extraction of cepstral coefficients have been applied for speech/ audio signal processing application in the recent past. Kumar et al. (2018) have shown the impact of Bark and Mel frequency for speaker identification system. (Liu, Li, & Kuo, 2018) have shown the importance of infant cries pattern recognition using various cepstral coefficient analysis. Lubis and Gondawijaya (2019) have shown the usage of BFCC and MFCC for heart sound diagnosis. Sengupta et al. (2016) made an attempt to extract cepstral based statistical features for lung sound classification. Liw et al. (2019) have made an experimental analysis to understand the cry language. A special study was carried out to understand the vowel and text-based cepstral analysis of chronic hoarseness. (Moers et al., 2012). Ghosh et al. (2013) have shown the FPGA based cepstral coefficients implementation using VHDL and Xlinx platform. Sharma et al. (2015) have employed Bark and Mel Frequency scale wrapped features for vocal track length normalization applications.

Liu, Li, & Kuo (2018) have used the audio features such as linear predictive coding (LPC), linear predictive cepstral coefficients (LPCC), bark frequency cepstral coefficients (BFCC) and mel frequency cepstral coefficients (MFCC) to classify attention and wet diaper cry using neural network and nearest neighbour approach. Tuduce, Cucu, & Burileanu (2018) have focused on creating an automatic distinguish system to identify different needs of neonate based on crying. They have used paralinguistic features and have applied rule-based or statistical classifiers. Tejaswini et al. (2019) classified the preterm neonate's physiological needs such as hunger, discomfort and pain using Bark frequency features and Recurrent Elman Neural Network and Support Vector Machine Classification. Cry recordings collected from preterm neonates were pre-processed and segmented into windowing length of 30 seconds. For each segment BFCC is estimated and mean value was considered for pattern classification. Two neural network modules, Support Vector Machine and Recurrent Elman Neural Network was employed for binary classification (hunger vs discomfort, hunger vs pain and discomfort vs pain) and experimental study reveals the 94.58% of classification accuracy with Recurrent Elman neural network.

Tejaswini et al. (2016) have applied wavelet derived Mel Frequency features for infant cries recognition. A cloud-based framework was proposed for pain scale assessment recently (Tejaswini et al., 2018). A portable device framework was proposed to record and interpret the infant cries in a typical NICU environment (Sriraam et al., 2016). Sriraam et al. (2014) have made a pilot study on detecting infant cries and assess the level of pain by making use of AI based supervised learning techniques.

This proposed study uses four clinical condition two Low Risk (LR) and two High Risk (HR), LR1- Appropriate Gestational Age (AGA), LR2- Intrauterine Growth Restriction (IUGR), HR1-Respiratory Distress Syndrome (RDS) and HR2- Premature Rupture of Membranes (PROM) cry data. The extracted cry was preprocessed and silence was removed from the cry signal. The Bark Frequency Cepstral Coefficients (BFCC) was estimated using three methods, B1: Schroeder method, B2: Zwicker and Terhardt and B3: Transmiller method. Then support vector machine classifier was employed for classification of High risk and low risk cries.

MATERIALS AND METHODS

Recording Protocol

Cry recordings were recorded in quiet environment of NICU unit in M. S. Ramaiah Memorial Hospital, Bangalore, India. Parent consent from preterm neonate was obtained to participate in this study. The inclusion criteria for the database collection are relatively stable neonate in NICU and the neonates on ventilators, Continuous Positive Airway Pressure (CPAP), major malfunction conjugate heart disease, sedation and anticoagulant therapy were excluded from recording.

A unidirectional SONY voice recorder was positioned at fixed distance of 20 cm from neonate's mouth for recording cry. the recordings stored in recorder was transferred to the data base system with sampling rate was Fs= 44KHz with 16-bit resolution. Each recording lasts for 30 to 60 seconds trials for each neonate.

We recorded 80 preterm infants with gestation age of preterm neonates between 37 weeks and 34 weeks; weight was between 1.2 kg to 2.5 kg; age of infants was 0 to 3 months. Four clinical condition two Low Risk (LR) and two High Risk (HR), LR1- Appropriate Gestational Age (AGA), LR2- Intrauterine Growth Restriction

(IUGR), HR1-Respiratory Distress Syndrome (RDS) and HR2- Premature Rupture of Membranes (PROM) were considered. An overall cry unit of 800 (n=20 per condition) was used for the proposed study. Table 1 shows the study database details.

Figure 1 shows the overall framework for the pattern recognition of high risk and low risk neonates at NICU environment.

Pre-Processing

The recorded cry signals were pre-processed to separate the silence portion using a threshold-based technique. This operation is very important to estimate/ extract acoustic features from the cry recordings to recognize patterns that convey meaningful information. An automated hamming windowing functions with segmentation length of 30s was applied and feature calculation was applied. (Muthusamy, Polat, & Yaacob, 2015). Figure 2a and 2b shows the sample cry recordings and the corresponding silence removal time series data.

Table 1. Database details

Condition	Condition Type	Duration (seconds)	No. of Cry Units
Low risk	LR1- AGA	200	400
	LR2- IUGR	200	400
High risk	HR1-RDS	200	400
	HR2- PROM	200	400

Figure 1. Proposed framework for cry pattern recognition

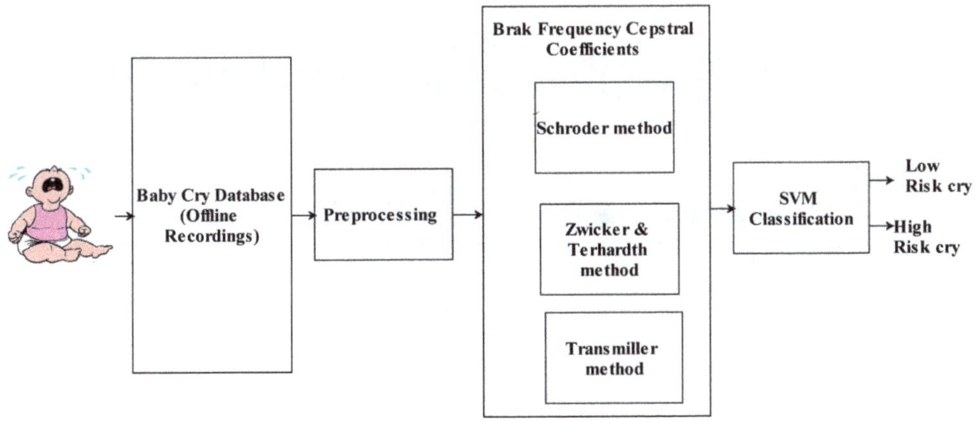

Figure 2a. Sample cry recordings with low risk and high risk conditions

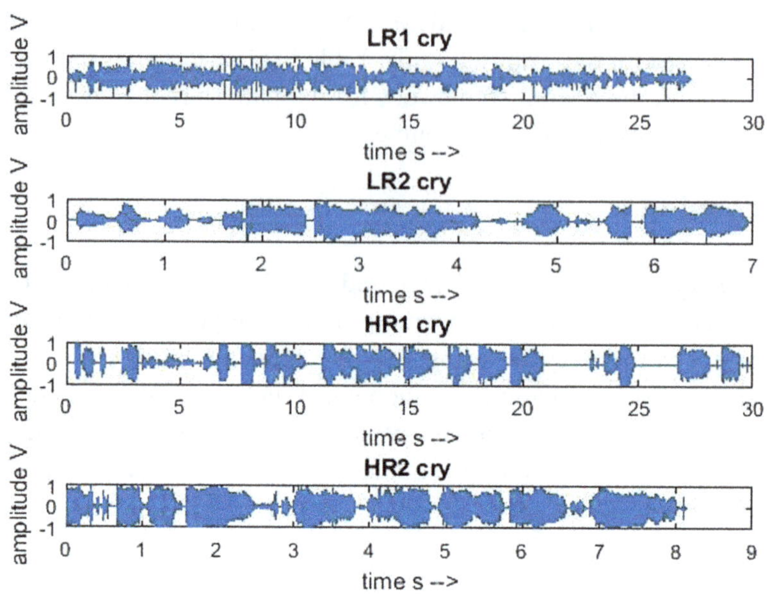

Figure 2b. Recordings with removal of silence region for high risk and low risk conditions

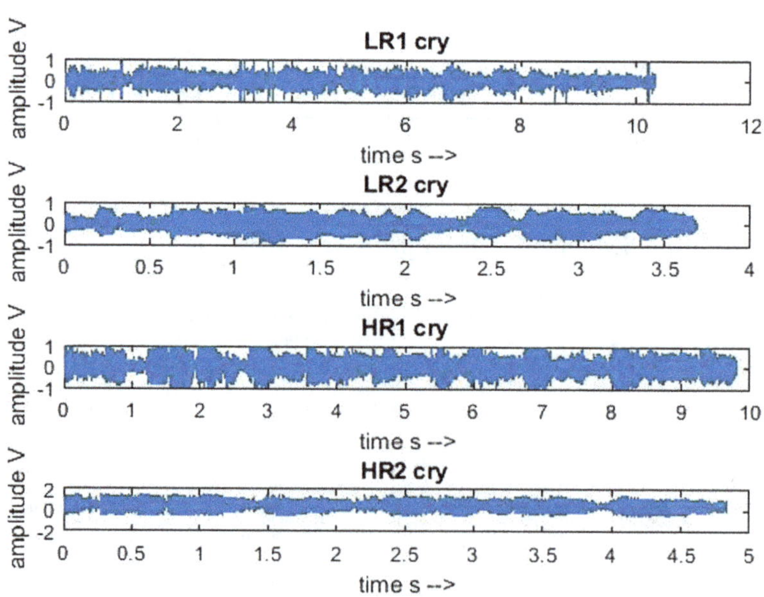

Estimation of Bark Frequency Cepstral Coefficients

The Bark scale is a psychoacoustic measure of frequency and it is well known fact that the bark scale makes the given audible spectrum into 24 critical bands that imitates the typical frequency response of the ear (Zwicker, 1961; Herrera & Fernando, 2010). The Bark scale filter bank has been found to be a promising tool for speaker recognition as well as speech processing applications (Liu, Li, and Kuo 2018), (Tuduce, Cucu, & Burileanu, 2018). The cepstral coefficients were found to provide a distinguishable feature bands which can be well exploited for pattern recognition problems.

In speech processing, the Bark frequency cepstrum is depiction of the short time power spectrum of a signal based on linear cosine transform of a log spectrum on a non-linear Bark scale of frequency. Bark Frequency Cepstral Coefficients (BFCC) is another method for extracting the features from the speech signal. This method is similar to Mel Frequency Cepstral Coefficients (MFCC). Implementation of bark scale filters in place of mel filters is quite obvious. The frequency segment of the spectrum is mapped to Bark scale perceptual filter bank. (Liu, Li, & Kuo, 2018b) Three bark filters were used namely B1- Schroeder(Gulzar, Singh, and Sharma 2014), B2- Zwicker and Terhardt (Shannon & Paliwal, 2003) and B3- Transmiller method (Mukhedkar & Alex, 2014). In this study, the coefficients were estimated based on the following.

$$B1 : bark\left(f\right) = 7 * a\sinh\left(\frac{f}{650}\right) \tag{1}$$

$$B2 : bark\_1\left(f\right) = 13\arctan\left(0.76 * f\right) + 3.5\ \arctan\left(\left(\frac{f}{7.5}\right)^2\right) \tag{2}$$

$$B3 : bark_{1(f)} = 26.81. \Big/ \left(1 + \left(\frac{1960.}{f}\right)\right) \tag{3}$$

Equation 1, 2, and 3 are Schroeder, Zwicker, and Terhardt and Transmiller method respectively. Where b denotes bark frequency and f is frequency in Hertz. The mapped Bark frequency was passed through 18 triangle band pass filters. The filter outputs were weighted according to the equal-loudness curve that uses the approximates of sensitivity of human hearing. The signal was then compressed under the intensity-loudness power law where the amplitude of the signal is compressed by the cubic root to match the non-linear relationship between intensity of sound and perceived loudness. Finally, signal is first compressed through the logarithmic function and DCT was used to decorrelate the features as in case of MFCC (Liu, Kuo, & Kuo, 2013).

Statistical Analysis

Statistical tests often are in the form of 'parametric tests' which, by definition test a hypothesis about the parameters of the probability distribution function (PDF) of a sample of data. Conversely, a non-parametric test does not require any formulation of the parameters of the pdf. The tests used in the present work, for the comparison of time series, are two tests for the analysis of the variance: The Kruskal-Wallis and the Friedman test. The Kruskal-Wallis test is used for analyzing multiple independent samples: it is the nonparametric version of one-way ANOVA, and a generalization of the Wilcoxon test for two independent samples. All the samples are combined into one large sample; the values are sorted from the smallest to the largest and transformed into their ranks. The original samples are then reconstructed, and the analysis is performed on the ranks, relative to all the samples merged together. The null hypothesis is that the means of the separate samples have the same value, whereas the alternate hypothesis is that the means have different values (Tantaratana et al., 1981)

Support Vector Machine (SVM) Classifier

SVM classifies cases using hyper plane as a decision boundary to differentiate cases with maximum margin. This margin is placed after training data mapped into high dimensional space. Basically, this hyper plane is created with supported by the training points called support vector. Kernel function is used to transform into space. Optimal model of SVM can be achieved by choosing right kernel and the hyper plane that has maximum margin between the points. We have used Fine Fine Gaussian and Fine and medium Gaussian kernel for classifying our cry data. The input to the SVM classifier was low-risk and high-risk bark frequency features. The classification was preformed between each Bark frequency methods and

In order to evaluate the performance of the neural network, the entire datasets were divided into training and testing patterns. 1680 patterns were used for training and testing using 10-fold cross validation procedure was adopted to validate the entire dataset.

Figure 3a. BFCC Schroeder method for low risk 1 and high risk 1 cries

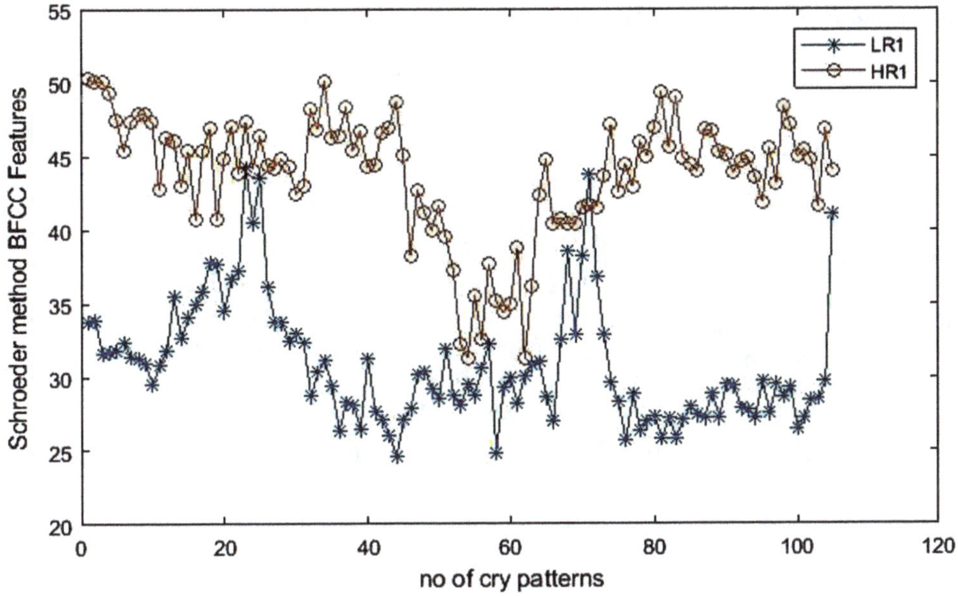

The performance of the SVM classifier is evaluated in terms of three parameters such as sensitivity, specificity and classification Accuracy (CA).

$$sesnitivity = \frac{No.of\ correctly\ identified\ Low\ risk\ pattern}{Total\ no.\ of\ low\ risk\ pattern} \tag{4}$$

$$specificity = \frac{No.\ of\ correctly\ rejected\ low\ risk\ pattern}{Total\ no.\ of\ low\ rsik\ patterns\ in\ the\ database} \tag{5}$$

$$CA = \frac{Total\ No.\ of\ correctly\ detected\ low\ risk\ pattern}{Total\ no.\ of\ applied\ pattern} \tag{6}$$

Figure 3b. BFCC Schroeder method for low risk 1 and high risk 2 cries

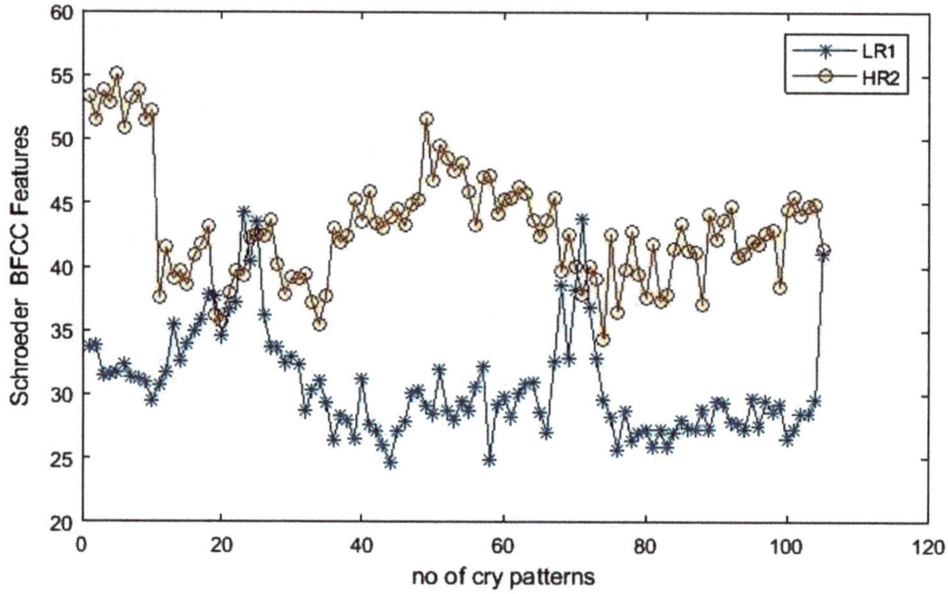

Figure 3c. BFCC Schroeder method for low risk 2 and high risk 1 cries

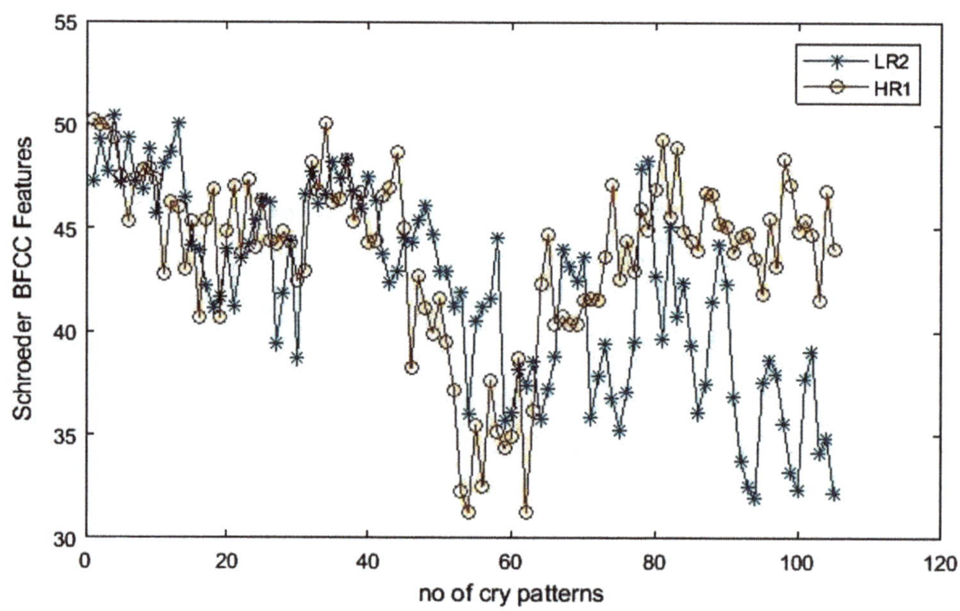

Figure 3d. BFCC Schroeder method for low risk 2 and high risk 2 cries

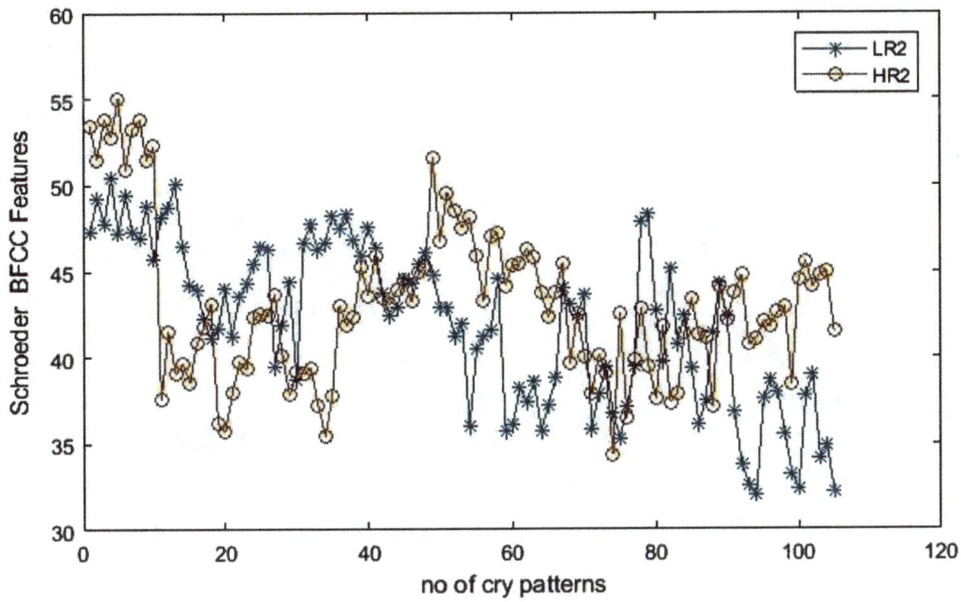

Figure 4a. BFCC Zwicker and Terhardt method for low risk 1and high risk 1 cries

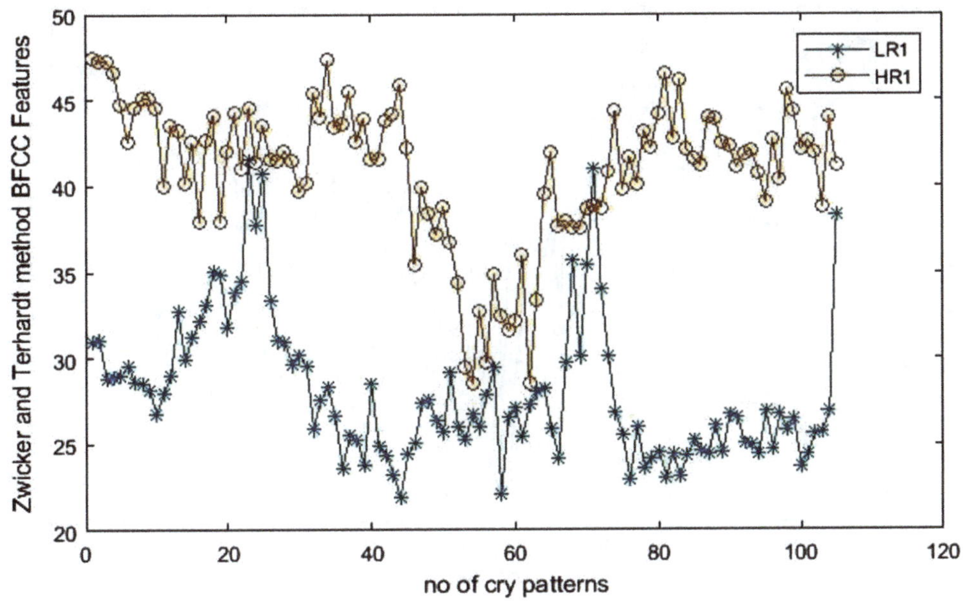

Figure 4b. BFCC Zwicker and Terhardt method for low risk 1 and high risk 2 cries

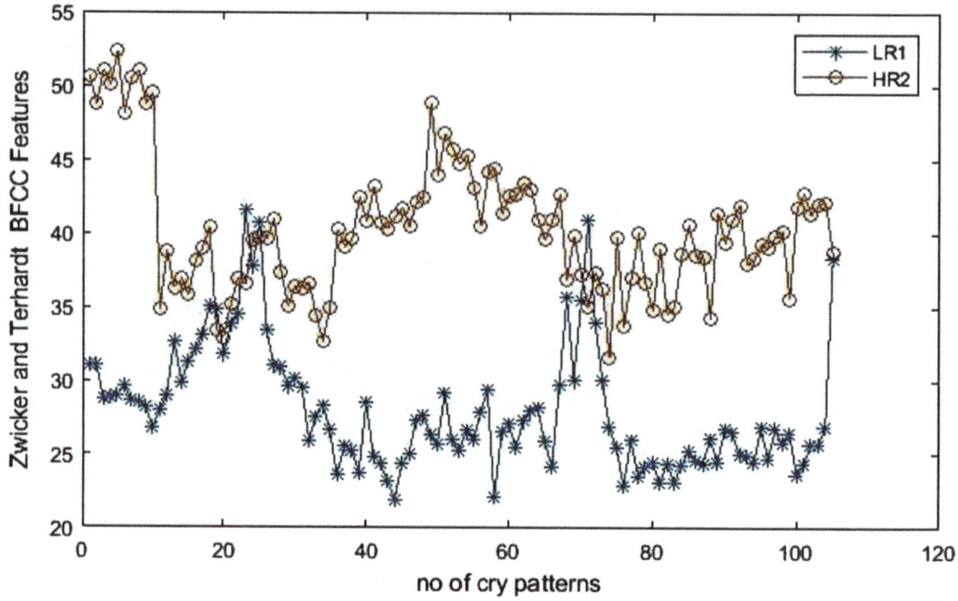

Figure 4c. BFCC Zwicker and Terhardt method for low risk 2 and high risk 1 cries

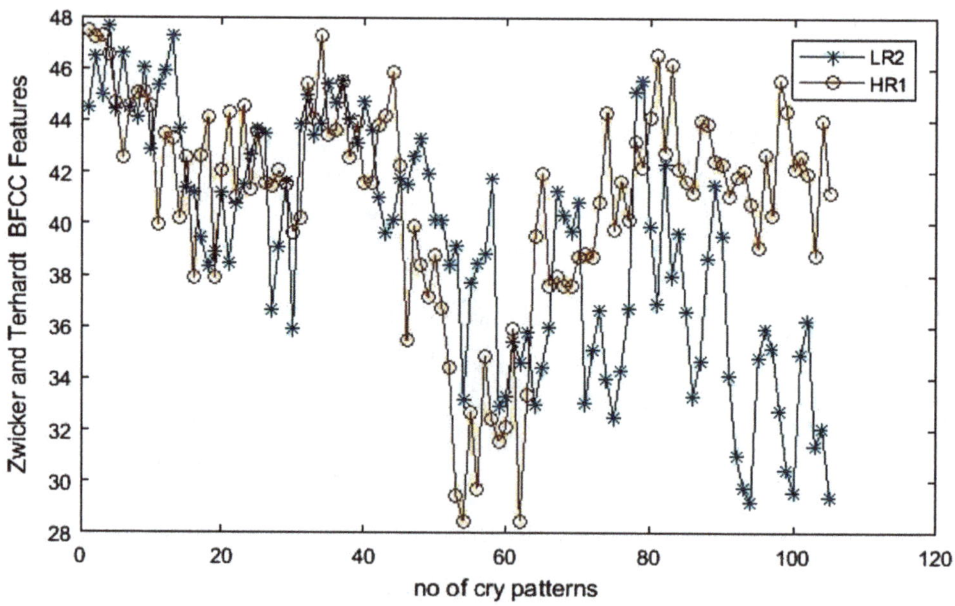

Figure 4d. BFCC Zwicker and Terhardt method for low risk 2 and high risk 1 cries

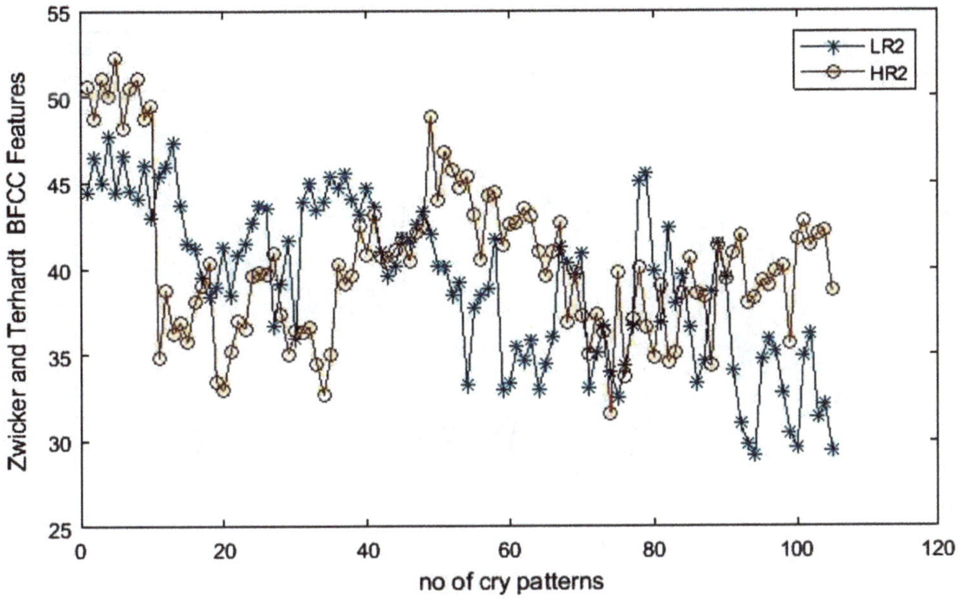

Figure 5a. BFCC Traunmiller method for low risk 1 and high risk 2 cries

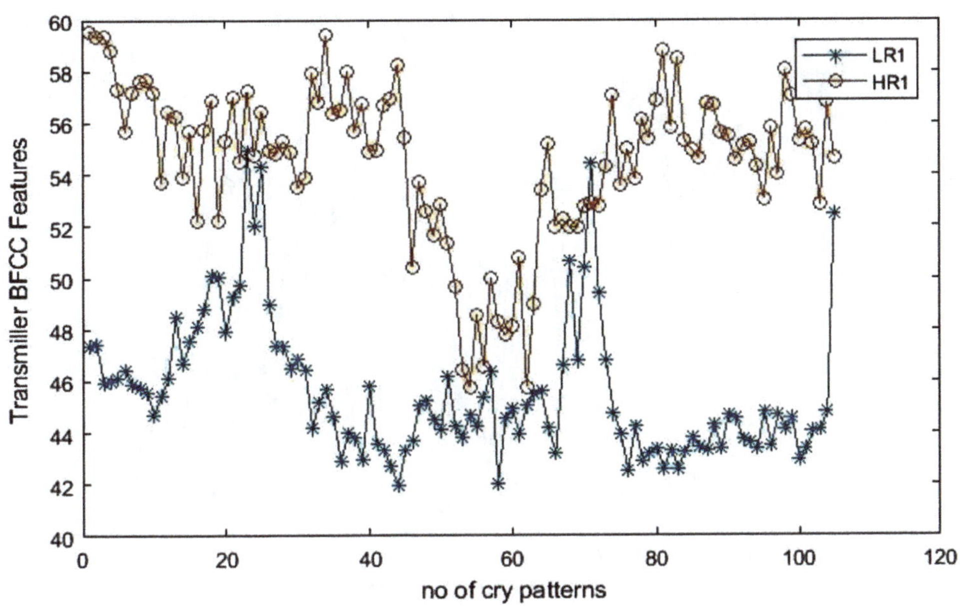

Figure 5b. BFCC Traunmiller method for low risk 1 and high risk 2 cries

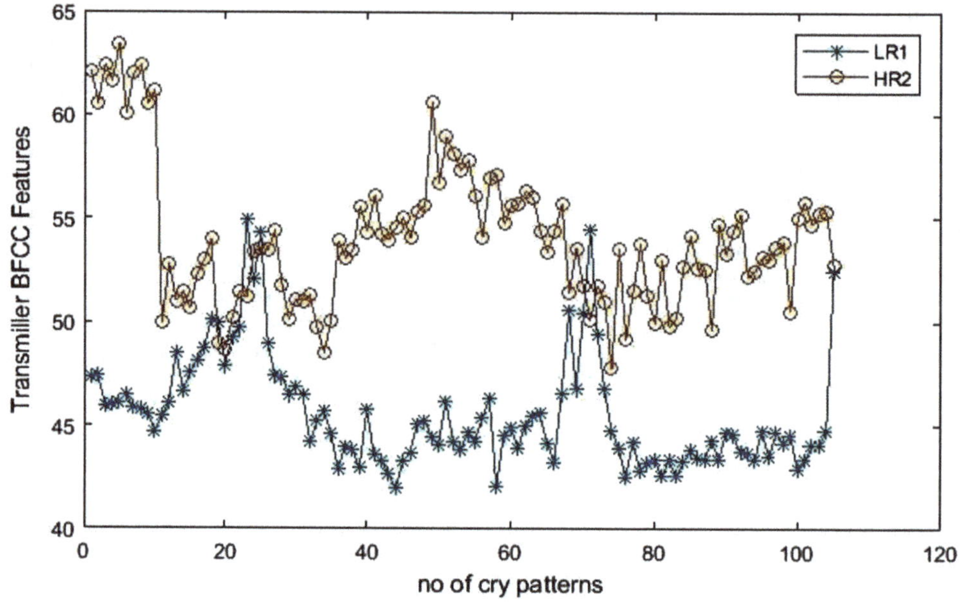

Figure 5c. BFCC Traunmiller method for low risk 2 and high risk 1 cries

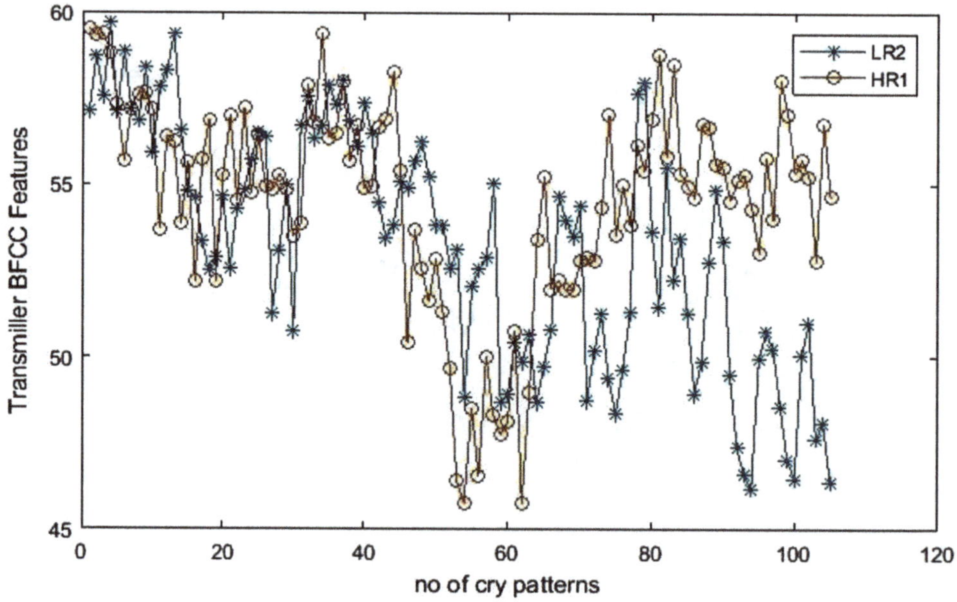

Figure 5d. BFCC Traunmiller method for low risk 2 and high risk 2 cries

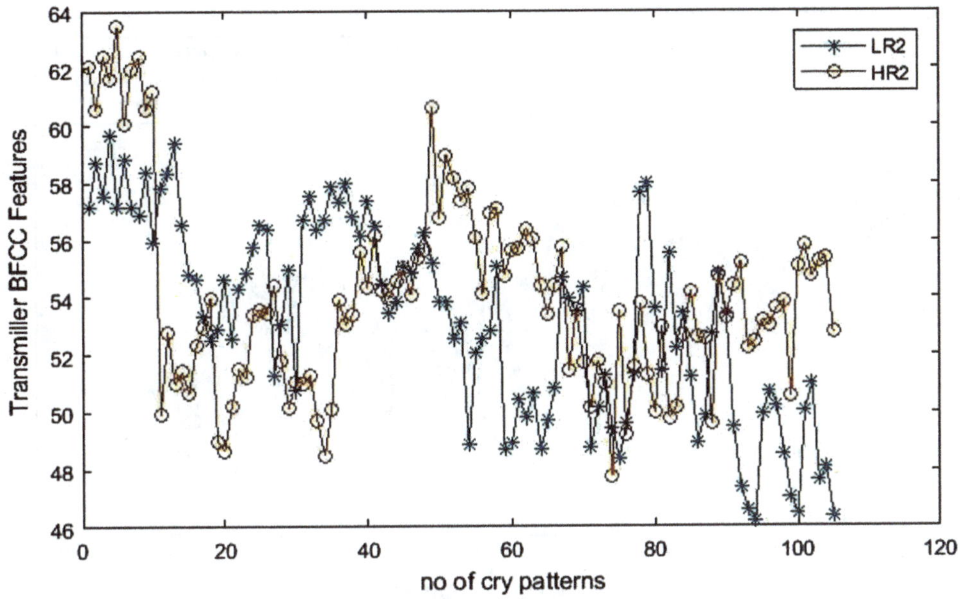

Figure 6a. Low risk 1 BFCC features for three methods

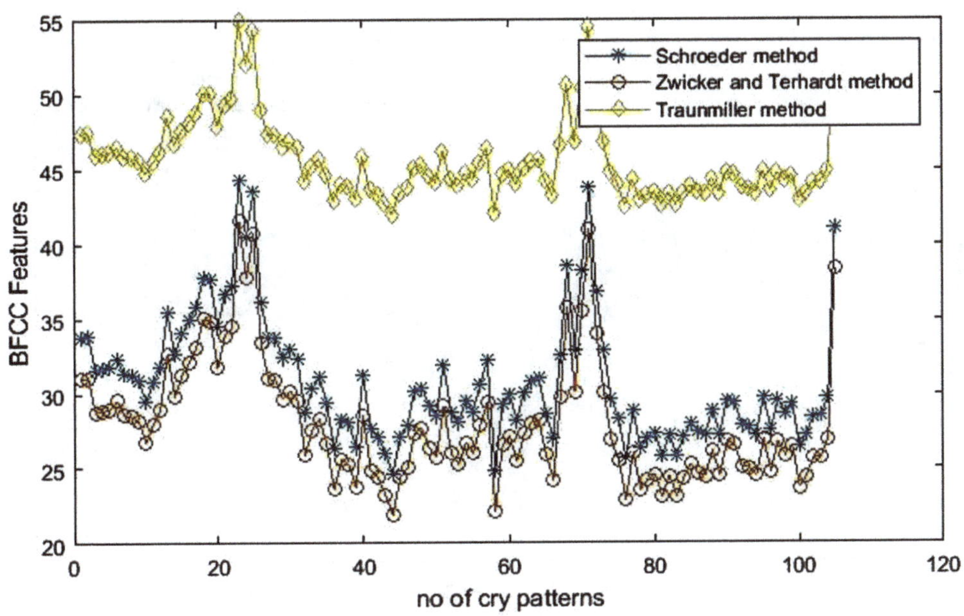

Figure 6b. Low risk 2 BFCC features for three methods

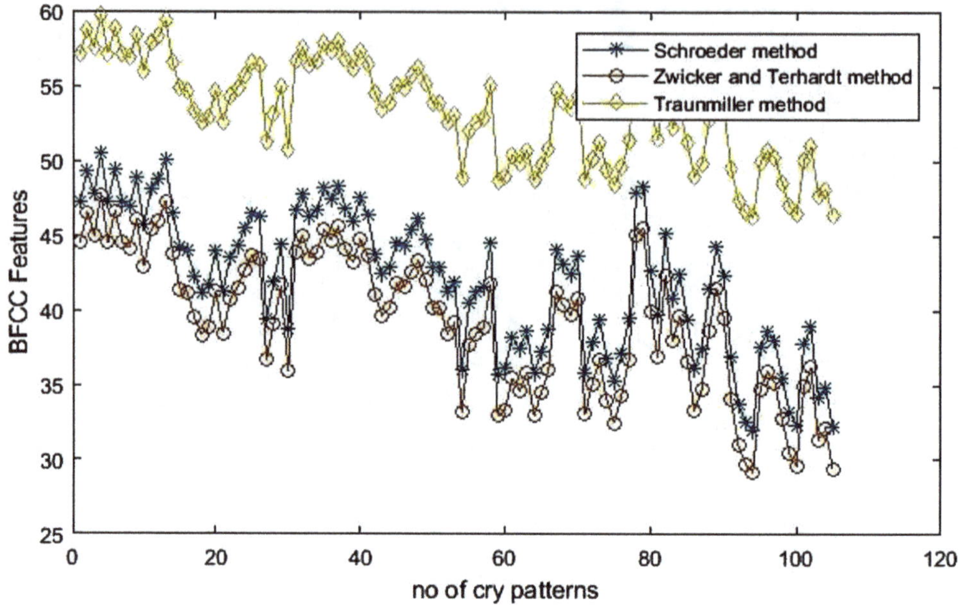

Figure 6c. High risk 1 BFCC features for three methods

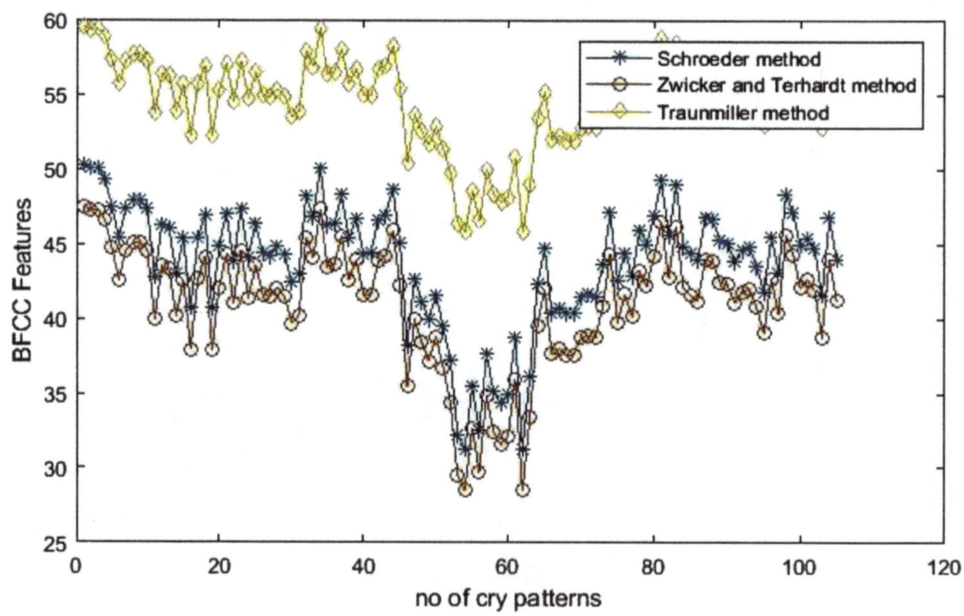

Figure 6d. High risk 2 BFCC features for three methods

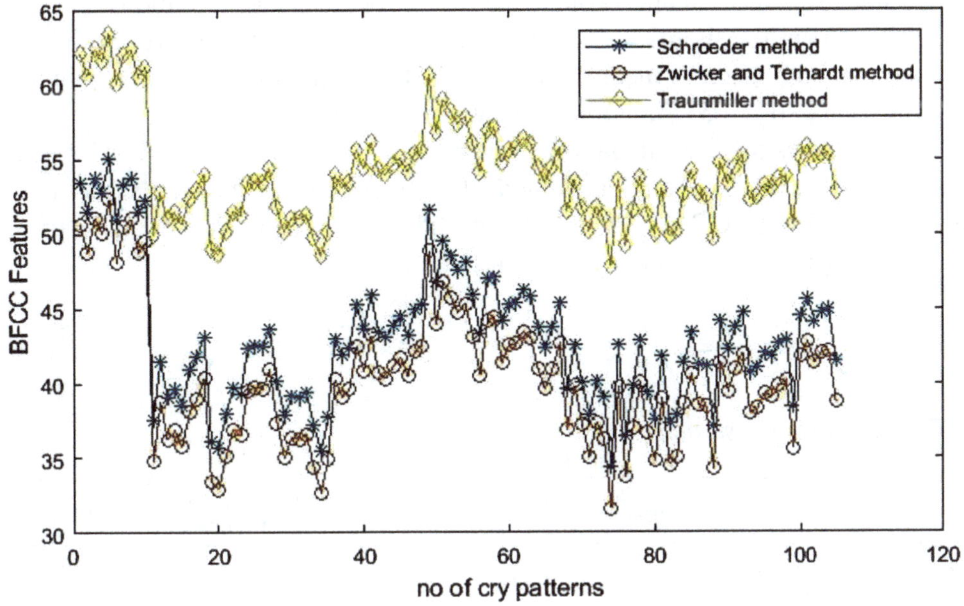

Evaluation

This section shows the BFCC features for all the three methods for low risk and high risk conditions of neonate cries. It also discusses the statistical analysis results and pattern classifier performance.

Figures 3a- 3d shows the BFCC features for high risk vs low risk for the bark filters using Schroeder method.

Figures 4a- 4d show the BFCC features for high risk vs Low risk for the bark filters using Zwicker and Terhardt method.

Figures 5a- 5d show the BFCC features for high risk vs Low risk for the bark filters using Traunmiller method.

It can be observed from Figures 3-5 that the proposed Bark frequency cepstral coefficients found to be potential acoustic features to discriminate low-risk and high-risk neonates. This feature plot holds good for all high-risk condition with significant discrimination band.

Figure 6a- 6d show the low-risk and high-risk conditions using bark filters all the three method. Among the three methods was found to provide very distinguishable band difference compared to other two methods for low and high-risk conditions which was also evident from figure 5.

Table 2 shows the descriptive analysis of BFCC features such as mean, median, mode, standard deviation and variance for all the methods and conditions.

Table 3 shows the significance value of each method when compared with high and low risk and different methods.it can be noted all the methods were found to be significance ($p<0.05$) for automated pattern classifier.

Table 4 shows the overall classification results of low risk and high-risk cry. It can be seen that B3: Transmiller Method BFCC feature yields better classification performance. The BFCC features for classifying low and high risk uses all the three B1, B2, B3 features considered for the classifier.

Table 2. Descriptive statistics

	Mean	Median	Mode	Standard Deviation	Variance
Schroder method BFCC feature: LR1	32.83	29.63	24.65	4.14	17.15
Schroder method BFCC feature: LR2	42.06	42.46	31.96	4.73	22.42
Schroder method BFCC feature: HR1	43.74	44.73	31.26	4.18	17.52
Schroder method BFCC feature: HR2	43.11	42.62	34.37	4.52	20.45
Zwicker and Terhardth method BFCC feature: LR1	28.05	26.85	21.87	4.14	17.15
Zwicker and Terhardth method BFCC feature: LR2	39.28	39.69	29.18	4.73	22.42
Zwicker and Terhardth method BFCC feature: HR1	40.96	41.95	28.48	4.18	17.52
Zwicker and Terhardth method BFCC feature: HR2	40.34	39.84	31.59	4.52	20.45
Transmiller method BFCC feature: LR1	45.60	44.76	41.94	2.69	7.24
Transmiller method BFCC feature: LR2	53.29	53.50	46.20	3.47	12.05
Transmiller method BFCC feature: HR1	54.53	55.20	45.76	3.03	9.42
Transmiller method BFCC feature: HR2	54.06	53.61	47.77	3.43	11.80

Table 3. Significance value using ANOVA

Condition	Significance P Value
Schroder method BFCC feature: LR1vs HR1	0.00
Schroder method BFCC feature: LR1 vs HR2	0.00
Schroder method BFCC feature: LR2 vs HR1	0.00
Schroder method BFCC feature: LR2 vs HR2	0.00
Zwicker and Terhardth method BFCC feature: LR1vs HR1	0.00
Zwicker and Terhardth method BFCC feature: LR1 vs HR2	0.00
Zwicker and Terhardth method BFCC feature: LR2 vs HR1	0.00
Zwicker and Terhardth method BFCC feature: LR2 vs HR2	0.00
Transmiller method BFCC feature: LR1vs HR1	0.01
Transmiller method BFCC feature: LR1 vs HR2	0.01
Transmiller method BFCC feature: LR2 vs HR1	0.02
Transmiller method BFCC feature: LR2 vs HR2	0.02
Low risk all methods vs high risk all methods	0.00

CONCLUSION

For this study, four conditions such as two low risk conditions of preterm such as LR1- Appropriate Gestational Age (AGA) and LR2- Intrauterine Growth Restriction (IUGR) and two high risk conditions such as HR1-Respiratory Distress Syndrome (RDS) and HR2- Premature Rupture of Membranes (PROM) was considered. Each condition 20 cries were considered approximately 800 seconds of cry for LR1, LR2, HR1 and HR2 was considered. For all the conditions Bark Frequency Cepstral Coefficients using three methods such as Schroeder method, Zwicker

Table 4. Classification Results of Low risk and High Risk cry

Sl. No	Classification	Kernel	Sensitivity%	Specificity%	Accuracy%
1.	B1: LR vs HR	Fine gaussian	90.47	90.47	90.5
2.	B2: LR vs HR	Fine and medium Gaussian	91.42	91.42	92.4
3.	B3: LR vs HR	Fine Gaussian	91.9	91	91
4.	BFCC LR vs HR (All methods	Fine Gaussian	90.47	91.42	92.9

and Terhardt Method and Traunmiller method features was extracted for each cry. Support Vector Machine (SVM) binary classification was performed for each BFCC method between high risk and low risk features and also combined BFCC features for binary classification of low risk and high risk conditions. The classification accuracy, sensitivity and specificity for Schroeder BFCC method was 90.5%, 90.47% and 90.47% respectively. The classification accuracy, sensitivity and specificity for Zwicker and Terhardt BFCC method was 92.4%, 91.42% and 91.42% respectively. The classification accuracy, sensitivity and specificity for Traunmiller BFCC method was 90.9%, 91% and 91% respectively. Binary classification accuracy, sensitivity and specificity of all the methods was 92.9%, 91.47% and 91.42% respectively.

ACKNOWLEDGMENT

The authors would like to thank Department of Science and Technology (DST), Government of India for their financial support to carry out this research project (TDP/BDTD/22/2019).

REFERENCES

Abou-Abbas, L., Tadj, C., & Fersaie, H. A. (2017). A fully automated approach for baby cry signal segmentation and boundary detection of expiratory and inspiratory episodes. *The Journal of the Acoustical Society of America*, *142*(3), 1318–1331. doi:10.1121/1.5001491 PMID:28964073

Da Motta, G. D. C. P., Schardosim, J. M., & Da Cunha, M. L. C. (2015). Neonatal infant pain scale: Cross-cultural adaptation and validation in Brazil. *Journal of Pain and Symptom Management*, *50*(3), 394–401. doi:10.1016/j.jpainsymman.2015.03.019 PMID:26025270

Ghosh, D., Debnath, D. S., & Bose, S. (2012). A Comparative Study of Performance of Fpgabased Melfilter Bank & Bark Filter Bank. *International Journal of Artificial Intelligence & Applications*, *3*(3), 37–54. doi:10.5121/ijaia.2012.3304

Gulzar, T., Singh, A., & Sharma, S. (2014). Comparative Analysis of LPCC, MFCC and BFCC for the Recognition of Hindi Words Using Artificial Neural Networks. *International Journal of Computers and Applications*, *101*(12), 22–27.

Herrera, A., & Del Rio, F. (2010). Frequency bark cepstral coefficients extraction for speech analysis by synthesis. *The Journal of the Acoustical Society of America*, *128*(4), 2290. doi:10.1121/1.3508042 PMID:20370010

Kamińska, D., Sapiński, T., & Pelikant, A. (2013). *Comparison of Perceptual Features Efficiency for Automatic Identification of Emotional States from Speech* (pp. 210–213). doi:10.1109/HSI.2013.6577824

Kumar, C., ur Rehman, F., Kumar, S., Mehmood, A. & Shabir, G. (2018). Analysis of MFCC and BFCC in a speaker identification system. In *Proceedings of 2018 International Conference on Computing, Mathematics and Engineering Technologies (iCoMET),* Sukkur, Pakistan, pp. 1-5. doi:10.1109/ICOMET.2018.8346330

Liu, L., Li, Y., & Kuo, K. (2018). Infant cry signal detection, pattern extraction and recognition. In *Proceedings of 2018 International Conference on Information and Computer Technologies (ICICT)*, DeKalb, IL, pp. 159-163. 10.1109/INFOCT.2018.8356861

Liu, L., Li, W., Wu, X., & Zhou, B. X. (2019). Infant cry language analysis and recognition: an experimental approach. *IEEE/CAA Journal of Automatica Sinica.* pp. 1-11. doi:. doi:10.1109/JAS.2019.1911435

Lubis, C., & Gondawijaya, F. (2019). Heart Sound Diagnose System with BFCC, MFCC, and Backpropagation Neural Network. *IOP Conference Series. Materials Science and Engineering*, *508*, 012119. doi:10.1088/1757-899X/508/1/012119

Moers, C., Möbius, B., Rosanowski, F., Nöth, E., Eysholdt, U., & Haderlein, T. (2012). Vowel- and Text-Based Cepstral Analysis of Chronic Hoarseness. *Journal of Voice*, *26*(4), 416–424. doi:10.1016/j.jvoice.2011.05.001 PMID:21940144

Muthusamy, H., Polat, K., & Yaacob, S. (2015). Particle Swarm Optimization Based Feature Enhancement and Feature Selection for Improved Emotion Recognition in Speech and Glottal Signals. *PLoS One*, *10*(3). doi:10.1371/journal.pone.0120344 PMID:25799141

Illingworth, R. S. (1972). The Normal Child and Some Problems of the Early Years and Their Treatment (10th ed.). Philadelphia, PA: W. B. Saunders Co.

Sengupta, N., Sahidullah, M., & Saha, G. (2016). Lung sound classification using cepstral-based statistical features. *Computers in Biology and Medicine*, *75*, 118–129. doi:10.1016/j.compbiomed.2016.05.013 PMID:27286184

Shannon, B. J. & Paliwal, K. K. (2003). A Comparative Study of Filter Bank Spacing for Speech Recognition. In *Microelectronic Engineering Research Conference 41:* 310–12. Retrieved from https://maxwell.ict.griffith.edu.au/spl/publications/papers/merc03_ben.pdf

Sharma, S., & Patil, H. A. (2015). Combining Evidences from Bark Scale and Mel Scale Warped Features for VTLN. In *Proceedings of the 2nd International Conference on Perception and Machine Intelligence (PerMIn '15)*. ACM, New York, NY, 133-136.

Sriraam, N., & Tejaswini, S. (2014). Infant Cry Detection and Pain Scale Assessment: A Pilot Study. *International Journal of Biomedical and Clinical Engineering*, *3*(1), 42–51. doi:10.4018/ijbce.2014010104

Sriraam, N., Tejaswini, S., & Chavan, A. A. (2016). Development of Portable Medical Electronic Device for Infant Cry Recognition: A Primitive Experimental Study. *International Journal of Biomedical and Clinical Engineering*, *5*(2), 53–63. doi:10.4018/IJBCE.2016070104

Tantaratana, S., & Thomas, J. B. (1981). A Class of Nonparametric Sequential Tests. *IEEE Transactions on Information Theory*, *27*(5), 596–606. doi:10.1109/TIT.1981.1056401

Tejaswini, S., Sriraam, N. & Pradeep, G. C. M. (2016). Recognition of infant cries using wavelet derived mel frequency feature with SVM classification. In *Proceedings of 2016 International Conference on Circuits, Controls, Communications and Computing (I4C),* Bangalore, India, pp. 1-4. 10.1109/CIMCA.2016.8053313

Tejaswini, S., Sriraam, N., & Pradeep, G. C. M. Cloud-Based Framework for Pain Scale Assessment in NICU- A Primitive Study with Infant Cries. In *Proceedings of 2018 3rd International Conference on Circuits, Control, Communication and Computing (I4C),* Bangalore, India, pp. 1-4. 10.1109/CIMCA.2018.8739712

Tejaswini, S., Sriraam, N., & Pradeep, G. C. M. (2019). Preterm Neonates Cry Pattern Recognition Using Bark Frequency Cepstral Coefficients. In *Proceedings of 2019 1st International Conference on Advanced Technologies in Intelligent Control, Environment, Computing and Communication Engineering,* Bangalore, India.

Tuduce, R. I., Cucu, H., & Burileanu, C. (2018). Why Is My Baby Crying? An In-Depth Analysis of Paralinguistic Features and Classical Machine Learning Algorithms for Baby Cry Classification. In *2018 41st International Conference on Telecommunications and Signal Processing, TSP 2018:* 1–4. 10.1109/TSP.2018.8441363

Chapter 8
Effect of Age on Heart Rate Variability Analysis in Breast Cancer Patients:
Heart Rate Variability in Breast Cancer

Reema Shyamsunder Shukla
Birla Institute of Technology, India

Yogender Aggarwal
Birla Institute of Technology, India

Rakesh Kumar Sinha
Birla Institute of Technology, India

Shreeniwas S. Raut
HCG Abdur Razzaque Ansari Cancer Center, India

ABSTRACT

Breast Cancer (BC) is the leading cause of death in women, worldwide. The Eastern Cooperative Oncology Group (ECOG) Performance Status (PS) of BC can be studied using HRV measures. The main purpose of this chapter is to give an insight to clinicians via HRV measures with respect to age to make them understand the PS of patients. Data from 114 BC patients was segregated into two age groups, G1 (20 to 40 years) and G2 (41 to 75 years). The 5-minute electrocardiogram of the subjects was taken and HRV measures were extracted. One-way ANOVA with Posthoc Tukeys' HSD test was done. Triangular Index, Ratio of standard deviation of poincare plot perpendicular to the line of identity to the standard deviation along line of identity, Detrended Fluctuation Analysis descriptors, Approximate Entropy,

DOI: 10.4018/978-1-7998-0326-3.ch008

Sample Entropy and Correlation Dimension significantly decreased from ECOG0 to 4 and from G1 to G2. The sympathetic activity increased with vagal withdrawal as age advanced.

INTRODUCTION

Cancer belongs to various classes of diseases which occurs due to the uncontrolled growth of cells. The type of cancer is solely dependent on the cell type or organ from which they evolve. Due to invasion, tumor spreads in various parts of the body (Hanahan & Weinberg, 2000). Human breast cancer (BC) is one such type which arises due to variation in genes of somatic cells but is mostly found to acquire from their ancestors found mainly in woman (Hall et al., 1990). Several factors leading to BC includes 5% to 10% due to family history, hormonal, full term pregnancy after 30 years of age, breast density of more than 75%, exposure to ionizing radiation etc. (King et al., 2013). The screening mammography or magnetic resonance imaging (MRI) and then confirmed findings from biopsy or fine needle aspiration leads to final diagnosis of BC (Berry et al., 2005; de la Rochefordiere et al., 1992). Several types of BC includes ductal carcinoma in situ, lobular neoplasia, Paget's disease of nipple and metastatic breast cancer (DeVita et al., 2015). The staging of the BC is given in Table 1a and Table 1b, respectively. Various optimized options are chosen to provide quality improvement in the treatment of BC patients (Giuliano et al., 2017; NCCN, 2003). The age has been considered a confounder while giving the treatment (Silliman et. al., 1989).

Heart Rate Variability (HRV) studies have been done in BC survivors and has been found to be of decreased value with more fatigue (Meersman, 1993). Performance Status (PS) evaluation using Eastern Cooperative Oncology Group (ECOG) Scale is commonly used in treating cancer patients which is explained in detail in Table 2 (Shukla and Aggarwal, 2018e; Blagden et al., 2003). Age and sex factors in analyzing HRV time, frequency and nonlinear analysis were not significant in patients with cardiac disorder and depression (Stapelberg et al., 2017). The HRV analysis of hypertensive patient was done by segmenting the overnight electrocardiogram (ECG) into various scales and extracting HRV features and then reducing feature dimensions using the temporal pyramid pooling method (Hratmann et al., 2019). In HRV biofeedback, patients can observe their HRV on computer screen and attempt to increase HRV and restore autonomic balance (Rourke et al., 2017). The HRV measures decreased in male BC patients as compared to their female counterparts which proves autonomic dysfunction (Shukla and Aggarwal, 2017). Heart rate variability analysis was of prognostic value in classifying the performance status in lung cancer patients (Park et al., 2018).

Foetal HRV is an essential biomarker for health and disease which depicts the vagus nerve functionality in foetus (Herry et al., 2019). The decreased values of HRV was observed in several cardiovascular risk factors such as hypertension (HTN), diabetes mellitus (DM), congestive heart failure, coronary artery disease (CAD) and acute myocardial infarction (AMI). Yoga therapy in ASD autism spectrum disorder children can upgrade parasympathetic activity and can normalize physiological as well as psychological balance (Vidyashree et al., 2019).

Breast Cancer has become the very commonly known cancer in both developing and developed countries (Hadjiiski et al., 2006). Micro-calcifications and masses are the two most significant signs of malignancy (Mousa et al., 2005). Women and 1% of men die due to BC across the globe (Youlden et al., 2012; Ottini et al., 2010). Mammography, MRI, computed tomography, ultrasound, electrical impedance tomography, thermography, positron emission tomography (PET), scintimammography, open surgical biopsy, fine needle aspiration (FNA), needle biopsy, core needle biopsy are the different techniques to confirm the occurrence of cancer (Vazquez et al., 2009; Prasad and Houserkova, 2007).

It has been hypothesized that the performance status in BC patients can be evaluated with HRV analysis where age can be considered as a confounder. It is novel and can give a vital feedback to the clinicians to plan appropriate treatment to their patients to improve their quality of living.

PARTICIPANTS AND METHOD

Patients

One hundred twenty-five adult BC patients or subjects were selected consecutively and evaluated in the study. The exclusion criteria were diabetes, mental illness, cardiovascular disorder, infection, anaemia or any nutritional deficiency, hypertension, atrial fibrillation and fibroadenosis. Of 125, 114 subjects were evaluable. Of 114 subjects, 4 were men and 110 were women. The ECG acquisition was done between 01/06/2015 and 01/12/2015. The histopathological report and other medical history reports were checked before collecting the information of each patient. Cancer stages and clinical history was obtained with their signed consent. The ECOG PS was noted by interrogating them and their helpers about their ease in performing daily day to day activities by medical oncologists. The demographics of the BC patients is given in Table 3. The minimum age of the BC survivor subject was 25 years and maximum age found was 75 years. The age group in BC patients was segregated

Table 1a. Nomenclature of Tumor size (T)

T Category	T Criteria
TX	Primary tumor cannot be evaluated
T0	No trace of primary tumor
Tis (DCIS)a	Ductal carcinoma in situ (DCIS)
Tis (Paget)	Paget disease of the nipple not related with malignant carcinoma and/or carcinoma in situ (DCIS) in the underlying breast
T1	Tumor≤20mm
T1mi	Tumor≤1mm
T1a	Tumor>1mm but ≤5mm (round any measurement from >1.0-1.9mm to 2 mm)
T1b	Tumor>5mm but≤10mm
T1c	Tumor>10mm but≤20mm
T2	Tumor>20mm but≤50mm
T3	Tumor>50mm
T4	Tumor of any size with invasion to the chest wall and/or to the skin
T4a	Invasion to the chest wall; invasion to pectoralis muscle and invasion of chest wall
T4b	Ulceration and/or ipsilateral macroscopic satellite nodules and/or Oedema of the skin
T4c	Both T4a and T4b are present
T4d	Inflammatory carcinoma

into two groups G1: 20 to 40 years and G2: 41 to 75 years. The segregation of age groups was done on the basis of maximum availability of patients in each group. In G1, of 44 subjects, the subjects in ECOG0 were 5, ECOG1 were 3, ECOG2 were 12, ECOG3 were 12 and ECOG4 were 12. In G2, of 70 subjects, the subjects in ECOG0 were 7, ECOG1 were 5, ECOG2 were 12, ECOG3 were 20 and ECOG4 were 26. The non-invasive data collection was done as per the ethical standards of Declaration of Helsinki and a signed consent was obtained from the participants.

Processing of ECG Signal

The 5-minute ECG of the subjects was taken from 11 a.m. to 12 noon in supine position at 24°C and HRV measures were extracted. The signals with movement artifacts were visually observed and discarded. The patients were asked to rest for 30 minutes in a cosy environment with a controlled breathing rate before acquiring the signal. Infinite impulse response high pass filter (IIR HPF) at 3Hz was applied after the recording of ECG. The signal was sampled at 200 samples/second. The

Table 1b. Stages as per tumor size, nodes present and occurrence of metastases

T	N	M	Stage
Tis	N0	M0	0
T1	N0	M0	IA
T0	N1	M0	IB
T1	N1mi	M0	IB
T0	N1	M0	IIA
T1	N1	M0	IIA
T2	N0	M0	IIA
T2	N1	M0	IIB
T3	N0	M0	IIB
T1	N2	M0	IIIA
T2	N2	M0	IIIA
T3	N1	M0	IIIA
T3	N2	M0	IIIA
T4	N0	M0	IIIB
T4	N1	M0	IIIB
T4	N2	M0	IIIB
Any T	N3	M0	IIIC
Any T	Any N	M1	IV

tachogram obtained from recorded signal with R-wave threshold level set at 0.5 was subjected to interpolation at a cubic-spline frequency of 8Hz and the ectopic beats were removed (Acknowledge 4.0 (Biopac Systems Inc., USA)). The RR interval

Table 2. Eastern Co-operative Oncology Group (ECOG) scale of Performance Status (PS)

ECOG	Meaning
0	Normal Activity
1	Exhibits symptoms and ambulatory
2	Less than 50% on bed but difficulty in carrying out day to day activities
3	More than 50% on bed
4	Bedridden
5	Death

(Blagden et al., 2003)

Table 3. Demographics of breast cancer patients

Documented History	Number (%)	Documented History	Number (%)
Gender		**Current Treatment**	
Male	4 (0.31)	Chemotherapy	80 (62.01)
Female	125 (96.89)	Radiation	31 (24.03)
		Surgery	52 (40.31)
Patient History		None	20 (15.5)
Diabetes	7 (5.42)	Hormone Therapy	10 (7.75)
Cardiac disease history	2 (1.55)		
Hypertension	2 (1.55)	**Performance Status**	
Fibroadenosis	4 (3.1)	ECOG 4	38 (29.45)
Smoking	3 (2.32)	ECOG 3	32 (24.8)
Tobacco	2 (1.55)	ECOG 2	24 (18.6)
Alcohol	0 (0)	ECOG 1	8 (6.2)
Cachexia	0 (0)	ECOG 0	12 (9.3)
Constipation	0 (0)		
Diarrhoea	0 (0)	**TNM Staging**	
Fever	2 (1.55)	0	1 (0.77)
Oedema	16 (12.4)	I	8 (6.2)
Vomiting	2 (1.55)	II	60 (46.51)
Anaemia	0 (0)	III	38 (29.45)
Ascitis	0 (0)	IV	7 (5.42)

(RRI) and power spectral density (PSD) plots were obtained from tachogram, which helped in further extraction of HRV features. The disposable Silver/Silver Chloride (Ag/AgCl) was used and placed as per Einthoven's triangle rule. The reference electrode (ground electrode) was placed on right leg, electrode with positive negative polarity was positioned on left leg and right arm, respectively. The Acknowledge 4.0 software was utilised to analyze ECG signal.

HRV Analysis

HRV is the physiological operation, in which there exists variation in time intervals between heartbeats. The variation in R to R interval gives a clue about the anomalies or cardiac disorder (Chuduc et al., 2013). The HRV measures are correlated with the disturbances found in the autonomic nervous system including sympathetic nervous system (SNS) and parasympathetic nervous system (PNS) where, vagal nerve controls the PNS activity (Aggarwal et al., 2014; Acharya et al., 2006). This method is analysed in time, frequency and nonlinear domain (Shukla and Aggarwal, 2018a-e; Shukla and Aggarwal, 2017a-b; Tarvainen et al., 2014).

The time-domain measures include mean RR interval (mRR), mean heart rate (mHR), standard deviation of normal to normal RR interval (SDNN), square root of the mean squared differences of successive RR intervals (RMSSD), triangular index (TI), triangular interpolation of RR intervals (TINN), standard deviation of heart rate (SDHR), number of successive RR intervals > 50ms (NN50) and proportion derived by dividing NN50 by the total number of RR intervals (pNN50).

The computation of time domain HRV measures are done as follows:

$$mRR(ms) = \frac{\sum_{y=1}^{N} RR_y}{N} \tag{1}$$

$$mHR(bpm) = \frac{\sum_{y=1}^{N} \frac{60000}{RR_y}}{N} \tag{2}$$

$$SDNN(ms) = \left(_{(y=1)}^{N} (RR_y - mRR)^2\right) / (N-1) \tag{3}$$

$$SDHR\left(bpm\right) = sqrt\left[\frac{\sum_{y=1}^{N} ((60000 / RR_y) - mHR)^2}{N-1}\right] \tag{4}$$

$$CVRR = \frac{SDRR * 100}{mRR} \tag{5}$$

$$RMSSD\left(ms\right) = sqrt\left(mean\left((RR_{y+1} - RR_y)^2\right)\right) \tag{6}$$

$$pNN20(\%) = \frac{Count\left(\left|RR_{y+1} - RR_{y}\right|\right)_{>20ms} * 100}{N-1} \tag{7}$$

$$pNN50(\%) = \frac{Count\left(\left|RR_{y+1} - RR_{y}\right|\right)_{>50ms} * 100}{N-1} \tag{8}$$

The PSD bands of very low frequency (VLF) (0.003 to 0.04 Hz), low frequency (LF) (0.04 to 15 Hz) and high frequency (HF) (0.15 to 4 Hz) was computed using fast fourier transformation (FFT) and autoregressive (AR) method with the order of 16. The normalized units (n.u.) computation was carried out by dividing each spectral component by the total power. LF/HF was obtained by dividing LF by HF (Tarvainen et al., 2014). All frequency domain measures considered are as follows (Boonnithi et al., 2011):

VLF (ms^2) = Power spectrum from 0.003 to 0.04Hz.
LF (ms^2) = Power spectrum from 0.04 to 0.15Hz.
HF (ms^2) = Power spectrum from 0.15to 0.4Hz.

$$Nlf(\%) = \frac{LF * 100}{VLF + LF + HF} \tag{9}$$

$$Nhf(\%) = \frac{HF * 100}{VLF + LF + HF} \tag{10}$$

The nonlinear studies of HRV is depicted by varied measures like poincare plot (PP), which includes standard deviation perpendicular to line of identity (LOI) known as SD_1, standard deviation along line of identity known as SD_2, approximate and sample entropy (ApEn; SampEn), detrended fluctuation analysis (DFA), which includes short term fluctuation (α_1, the range being 4 to 16), long term fluctuation (α_2, range being 17 to 64), correlation dimension (CD) and recurrence plots (RP) (Acharya et al., 2006).

Poincare Plot

One of the methods to evaluate non-linear properties of HRV is PP. It is pictorially represented in Figure 1. The ellipse is formed as per the line-of-identity (LOI) ($RR_y = RR_{y+1}$). The standard deviation of the dots perpendicular to the LOI shown by SD_1 explains short-term variability occurring due to Respiratory Sinus Arrythmia. SD_1 is linked with time-domain measure Standard Deviation of Successive Differences in RR Intervals (SDSD) as per

$$SD_1^2 = \frac{1}{2} SDSD^2 \tag{11}$$

The standard deviation along the line of identity shown by SD_2 explains the long-term variability, which is linked with time-domain measures SDNN and SDSD by (Brennan et al., 2001).

$$SD_2^2 = 2SDNN^2 - \frac{1}{2} SDSD^2 \tag{12}$$

Figure 1. Poincare plot

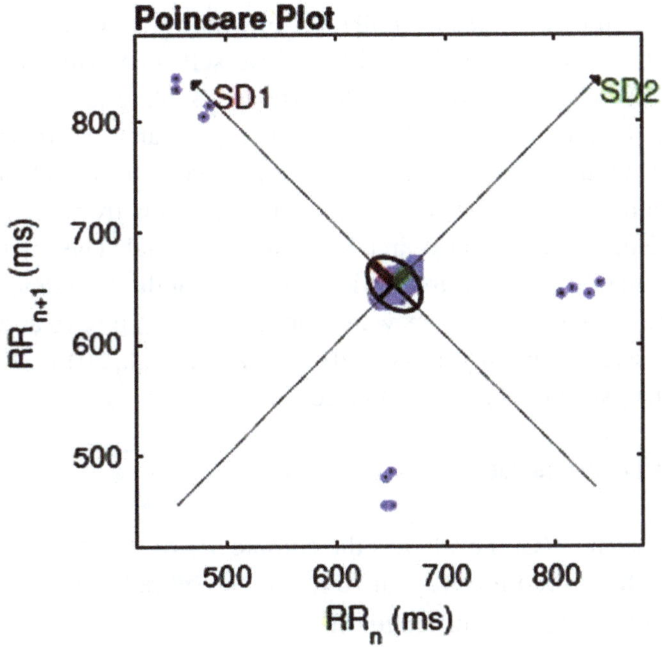

Detrended Fluctuation Analysis

The Detrended Fluctuation Analysis is upgradation of square root of the squares of the mean of RR intervals implemented to nonstationary signals for measuring the fractal grading properties of short RR interval signals. It evaluates the correlation within the signal. For various time scales, the correlation is given as (Acharya et al., 2002),

$$Z\left(x\right)=\sum_{i=1}^{x}[RR\left(y\right)-RR_{avg}],\text{ where x=1,2,......,N} \quad (13)$$

Where Z(x) is the xth value of the unified series, RR(y) is the yth interbeat interval, and the RR_{avg} is the mean of RR intervals along the entire series. The integrated time series is equally segregated into n windows in which a least-squares line is fitted to the RR interval data. The y coordinate of the straight-line segments is implicated by the regression line Zn(x), which is detrended in each window. The root-mean-square fluctuation denoted by F(n) is calculated using the equation:

$$F\left(n\right)=\sqrt{(\frac{1}{N}\sum_{w=1}^{N}[Z\left(x\right)-Z_{n}(x)]^{2})} \quad (14)$$

This calculation is reiterated over all sizes of window to acquire the association between F(n) and the size of window n. F(n) is inversely related to window size. Log F(n) is plotted against log(n) to obtain the exponent scaling factor (α). For Brown noise; integral of white noise, α is 1.5. For white Gaussian noise α is 0.5 (Acharya et al., 2006). Detrended Fluctuation Analysis prevents wrong detection of long-range correlations and eliminates constant or linear trends from the time series. It correlates to identify the similarity in non-stationary signal. The fluctuation (α.) is root-mean square of detrended time series, measured at different length. The short (α_1) and long (α_2) fluctuation slopes were calculated at $4 \leq n \leq 16$ and $16 \leq n \leq 64$ detrended time series segment, respectively (Tarvainen et al., 2014). The Detrended Fluctuation Analysis plot is given in Figure 2.

Correlation Dimension

Correlation dimension (CD) evaluates the complexity of the RR interval series. It conveys data on the lower limit on dynamic variables required to frame the underlying unit. Consider the vectors u_w of length m,

Figure 2. Detrended fluctuation analysis plot

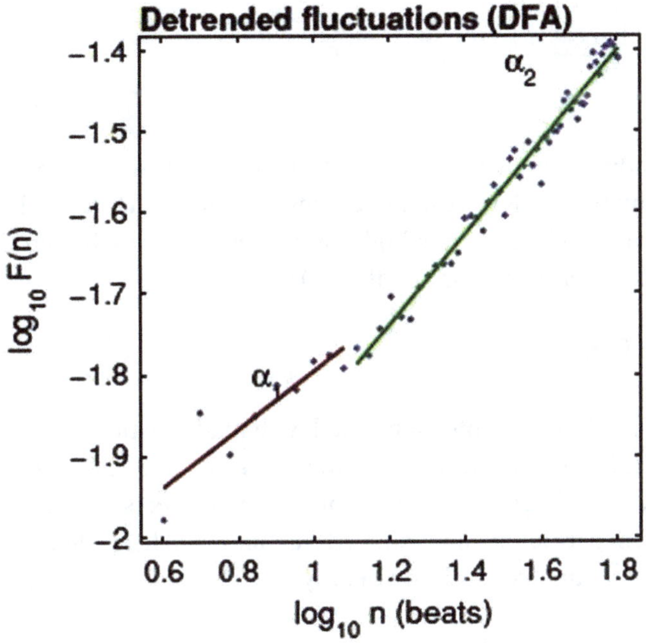

$$u_w = (R^{R_y}, R^{R_{y+1}}, \ldots. R^{R_{y+m-1}}),$$

Where, y = 1,2,...N-m+1

In order to compute the number of vectors u_z such that $d(u_y, u_z) \leq r$,

$$C_y^m(r) = \frac{nbr\left\{u_w \mid d(u_y, u_w) \leq r\right\}}{N-m+1} \forall w \text{, where}$$

$$d(u_y, u_w) = \sqrt{\sum_{l=1}^{m} (u_y(l) - u_w(l))^2}$$

CD integral is taking the average of the following:

$$C^m(r) = \frac{1}{N-m+1} \sum_{y=1}^{N-m+1} C_y^m(r)$$

It is also given as:

$$CD = \lim_{r \to 0} \lim_{N \to \infty} \frac{\log C^m(r)}{\log(r)} \tag{15}$$

The regression curve slope (log r, log $C^m(r)$) gives us the approximate measure. When the fluctuation of RR signal becomes less, then CD value decreases and it increases for the chaotic data. It is high for normal sinus rhythm group and low for different cardiac diseases (Henry et al., 2001).

Recurrence Plot

Recurrence plot (RP) is a graphical method with mathematics, which helps to study the non-stationarity of time series. The diagonal line and less squares were found highlighting extreme fluctuation in case of healthy subjects. Whereas more squares indicated inherent periodicity and reduced fluctuation in heart rate in complete heart block and ischemic/dilated cardiomyopathy.

$$u_y = \left(RR_y, RR_{y+\tau}, \ldots\ldots, RR_{y+(m-1)\tau}\right), \text{ y=1,2,...N-(m-1)}\tau$$

where, 'm' is the embedding dimension and 'τ' the embedding lag. The vectors u_y implies the RR interval time series in m dimensional space. A RP is a symmetrical N-(m-1)τ X N-(m-1)τ matrix of zeros and ones. The element in the y'th row and w'th column of the RP matrix is 1 only when the point u_y on the trajectory is close to u_w, explained as:

$$RP(y,w) = \begin{Bmatrix} 1, d(u_y - u_w) \le r \\ 0, otherwise \end{Bmatrix}$$

$d(u_y, u_w)$ is the euclidean distance and r is a fixed threshold (Eckmann et al., 1987). Assuming, r= ($\sqrt{m}$) * SD, where SD depicts the standard deviation of the RR time series. The foremost quantitative measure of RP is the recurrence rate (REC) defined as the ratio of ones to zeros in the RP matrix (Trulla et al., 1996).

$$REC = \frac{1}{(N-m+1)^2} \sum_{y,w=1}^{N-m+1} RP(y,w) \tag{16}$$

Lyapunov Exponent (L_{MEAN}, L_{MAX})

Divergence (DIV) is defined as inverse of maximum line length l_{max} (number of diagonal lines parallel to line of identity, main diagonal)

$$DIV = \frac{1}{l_{\max}} \tag{17}$$

The mean diagonal line length (l_{mean}) is given by,

$$l_{mean} = \frac{\sum_{l=l_{\min}}^{l_{\max}} lN_l}{\sum_{l=l_{\min}}^{l_{\max}} N_l} \text{, where } N_l \text{ is the number of length lines.} \tag{18}$$

Determinism (DET)

The determinism is given as,

$$DET = \frac{\sum_{l=l_{\min}}^{l_{\max}} lN_l}{\sum_{y,w=1}^{N-m+1} RP(y,w)} \tag{19}$$

The Shannon information entropy of the line length is given as, $ShanEn = -n_l \ln n_l$, where, n_l is the count of length l lines given by,

$$n_l = \frac{N_l}{\sum_{l'=l_{\min}}^{l_{\max}} N_{l'}} \tag{20}$$

Approximate and Shannon Entropy

Approximate entropy (ApEn) mentions irregularity in the signal, which explains the 'extent of randomness' in sequences or time series (Bettermann et al., 2001). The aim was to examine binary sequences and study its pattern retaining the dynamic information. RR interval sequences obtained from electrocardiogram (ECG) recordings were changed to a sequence of binary digits thereby encoding the beat-to-beat rise or fall in the RR interval. Shannon entropy (ShanEn) in similar lines quantified the persistence of short binary symbols (length N5) measured in 10-min intervals. The repetition of the short binary patterns was studied as per ApEn. Shannon Entropy of the same sequences proved that the enhancement in irregularity determines decrease in occurrence of some patterns.

Figure 3 illustrates how beat-to-beat differences are measured. If there exists an increase in RR interval and decrease in Heart Rate (HR), the value will set to 1 and for decrease in RR interval and increase in HR, the value is set to 0. The binary sequences are measured by evaluation of two varied entropies: ApEn and ShanEn. Approximate Entropy measures irregularity in RR intervals, whereas ShanEn integrates its information. Approximate Entropy (m, r, N) (u) measures the logarithmic frequency with vectors with 'm' components stay (within resolution r<1) close, where, the number of vector components is increased by one. Approximate Entropy points regularity for small values and irregularity for large values in a time series 'u'. ShanEn gives a number that qualifies the probability that varied binary patterns of length N takes place. Few different patterns have been seen for a regular binary sequence. Thus, ShanEn results to be of lowered value because the probability for these patterns is high and extremely little data is contained in the whole sequence. When patterns are observed with the same probability for a random binary sequence, the information content is maximal. The probability of each pattern of length N is given as:

$$\hat{p}(s_1, s_2, \ldots, s_n) = \frac{n_{s1,\ldots,sn}}{n_{tot}}$$

Where, $n_{s1,\ldots\ldots,sn}$ is the number of occurrences of the pattern $s1,\ldots.,sn$ and n_{tot} is the total number of patterns.

The entropy estimation is defined as:

$$S(N) = -\frac{1}{N}\sum_{S_1}^{S_N} \hat{p}(s_1, s_2, \ldots, s_n) \log_2 \hat{p}(s_1, s_2, \ldots, s_n)$$

Figure 3. Electrocardiogram of human subject

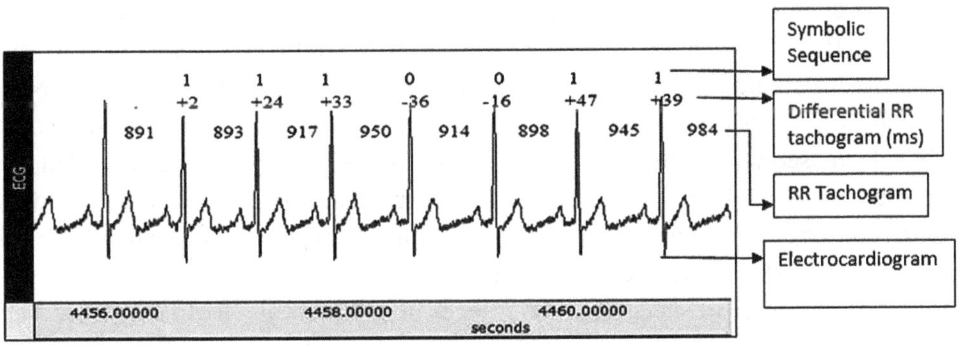

Shannon Entropy maximum value is always 1 (Cysarz et al., 2000). Sample Entropy evaluates the probability that sequences of patterns in a data set that are initially closely related stay close on the next incremental comparison, within known set of tolerance (Lake et al., 2002). It gives large values when the data is more complex while lower values indicates that the data is identical (Richman and Moorman, 2000).

Statistical Analysis

One-way analysis of variance (ANOVA) with posthoc Tukeys' honestly significant difference (HSD) test was conducted at statistical significance of $p \leq 0.05$.

RESULTS AND DISCUSSION

The present study showed that as the age increased HRV measures decreased with ECOG PS Scale of 0 to 4. As the age advances, the sympathetic activity increases and parasympathetic activity decreases, which worsens the condition of subjects. The frequency domain measures were evaluated but did not give significant results.

In our previous study in lung cancer subjects, there was no association between HRV measures and the cancer severity. The age groups consisted of varied combination of ECOG PS Scale patients, hence the sole effect of cancer severity with respect to age could not give any significant results. In the study of pulmonary metastases patients, the number of subjects being 24, the individual effect of age could not be studied (Shukla & Aggarwal, 2018c-e). The current study did not have any cachexia patients which could affect HRV and autonomic nervous system (Hundsberger et al., 2014).

Bonnemeier et al. (2003) have analysed that HRV measures decrease with age. Standard deviation of normal to normal RR intervals (SDNN) decreased from G1 *(F=10.37, P=8.1e-06)* to G2 *(F=28.11, P=1.45E-13)* in ECOG0 and 4. It is in line with previous studies which showed that increasing age had a decline in SDNN in lung cancer patients (De Couck & Gidron, 2013). Greiser et al. (2009) showed that SDNN decreased with increase in age in women, whereas in men it decreased in the age group of 45 to 74 years but increased for more than 74 years. Literature studies also demonstrated that higher age groups and higher stages of cancer had lowered value of SDNN (De Couck & Gidron, 2013).

Root mean square of successive differences in RR intervals (RMSSD) decreased from G1 *(F=13.56, P=5.12E-07)* to G2 *(F=30.3, P=3.09E-14)* in ECOG0. Average of RR intervals (mRR) decreased from G1 to G2 *(F=3.765, P=0.00814)* in ECOG1, 2 and 4. Average of heart rate (mHR) increased from G1 to G2 *(F=3.108, P=0.021)* in ECOG1, 2 and 4. Although, Mean Heart Rate was suggested to be higher in healthy women in comparison with age-matched healthy men (Moodithaya et al., 2012; Agelink et al., 2001). Morever, higher values of frequency domain parameters that increases with age was also suggested (Piskorski et al., 2010; Galeev et al., 2002). Standard deviation of heart rate (SDHR) increased from G1 *(F=5.1, P=0.00211)* to G2 *(F=15.12, P=8.63E-09)* in ECOG1, 2 and 4. Number of successive NN interval > 50ms (NN50) decreased from G1 *(F=5.213, P=0.00184)* to G2 *(F=5.884, P=0.000419)* in ECOG0 and 3. The percentage of NN50 (pNN50) decreased from G1 *(F=5.737, P=0.000991)* to G2 *(F=4.933, P=0.00155)* in ECOG0, 3 and 4. HRV Triangular Index (TI) decreased from G1 *(F=6.882, P=0.000272)* to G2 *(F=6.453, P=0.000195)* in ECOG1, 2, 3 and 4. Triangular Interpolation of RR intervals (TiNN) decreased from G1 *(F=4.921, P=0.00261)* to G2 *(F=10.21, P=1.78E-06)* in ECOG0.

Standard deviation of poincare plot perpendicular to line of identity (SD_1) decreased from G1 *(F=12.18, P=1.61E-06)* to G2 *(F=29.96, P=3.9E-14)* in ECOG0. Standard deviation of poincare plot along the line of identity (SD_2) decreased from G1 *(F=8.361, P=5.7E-05)* to G2 *(F=24.29, P=2.56E-12)* in 0 and 4. The ratio of SD_1 to SD_2 (SD_1/SD_2) increased from G1 *(F=3.14, P=0.0249)* to G2 *(F=4.818, P=0.00182)* in 1, 2, 3 and 4. Mean line length (L_{mean}) increased from G1 to G2 in ECOG1, 2, 3 and 4. In similar lines, SD_1/SD_2 increases with age in healthy controls but also in BC patients (Acharya et al., 2004). L_{max} decreased from G1 *(F=2.78, P=0.04)* to G2 in ECOG0 and 4. Recurrence Rate (REC) decreased in 0 and 1. Determinism (DET) decreased in ECOG0, 1 and 3. Shannon Entropy (ShanEn) decreased in ECOG0 and 1. Detrended fluctuation analysis long term fluctuation slope (α_2) is more than short term detrended fluctuation slope (α_1) in G2 than G1 in ECOG4. It is also more in ECOG2 and ECOG3 than α_1. α_2 decreased from G1 *((F=5.376, P=0.00151)* to G2 *(F=6.345, P=0.000225)* and α_1 as well in all PS states.

Table 4. Heart Rate Variability (HRV) measures of time domain, frequency domain and non-linear measures in age group of G1: 20 to 40 years and G2: >40 years as per Eastern Cooperative Oncology (ECOG) Performance Status (PS) Scale

HRV Analysis	PS	ECOG0		ECOG1		ECOG2		ECOG3		ECOG4	
	Age Group	G1	G2	G1	G2	G1	G2	G1	G2	G1	G2
Time domain	mRR (ms)	610.20± 72.71	627.91± 18.45	831.36± 93.22	697.73± 55.02	665.67± 27.32	639.49± 31.84	716.09± 32.26	756.15± 28.98	666.38± 32.26	636.22± 22.54
	SDNN (ms)	34.09± 19.54	14.91± 1.48	93.32± 16.04	152.35± 39.2	24.95± 4.97	31.41± 6.97	41.04± 2.84	43.62± 4.59	19.36± 2.84	18.47± 1.29
	mHR (bpm)	103.46± 10.32	96.10± 2.77	75.03± 7.22	90.89± 6.72	91.91± 3.54	96.65± 4.77	85.83± 3.51	82.14± 3.59	91.66± 3.51	97.29± 3.16
	SDHR (bpm)	3.74± 1.41	2.29± 0.27	10.49± 4.56	12.62± 3.35	3.63± 0.72	4.07± 0.78	5.63± 0.73	4.87± 0.49	2.87± 0.73	2.96± 0.29
	RMSSD (ms)	30.63± 22.25	9.29± 1.49	108.72± 17.64	208.89± 50.89	16.76± 3.94	30.22± 9.98	40.06± 5.38	45.64± 7.37	13.91± 5.38	16.88± 2.1
	NN50	1.8± 1.8	0± 0	62.33± 31.49	79.2± 35.31	8.5± 8.06	23.08±16.55	47± 13.64	27.25± 6.82	2.58± 13.64	3.23± 0.79
	pNN50	0.32± 0.32	0± 0	19.37± 11.41	20.19± 10.12	1.84± 1.71	5.85± 4.55	11.54± 3.41	7.51± 2.05	0.55± 3.41	0.69± 0.17
	TI	3.53± 0.45	3.69± 0.38	8.14± 1.53	5.68± 2.07	5.29± 0.72	4.73± 0.61	7.97± 0.69	6.82± 0.57	4.5± 0.69	3.69± 0.28
	TINN (ms)	188± 117.22	70± 6.07	453.33± 31.79	535± 70.19	134.17± 36.48	201.25± 60.11	245± 35.02	303.25± 36.61	122.5± 35.02	159.42± 22.59
Non-Linear	SD1 (ms)	21.68± 15.75	6.58± 1.05	76.98± 12.5	147.88± 36.02	17.81± 3.55	21.39± 7.07	28.36± 3.81	30.89± 5.32	9.85± 3.81	11.95± 1.49
	SD2 (ms)	42.62± 22.96	19.77± 2.24	106.77± 20.56	156.57± 42.58	36.15± 6.42	37.73± 7.47	49.91± 2.88	50.72± 4.73	25.31± 2.88	22.46± 1.62
	SD1/SD2	0.37± 0.07	0.36± 0.08	0.74± 0.11	0.99± 0.07	0.43± 0.06	0.47± 0.08	0.55± 0.06	0.58± 0.05	0.40± 0.06	0.56± 0.06
	Lmean	39.29± 24.18	16.73± 3.33	29.75± 8.88	38.13± 16.89	19.86± 1.79	23.08± 4.18	15.53± 1.67	22.95± 4.19	16.03± 1.67	25.89± 5.29
	Lmax	376.±8 41.87	358.43± 75.79	157± 48.01	188.2± 65.66	311.92± 41.49	323.08± 44.51	206.92± 25.41	230.9± 24.72	302.67± 25.41	299.77± 21.11
	REC (%)	51.70± 11.05	38.83± 5.38	68.51± 7.36	60.81± 13.88	47.14± 3.72	51.20± 4.49	40.17± 3.98	49.27± 5.22	42.35± 3.98	51.17± 3.62
	DET (%)	99.21± 0.27	98.44± 0.65	99.58± 0.16	98.64± 1.11	98.91± 0.36	99.04± 0.22	98.63± 0.38	98.49± 0.34	98.76± 0.38	99.05± 0.17
	ShanEn	3.67± 0.21	3.5± 0.21	3.82± 0.34	3.47± 0.26	3.62± 0.12	3.734± 0.12	3.46± 0.12	3.52± 0.11	3.47± 0.12	3.69± 0.09
	α1	1.19± 0.09	1.11± 0.12	0.75± 0.14	0.64± 0.08	0.98± 0.08	0.95± 0.07	0.93± 0.08	0.87± 0.07	1.09± 0.08	0.92± 0.09
	α2	0.98± 0.08	0.99± 0.05	0.51± 0.08	0.41± 0.16	0.99± 0.05	0.99± 0.08	0.93± 0.05	0.88± 0.04	0.96± 0.05	0.93± 0.05
	ApEn	0.89± 0.22	1.17± 0.04	0.78± 0.21	0.48± 0.16	1.05± 0.05	1.06± 0.05	1.07± 0.05	0.99± 0.06	1.16± 0.05	1.04± 0.05
	SampEn	1.27± 0.36	1.57± 0.15	0.76± 0.23	0.57± 0.36	1.57± 0.13	1.49± 0.16	1.36± 0.12	1.31± 0.12	1.55± 0.12	1.42± 0.11
	CD	0.07± 0.02	0.11± 0.07	1.96± 0.84	0.86± 0.59	0.55± 0.24	0.62± 0.36	1.67 0.37	1.38± 0.34	0.19± 0.37	0.14± 0.03

The findings of the study is similar to previous study which shows that DFA values decrease as age advances (Francesco et al., 2010). Approximate Entropy (ApEn) and Sample Entropy (SampEn) decreased from G1 to G2 *(F=6.86, P=0.000114; F=3.167, P=0.0193)* in ECOG1, 2, 3 and 4. Morever, Kaplan et al. (1991) also stated that as the age advances, ApEn reduces which is similar to current study. Previous study also suggested not only decrease of DFA and ApEn values but also reduction in complexity occurs with increase in age (Porta et al., 2007; Yeragani et al., 1997).

Correlation dimension (CD) decreased from G1 *(F=6.696, P=0.000334)* to G2 *(F=4.663, P=0.00227)* in ECOG1, 3 and 4. All the values are given in mean±standard error form in [Table 4]. There also exists correlation within the ECOG PS States in G1 and G2 respectively, shown in [Figure 4a, Figure 4b and Figure 5]. In the Figure, A represents ECOG0, B represents ECOG1, C represents ECOG2, D represents ECOG3 and E represents ECOG4, respectively. Our study is in line with published work which states that the complexity of the signal reduces with increase in age (Porta et al., 2007). Decrease in non-linear measures with advancing age has been found (Yeragani et al., 1997).

CONCLUSION

Heart rate variability measures decreased in the studied cancer patients as the severity of cancer determined by ECOG PS Scale progressed. The decrease in HRV determined that the status of BC patients was very critical. The age was such

Figure 4a. Posthoc Tukeys' HSD test for nonlinear analysis for age group of >40 years in breast cancer patients

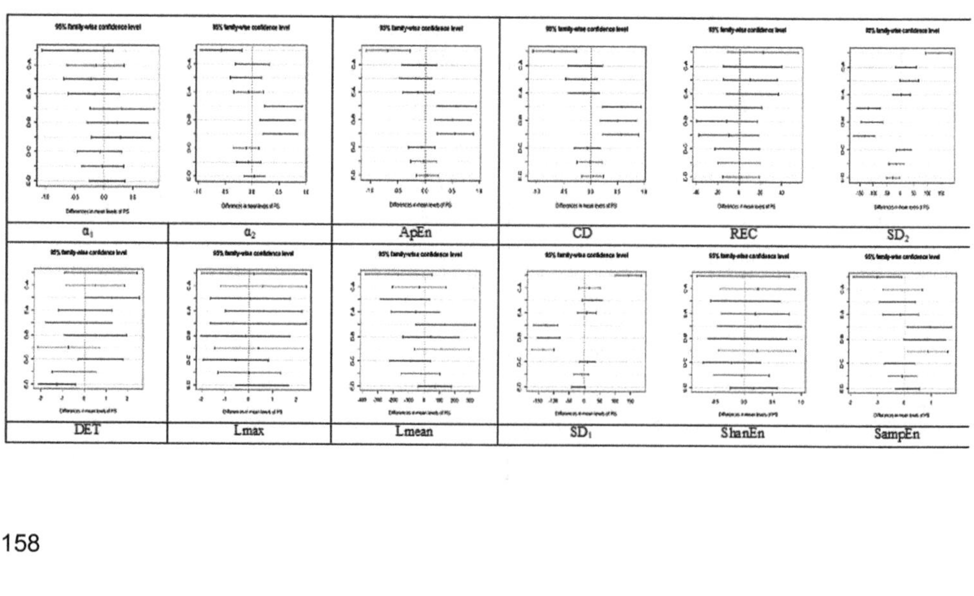

Figure 4b. Posthoc Tukeys' HSD test for time domain analysis for the age group of >40 years in breast cancer patients

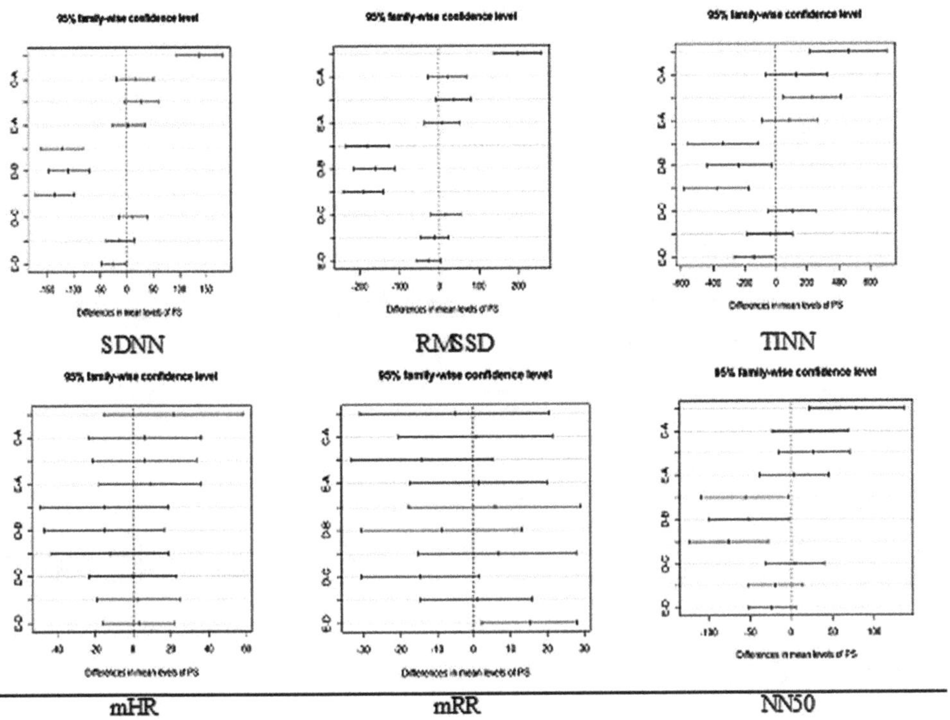

an important factor which was categorized with respect to ECOG PS Scale. It was found that as the age increased in BC patients, the time-domain measures of mRR, mHR, SDHR and TiNN indicated that PS deteriorated from ECOG0 to 4. The chaotic status of the signal decreased which was implied by the non-linear measures of SD_1/SD_2, ApEn, SampEn, α_1, α_2 and CD. The frequency domain measures did not give any significant results. Overall, as the age increased, the critical state of BC patients deteriorated from ECOG0 to ECOG4. This can give a better understanding to the clinicians to improve the quality of treatment to their patients wherein age can be considered as a confounder.

Figure 5. Posthoc Tukeys' test of time domain and non-linear measures for the age group of <40 years in breast cancer patients

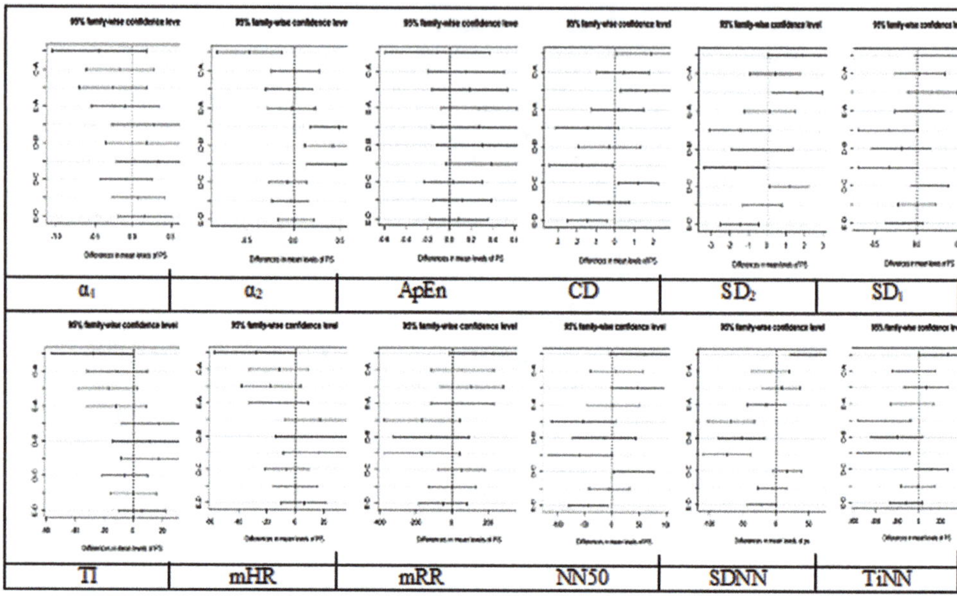

ACKNOWLEDGMENT

Conflict of Interest

This research received no specific grant from any funding agency in the public, commercial, or not-for-profit sectors.

REFERENCES

Abdelnabi, M. H. (2019). Cardiovascular clinical implications of heart rate variability. *International Journal of the Cardiovascular Academy*, *5*(2), 37. doi:10.4103/IJCA.IJCA_36_18

Acharya, R., Kannathal, N., Sing, O. W., Ping, L. Y., & Chua, T. (2004). Heart rate analysis in normal subjects of various age groups. *Biomedical Engineering Online*, *3*(1), 24. doi:10.1186/1475-925X-3-24 PMID:15260880

Acharya, R. U., Lim, C. M., & Joseph, P. (2002). Heart rate variability analysis using correlation dimension and detrended fluctuation analysis. *ITBM-RBM*, *23*(6), 333–339. doi:10.1016/S1297-9562(02)90002-1

Acharya, U. R., Joseph, K. P., Kannathal, N., Lim, C. M., & Suri, J. S. (2006). Heart rate variability: A review. *Medical & Biological Engineering & Computing*, *44*(12), 1031–1051. doi:10.100711517-006-0119-0 PMID:17111118

Agelink, M. W., Malessa, R., Baumann, B., Majewski, T., Akila, F., Zeit, T., & Ziegler, D. (2001). Standardized tests of heart rate variability: Normal ranges obtained from 309 healthy humans, and effects of age, gender, and heart rate. *Clinical Autonomic Research*, *11*(2), 99–108. doi:10.1007/BF02322053 PMID:11570610

Aggarwal, Y., Singh, N., Ghosh, S., & Sinha, R. K. (2014). Eye Gaze–Induced Mental Stress Alters the Heart Rate Variability Analysis. *Journal of Clinical Engineering*, *39*(2), 79–89. doi:10.1097/JCE.0000000000000023

Antoch, G., Stattaus, J., Nemat, A. T., Marnitz, S., Beyer, T., Kuehl, H., ... Freudenberg, L. S. (2003). Non–small cell lung cancer: Dual-modality PET/CT in preoperative staging. *Radiology*, *229*(2), 526–533. doi:10.1148/radiol.2292021598 PMID:14512512

Berry, D. A., Cronin, K. A., Plevritis, S. K., Fryback, D. G., Clarke, L., Zelen, M., & Feuer, E. J. (2005). Effect of screening and adjuvant therapy on mortality from breast cancer. *The New England Journal of Medicine*, *353*(17), 1784–1792. doi:10.1056/NEJMoa050518 PMID:16251534

Bettermann, H., Kröz, M., Girke, M., & Heckmann, C. (2001). Heart rate dynamics and cardiorespiratory coordination in diabetic and breast cancer patients. *Clinical Physiology and Functional Imaging*, *21*(4), 411–420. PMID:11442574

Blagden, S. P., Charman, S. C., Sharples, L. D., Magee, L. R. A., & Gilligan, D. (2003). Performance status score: Do patients and their oncologists agree? *British Journal of Cancer*, *89*(6), 1022–1027. doi:10.1038j.bjc.6601231 PMID:12966419

Bonnemeier, H., Wiegand, U. K., Brandes, A., Kluge, N., Katus, H. A., Richardt, G., & Potratz, J. (2003). Circadian profile of cardiac autonomic nervous modulation in healthy subjects. *Journal of Cardiovascular Electrophysiology*, *14*(8), 791–799. doi:10.1046/j.1540-8167.2003.03078.x PMID:12890036

Boonnithi, S., & Phongsuphap, S. (2011, September). Comparison of heart rate variability measures for mental stress detection. IEEE. *Computers in Cardiology, 2011*, 85–88.

Brennan, M., Palaniswami, M., & Kamen, P. (2001). Do existing measures of Poincare plot geometry reflect nonlinear features of heart rate variability? *IEEE Transactions on Biomedical Engineering*, *48*(11), 1342–1347. doi:10.1109/10.959330 PMID:11686633

ChuDuc, H., Stein, P. K., & PhamManh, H. (2013). Effect of calculation algorithm on heart rate variability by chaos theory. *International Journal of Electronics and Electrical Engineering*, *1*(3), 145–148. doi:10.12720/ijeee.1.3.145-148

Cysarz, D., Bettermann, H., & van Leeuwen, P. (2000). Entropies of short binary sequences in heart period dynamics. *American Journal of Physiology. Heart and Circulatory Physiology*, *278*(6), H2163–H2172. doi:10.1152/ajpheart.2000.278.6.H2163 PMID:10843917

De Couck, M., & Gidron, Y. (2013). Norms of vagal nerve activity, indexed by Heart Rate Variability, in cancer patients. *Cancer Epidemiology*, *37*(5), 737–741. doi:10.1016/j.canep.2013.04.016 PMID:23725879

de la Rochefordière, A., Abner, A. L., Silver, B., Vicini, F., Recht, A., & Harris, J. R. (1992). Are cosmetic results following conservative surgery and radiation therapy for early breast cancer dependent on technique?. *International Journal of Radiation Oncology* Biology* Physics, 23*(5), 925-931.

DeVita, V. T., Lawrence, T. S., & Rosenberg, S. A. (2015). *Cancer of the Skin: Cancer: Principles & Practice of Oncology*. Philadelphia, PA: Lippincott Williams & Wilkins.

Eckmann, J. P., Kamphorst, S. O., & Ruelle, D. (1987). Recurrence plots of dynamical systems. *Europhysics Letters*, *4*(9), 973–977. doi:10.1209/0295-5075/4/9/004

Francesco, B., Maria Grazia, B., Emanuele, G., Valentina, F., Sara, C., Chiara, F., & Francesco, F. (2012). Linear and nonlinear heart rate variability indexes in clinical practice. *Computational and Mathematical Methods in Medicine*. PMID:22400047

Galeev, A. R., Igisheva, L. N., & Kazin, E. M. (2002). Heart rate variability in healthy six-to sixteen-year-old children. *Human Physiology*, *28*(4), 428–432. doi:10.1023/A:1016529931519 PMID:12187882

Giuliano, A. E., Connolly, J. L., Edge, S. B., Mittendorf, E. A., Rugo, H. S., Solin, L. J., & Hortobagyi, G. N. (2017). Breast cancer—major changes in the American Joint Committee on Cancer eighth edition cancer staging manual. CA: A Cancer Journal for Clinicians, 67(4), 290-303.

Greiser, K. H., Kluttig, A., Schumann, B., Swenne, C. A., Kors, J. A., Kuss, O., & Werdan, K. (2009). Cardiovascular diseases, risk factors and short-term heart rate variability in an elderly general population: The CARLA study 2002–2006. *European Journal of Epidemiology*, *24*(3), 123–142. doi:10.100710654-009-9317-z PMID:19199053

Hadjiiski, L., Sahiner, B., Helvie, M. A., Chan, H. P., Roubidoux, M. A., Paramagul, C., ... Foster, M. (2006). Breast masses: Computer-aided diagnosis with serial mammograms. *Radiology*, *240*(2), 343–356. doi:10.1148/radiol.2401042099 PMID:16801362

Hall, J. M., Lee, M. K., Newman, B., Morrow, J. E., Anderson, L. A., Huey, B., & King, M. C. (1990). Linkage of early-onset familial breast cancer to chromosome 17q21. *Science*, *250*(4988), 1684–1689. doi:10.1126cience.2270482 PMID:2270482

Hanahan, D. & Weinberg, R. A. (2000). The hallmarks of cancer. *cell, 100*(1), 57-70.

Henry, B., Lovell, N., & Camacho, F. (2001). Nonlinear dynamics time series analysis. In Nonlinear Biomedical Signal Processing: Dynamic Analysis and Modeling (pp. 1–39). New York, NY: IEEE.

Herry, C. L., Burns, P., Desrochers, A., Fecteau, G., Durosier, L. D., Cao, M. . . . Frasch, M. G. (2019). Decoding vagal contributions to fetal heart rate variability. *arXiv*:1901.06431.

Housa, R., Munib, Q., & Moussa, A. (2005). Breast cancer diagnosis system based on wavelet analysis and fuzzy-neural. *Expert Systems with Applications*, *28*(4), 713–723. doi:10.1016/j.eswa.2004.12.028

Hundsberger, T., Omlin, A., Haegele-Link, S., Vehoff, J., & Strasser, F. (2014). Autonomic dysfunction in cancer cachexia coincides with large fiber polyneuropathy. *Journal of Pain and Symptom Management*, *48*(4), 611–618. doi:10.1016/j.jpainsymman.2013.11.018 PMID:24709363

Kaplan, D. T., Furman, M. I., Pincus, S. M., Ryan, S. M., Lipsitz, L. A., & Goldberger, A. L. (1991). Aging and the complexity of cardiovascular dynamics. *Biophysical Journal*, *59*(4), 945–949. doi:10.1016/S0006-3495(91)82309-8 PMID:2065195

King, T. A., Muhsen, S., Patil, S., Koslow, S., Oskar, S., Park, A., & Morrow, M. (2013). Is there a role for routine screening MRI in women with LCIS? *Breast Cancer Research and Treatment*, *142*(2), 445–453. doi:10.100710549-013-2725-5 PMID:24141896

Lake, D. E., Richman, J. S., Griffin, M. P., & Moorman, J. R. (2002). Sample entropy analysis of neonatal heart rate variability. *American Journal of Physiology. Regulatory, Integrative and Comparative Physiology*, *283*(3), R789–R797. doi:10.1152/ajpregu.00069.2002 PMID:12185014

Massaro, S., & Pecchia, L. (2019). Heart rate variability (HRV) analysis: A methodology for organizational neuroscience. *Organizational Research Methods*, *22*(1), 354–393. doi:10.1177/1094428116681072

Moodithaya, S., & Avadhany, S. T. (2012). Gender differences in age-related changes in cardiac autonomic nervous function. *Journal of Aging Research*. PMID:22187649

National Comprehensive Cancer Network. (2003). Breast cancer Clinical Practice Guidelines in Oncology. *Journal of the National Comprehensive Cancer Network: 1*(2), 148. doi:10.6004/jnccn.2003.0016 PMID:19768876

Ottini, L., Palli, D., Rizzo, S., Federico, M., Bazan, V., & Russo, A. (2010). Male breast cancer. *Critical Reviews in Oncology/Hematology*, *73*(2), 141–155. doi:10.1016/j.critrevonc.2009.04.003 PMID:19427229

Park, H., Oh, S., Noh, Y., Kim, J. Y., & Kim, J. H. (2018). Heart rate variability as a marker of distress and recovery: The effect of brief supportive expressive group therapy with mindfulness in cancer patients. *Integrative Cancer Therapies*, *17*(3), 825–831. doi:10.1177/1534735418756192 PMID:29417836

Piskorski, J., Guzik, P., Krauze, T., & Żurek, S. (2010). Cardiopulmonary resonance at 0.1 Hz demonstrated by averaged Lomb-Scargle periodogram. *Central European Journal of Physics*, *8*(3), 386–392.

Porta, A., Gnecchi-Ruscone, T., Tobaldini, E., Guzzetti, S., Furlan, R., & Montano, N. (2007). Progressive decrease of heart period variability entropy-based complexity during graded head-up tilt. *Journal of Applied Physiology*, *103*(4), 1143–1149. doi:10.1152/japplphysiol.00293.2007 PMID:17569773

Porta, A., Guzzetti, S., Furlan, R., Gnecchi-Ruscone, T., Montano, N., & Malliani, A. (2007). Complexity and nonlinearity in short-term heart period variability: Comparison of methods based on local nonlinear prediction. *IEEE Transactions on Biomedical Engineering*, *54*(1), 94–106. doi:10.1109/TBME.2006.883789 PMID:17260860

Prasad, N., & Houserkova, D. (2007). The role of various modalities in breast imaging. *Biomedical Papers of the Medical Faculty of the Palacky University, Olomouc*, Czech Republic, *1519*(2), 209–218. doi:10.5507/bp.2007.036 PMID:18345253

Richman, J. S., & Moorman, J. R. (2000). Physiological time-series analysis using approximate entropy and sample entropy. *American Journal of Physiology. Heart and Circulatory Physiology*, *278*(6), H2039–H2049. doi:10.1152/ajpheart.2000.278.6.H2039 PMID:10843903

Sheffield, D., Krittayaphong, R., Cascio, W. E., Light, K. C., Golden, R. N., Finkel, J. B., & Sheps, D. S. (1998). Heart rate variability at rest and during mental stress in patients with coronary artery disease: Differences in patients with high and low depression scores. *International Journal of Behavioral Medicine*, *5*(1), 31–47. doi:10.120715327558ijbm0501_3 PMID:16250714

Shukla, R. S., & Aggarwal, Y. (2017a). Heart Rate Variability Time-Domain Analysis in Pulmonary Metastasis to Assess Performance Status. *Indian Journal of Social Research*, *14*(2), 540–545.

Shukla, R. S., & Aggarwal, Y. (2017b). Spectral Analysis to Evaluate the Effect of Treatment on Autonomic Nervous System in Pulmonary Metastasis. *Journal of Cancer Research and Therapeutics*, 13.

Shukla, R. S., & Aggarwal, Y. (2018a). Electrocardiogram in Lung Cancer Patients Envisage as Pseudo-Myocardial Infarction and Ischemic Heart Disease. *Journal of Clinical Engineering*, *43*(1), 48–52. doi:10.1097/JCE.0000000000000252

Shukla, R. S., & Aggarwal, Y. (2018b). Heart Rate Variability in Male Breast Cancer. *Clinical Cancer Investigation*, *7*(3), 125. doi:10.4103/ccij.ccij_12_18

Shukla, R. S., & Aggarwal, Y. (2018c). Nonlinear Heart Rate Variability based Analysis and Prediction of Performance Status in Pulmonary Metastases Patients. *Biomedical Engineering: Applications, Basis and Communications*, *16*(2), 145–155.

Shukla, R. S., & Aggarwal, Y. (2018d). Time-domain heart rate variability-based computer-aided prognosis of lung cancer. *Indian Journal of Cancer*, *55*(1), 61. doi:10.4103/ijc.IJC_395_17 PMID:30147095

Shukla, R. S., & Aggarwal, Y. (2018e). Nonlinear Heart Rate Variability based artificial intelligence in lung cancer prediction. *Journal of Applied Biomedicine*, *16*(2), 145–155. doi:10.1016/j.jab.2017.12.002

Silliman, R. A., Guadagnoli, E., Weitberg, A. B., & Mor, V. (1989). Age as a predictor of diagnostic and initial treatment intensity in newly diagnosed breast cancer patients. *Journal of Gerontology*, *44*(2), M46–M50. doi:10.1093/geronj/44.2.M46 PMID:2921470

Stapelberg, N. J., Neumann, D. L., Shum, B. H. K., McConnell, H., & Hamilton-Craig, I. (2018). The sensitivity of 38 heart rate variability measures to the addition of artifact in human and artificial 24-hr cardiac recordings. *Annals of Noninvasive Electrocardiology*, *23*(1). doi:10.1111/anec.12483 PMID:28670841

Tarvainen, M. P., Niskanen, J. P., Lipponen, J. A., Ranta-Aho, P. O., & Karjalainen, P. A. (2014). Kubios HRV–heart rate variability analysis software. *Computer Methods and Programs in Biomedicine*, *113*(1), 210–220. doi:10.1016/j.cmpb.2013.07.024 PMID:24054542

Trulla, L. L., Giuliani, A., Zbilut, J. P., & Webber, C. L. Jr. (1996). Recurrence quantification analysis of the logistic equation with transients. *Physics Letters. [Part A]*, *223*(4), 255–260. doi:10.1016/S0375-9601(96)00741-4

Vazquez, M., Carter, D., Brambilla, E., Gazdar, A., Noguchi, M., Travis, W. D., ... Henschke, C. I. (2009). Solitary and multiple resected adenocarcinomas after CT screening for lung cancer: Histopathologic features and their prognostic implications. *Lung Cancer (Amsterdam, The Netherlands)*, *64*(2), 148–154. doi:10.1016/j.lungcan.2008.08.009 PMID:18951650

Vidyashree, H. M., Maheshkumar, K., Sundareswaran, L., Sakthivel, G., Partheeban, P. K., & Rajan, R. (2019). Effect of yoga intervention on short-term heart rate variability in children with autism spectrum disorder. *International Journal of Yoga*, *12*(1), 73. doi:10.4103/ijoy.IJOY_66_17 PMID:30692787

von Rosenberg, W., Chanwimalueang, T., Adjei, T., Jaffer, U., Goverdovsky, V., & Mandic, D. P. (2017). Resolving ambiguities in the LF/HF ratio: LF-HF scatter plots for the categorization of mental and physical stress from HRV. *Frontiers in Physiology*, *8*, 360. doi:10.3389/fphys.2017.00360 PMID:28659811

Yeragani, V. K., Sobolewski, E., Kay, J., Jampala, V. C., & Igel, G. (1997). Effect of age on long-term heart rate variability. *Cardiovascular Research*, *35*(1), 35–42. doi:10.1016/S0008-6363(97)00107-7 PMID:9302345

Youlden, D. R., Cramb, S. M., Dunn, N. A., Muller, J. M., Pyke, C. M., & Baade, P. D. (2012). The descriptive epidemiology of female breast cancer: An international comparison of screening, incidence, survival and mortality. *Cancer Epidemiology*, *36*(3), 237–248. doi:10.1016/j.canep.2012.02.007 PMID:22459198

Chapter 9
Introduction to Motor Imagery-Based Brain-Computer Interface:
Time, Frequency, and Phase Analysis-Based Feature Extraction for Two Class MI Classification

Nitesh Singh Malan
Indian Institute of Technology (Banaras Hindu University), India

Shiru Sharma
Indian Institute of Technology (Banaras Hindu University), India

ABSTRACT

In this chapter, motor imagery (MI) based brain-computer interface (BCI) is introduced incorporating the explanation of key components required to design a practical BCI device. Its application to the medical and nonmedical sector is discussed in detail. In the experimental study, a feature extraction method using time, frequency, and phase analysis of Motor imagery EEG is presented. For the classification of MI task, EEG signals are decomposed using a dual-tree complex wavelet transform (DTCWT) and then time, frequency, and phase features are extracted. The validation of the proposed method is conducted using BCI competition IV dataset 2b. A Support vector machine (SVM) classifier is used to perform the classification task. Performance of the proposed method is compared with the standard feature extraction methods. The proposed scheme achieved a larger average classification accuracy of 82.81% which is better than that obtained by other methods.

DOI: 10.4018/978-1-7998-0326-3.ch009

INTRODUCTION

The system aims to develop a communication pathway between the brain, and a computer is popularly referred as brain-computer interface (BCI) system (Chaudhary, Birbaumer, & Ramos-Murguialday, 2016). Such direct interaction of the brain activities with the computer facilitates a human subject to control surrounding electronic devices. In other words, BCI translates the neural responses directly to the computer which signals the external devices to respond in accordance with the subject's intentions. These capabilities of BCI makes it a promising system to be used in many medical applications such as rehabilitation of stroke patients, reinstating motor functions of paralyzed patients, building up communication with locked-in patients, and augmenting cognitive and sensory processing (Bi, Fan, & Liu, 2013). Other than building an interface, researchers find the scope of BCI systems in the diagnosis of brain tumor, sleeping disorders, and brain diseases (Sharanreddy, 2013).

Apart from medical applications, researchers have widened the scope of BCIs to assist healthy users for faster hand-free control of devices (Rao & Scherer, 2010). By using BCI, they can control devices such as a robotic arm, smart home appliances or a wheelchair using their thoughts and cognitive power. However, designing of the BCI for use in the real environment involves challenges like poor information transfer rate (ITR), and long training sessions of the users (Navarro et al., 2011).

From the above discussion, it is notable that BCI research can benefit both abled-body as well as disabled-body users. However, designing an effective real-time BCI device is still a complex exercise. In general, the first step in the BCI system design is to capture electroencephalogram (EEG) patterns that represent the neural responses of a human subject while performing a specific mental task. The second step includes pattern recognition algorithms and machine learning approaches that work to define human's intentions. In the third step, researchers generate controlling commands to operate various devices. The commonly used EEG patterns are steady-state visual evoked potential (SSVEP) (Norcia, Appelbaum, Ales, Cottereau, & Rossion, 2015), sensorimotor rhythms (SMR) (Yuan & He, 2014), motor imagery (MI) (Gert Pfurtscheller & Neuper, 2001), and event-related potentials (ERP) (Sur & Sinha, 2009). These patterns are originated from the different areas of the brain depending on the type of stimulus being provided to the subject. This chapter mainly focuses on MI-based BCI.

In the MI-based BCI, the EEG signals of a subject are recorded while performing a motor movement mental task (Kawasaki, 2017). In the mental task, the subject has to think about the movement of either right hand or left hand. The recorded data are then analyzed using pattern recognition techniques (Grosse-Wentrup, Liefhold, Gramann, & Buss, 2009). In MI BCI signal analysis, Feature extraction plays a vital role as it provides the main information contained in the raw EEG signal (Gert

Pfurtscheller & Neuper, 2001). Common spatial pattern (Ramoser, Muller-Gerking, & Pfurtscheller, 2000) is an effective approach to differentiate between two classes of motor imagery EEG. However, spatial filtering using CSP is highly frequency band dependent. CSP gives poor classification results if the EEG is unfiltered or filtered in an unsuitable band of frequency (Novi, Guan, Dat, & Xue, 2007). Since MI EEG shows siginificant ERD/ERS patterns in 8-30 Hz frequency range (Gert Pfurtscheller & Neuper, 2001), a wider bandpass filtering is applied between 8 and 30 Hz before applying CSP on the EEG. As the EEG is subject specific, wider bandpass filter generally degrades the classification efficiency. (Ang, Chin, Zhang, & Guan, 2008) proposed a filter bank common spatial pattern (FBCSP) where EEG is decomposed into multiple bands of frequencies before applying the conventional CSP and mutual information is betwwen the sub bands is extracted to select the useful features for classification. However, overlapping of multiple frequency bands harms the raw EEG signal and thus, degrades the classification performance. For the analysis of complex time series signals like EEG, a few studies (Hsu, 2013; Xu & Song, 2008)] proposed the use of wavelet transform. In the work of (Xu & Song, 2008), feature extraction using wavelet transform has been proposed. It should be noted that wavelet transform faces the problem of aliasing and gives energy losses at transition bands (Peng, Jackson, Rongong, Chu, & Parkin, 2009). Dual-tree complex wavelet transform (DTCWT) overcomes these disadvantages of the wavelet transform. Also, DTCWT incorporates advantages like nearly shift invariant and perfect reconstruction of the signal (Chaudhury & Unser, 2010). However, a few studies (Bashar, Hassan, & Bhuiyan, 2015; Ming, Shaona, Haitao, Yuliang, & Yunyuan, 2015), have used DTCWT for decomposition of EEG time series signal to extract features for two class motor imagery classification and have reported that an improved classification performance was achieved, they have evaluated features either in time or frequency domain. In the work of (Song & Gordon, n.d.), use of instantaneous phase relationship between two channels of EEG has been proposed to discriminate between motor imagery tasks. Whereas, in most of the studies (Kim, Sun, Liu, Wang, & Paek, 2018; Gert Pfurtscheller & Da Silva, 1999), power spectral density of the mu and beta rhythms are widely investigated for feature extraction of MI EEG. Therefore, in this chapter authors have used a combination of different time, frequency and phase features to evaluate the classification performance of MI BCI. Further, EEG signals from sensory-motor cortex area, i.e., channel locations C3, Cz, and C4 are decomposed using DTCWT and features are extracted in time, frequency and phase domains. Then, the classification task is performed using a support vector machine (SVM) classifier to discriminate between two classes of motor imagery.

Following sections in this chapter introduce the motor imagery based BCI system and various aspects involved in the designing of a real-time performing BCI system.

The general block diagram and components of MI BCI system are briefly explained. A brief survey is presented of the state-of-art methods used and challenges involved in the development of a BCI system from the training of users to finally generated commands. Finally, authors have proposed a method for feature extraction and applied it on the public MI data. Results are compared with the standard signal processing methods widely used for the MI task feature extraction.

BACKGROUND: MOTOR IMAGERY BASED BCI

The imagination of movements of different body parts is known as motor imagery (Kamousi & and, 2005). The human brain originates rhythmic neural waves over different areas of the cortex while performing certain mental tasks (Penn & Shatz, 1999). Mu rhythms are one of such rhythms associated with the voluntary movement related mental tasks [ref]. These waves are mainly generated over sensorimotor cortex and have a frequency range between 8 and 12 Hz. The homunculus representation explains that each body part movement is controlled by the contralateral section in the motor cortex. For instance, if the subject is thinking about the movement of left-hand, significant changes in the mu rhythms are observed in the right hemisphere of the motor cortex and vice versa. Therefore, EEG acquired from contralateral section contains information about the movement of that body part. The mu rhythms are explained in (Gert Pfurtscheller & Da Silva, 1999) where the researcher explains the patterns of mu rhythm in accordance with the movement performed. The power of the mu rhythm gets attenuated when the person imagines or perform the motor movement. This attenuation in the mu rhythm is known as event-related desynchronization. Another important rhythmic pattern observed is beta rhythm. Unlike mu rhythms, the average power of the beta rhythms tends to increase when the motor imagery task ceases. The associated improvement in beta rhythms is known as event-related synchronization (ERS) (see Figure 1). With a sufficient amount of training, a user can control the ERD/ERS patterns of mu and beta rhythms. The learned ability to control ERD/ERS patterns is utilized by the BCI system to control external devices.

The observed variations in the EEG induced the idea of controlling the external devices employing a software module. In practice, signal conditioning of the EEG patterns during the motor imagery task can generate the controlling commands for the devices to take action following the user intention. This is the general idea of an MI- BCI system.

Figure 1. ERD/ERS pattern over the channel location C3 during right-hand motor imagery in the mu band

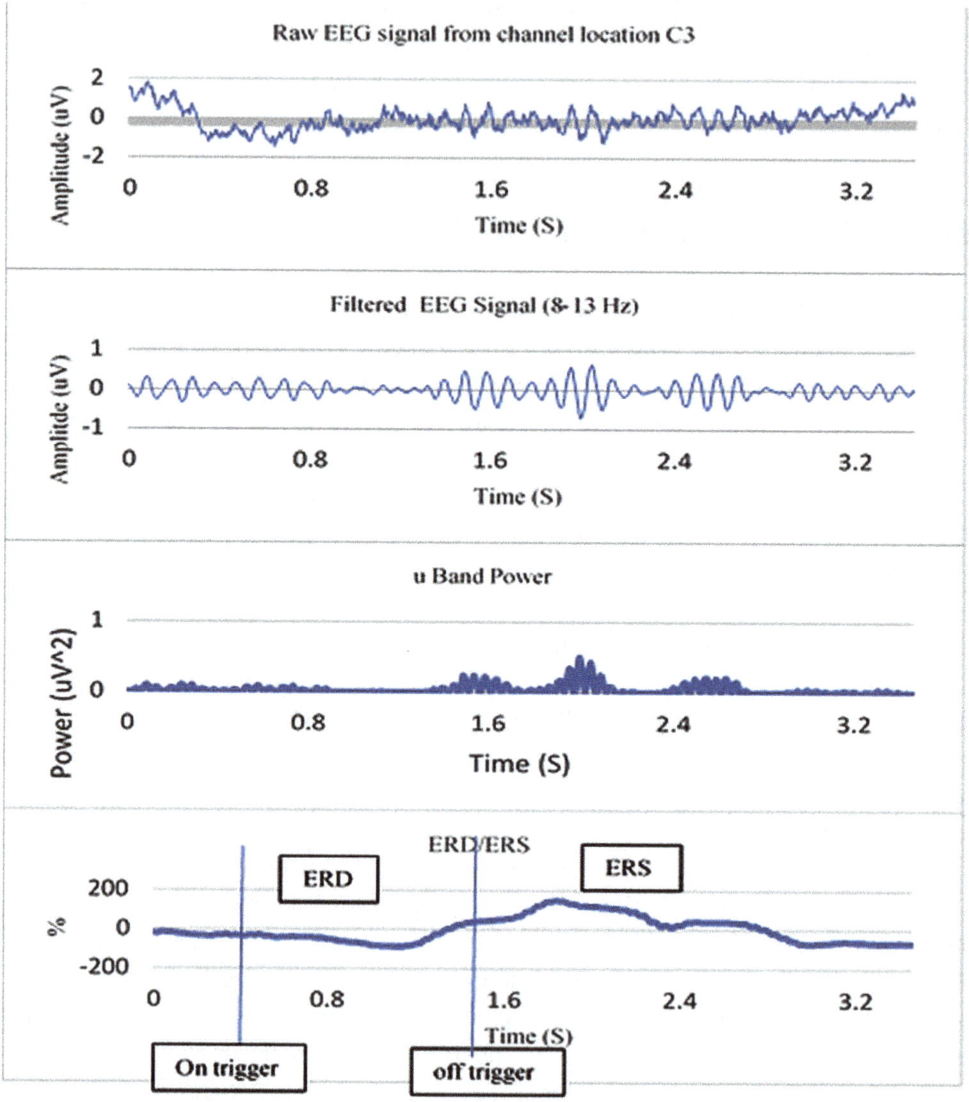

APPLICATIONS OF MOTOR IMAGERY BASED BCI

Research on MI BCI has spread its contribution in different fields including both medical and non-medical sectors. Figure 2 shows the general categorization of MI BCI applications. In the medical field, MI BCI research has investigated the use of brain signals of patients suffering from stroke to regain their motor functionality

Figure 2. Applications of motor imagery-based brain-computer interface systems

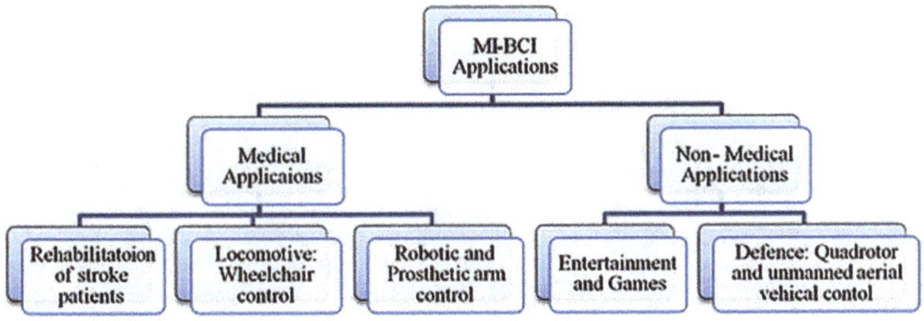

(Cantillo-Negrete, Carino-Escobar, Carrillo-Mora, Elias-Vinas, & Gutierrez-Martinez, 2018). Numerous studies have suggested that paralyzed patients or people with neuromuscular disorders can learn to control their brain waves associated with imagination of motor functionality and thus can instruct a locomotive device, a robotic arm, or a prosthetic arm to perform in accordance with their intentions (Abiyev, Akkaya, Aytac, Günsel, & Çağman, 2016; Mishchenko, Kaya, Ozbay, & Yanar, 2017). Non-medical applications of MI BCI includes controlling of unmanned aerial vehicles, various 2D and 3D games. In the work of (LaFleur et al., 2013), researchers have experimented on healthy users to control a quadrotor in three-dimensional space. Games and entertainment is another area explored by MI BCI researchers where they control the actions happening in the virtual world by the motor imagery EEG signals of users (Li, Zhang, Xue, & Wang, 2017). Apart from existing real-time performing systems, MI BCI research is still progressing. In (Yu et al., 2016) researchers have proposed a vehicle controlling scheme and hypothesize that the proposed system shows the potential of driving a car in real time. However, the implementation of such systems in the real world is yet to be explored further.

GENERAL BLOCK DIAGRAM OF A MOTOR IMAGERY BASED BCI DEVICE

The block diagram of an MI BCI system is shown in Figure 3. The major modules include stimulus generation to provide instructions to the user, signal acquisition device, signal processing unit, and feedback from the external devices. As it can be seen from the Figure 3 that the MI BCI is a closed loop system. Feedback is provided to the user in auditory or visual form. The user directly interacts with the device by looking at the function it is performing. If it is not performing the desired task which is associated with the thinking of the corresponding limb movement, then the user tries to control it again by focusing more on the motor imagery task.

Figure 3. Block diagram representing the components of the motor imagery-based brain-computer interface system

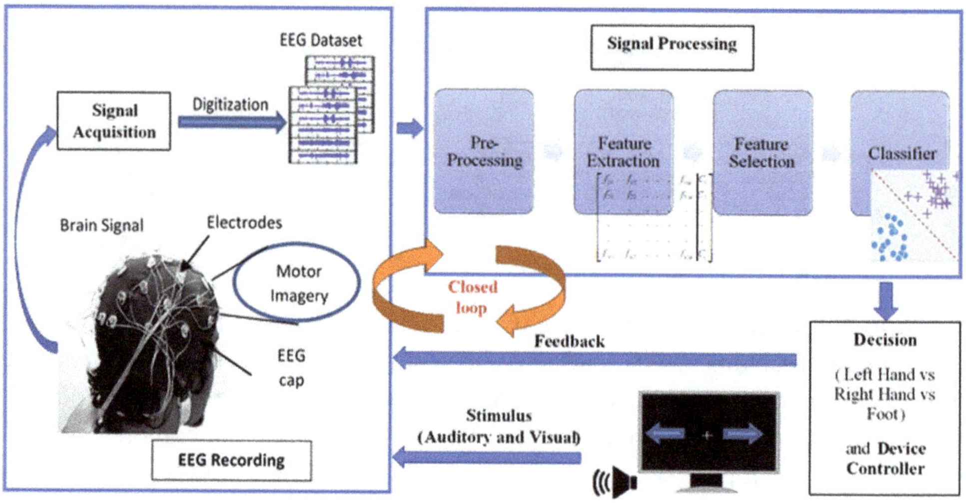

In this way, the user learns to control the device. Following sections give detail explanation about each module.

Motor Imagery Task

In BCI research, the most commonly used BCI datasets are provided by a series of BCI competitions such as BCI competition I, BCI competition II, BCI competition III, and BCI competition IV. Many of these datasets were recorded for motor imagery tasks (B. Blankertz et al., 2004; Tangermann et al., 2012). They have provided general guidelines to perform motor imagery. In general, during motor imagery, a user is instructed to think about the closing and opening of his fist of either left hand or right hand at a time. The decision of which hand movement the user has to make is made by the screen. The user sits relaxed on a comfortable armchair and looks at a monitor for instructions. Usually, auditory and visual instructions are given to the user. First, a black screen appears followed by a beep sound is made indicating the start of motor imagery. After one or two seconds, an arrow pointing either to the right or left is shown on the screen for about 4- 6 seconds. During this period the subject has to think about the movement of his right or left hand according to direction of the arrow, i.e., if the arrow indicated towards right then, the user thinks about the movement of his right hand and vice versa.

EEG Recording

The neural oscillations or brain waves are continuous time-varying patterns originate due to the mental activities in the central nervous system (CNS). During a mental activity, a neuron interacts with another neuron in the brain, and this induces an electrical current. The naturally induced brain current produces electric and magnetic fields which can be recorded using different modalities. The commonly used modalities to map brain activities are magnetoencephalography (MEG) (Mellinger et al., 2007), Electroencephalography (EEG) (G. Pfurtscheller, Flotzinger, Pregenzer, Wolpaw, & McFarland, 1995), positron emission tomography (PET) (Zhu et al., 2016), Electrocorticography (ECoG) (Schalk & Leuthardt, 2011), and Functional Near-Infrared Spectroscopy (fNIRS) (Naseer & Hong, 2015). A comparison of these acquisition devices is drawn in Table 1.

For BCI applications, EEG is widely used due to its characteristics like high temporal resolution, non-invasive acquisition, and portability. In EEG acquisition, biopotential signals are captured by the electrodes placed over the scalp according to the standard International 10- 20 system as shown in Figure 4. The silver/ silver-chloride or gold cup electrodes are generally used as they provide good conductivity. An electrolytic get is used to further enhance the conductivity and decrease the skin-electrode contact impedance.

- **Labeling of Electrodes in EEG:** The Brain is divided into six main lobes: pre-frontal, frontal, parietal, temporal, central, and occipital. According to 10-20 system electrodes are placed at a distance of either 10% or 20% of the total nasion-inion or right ear–left ear distance of the skull. As shown in the Figure 4, each electrode has a label in the form of a letter followed by a numeric value for example 'c3'. The letter is the electrode's identity given by the area of the brain where it is placed. For example, the letter 'O' stands for occipital lobe, 'F' represents frontal and so on. There is also 'Z' which represents the midline sagittal plane of the skull (Fz, Cz, Pz). The numbers after the letters electrode placement on the right or left side of the head. Even numbers are assigned to the right section of the head whereas odd numbers are used to represent electrodes at the left side of the head.
- **Acquisition device:** The amplitude of the EEG signal is in the range of 1-100 uV and needs to be amplified. The biopotential signal acquired over the skull is received by a bio-amplifier device. The first stage in the device is a patient protection circuitry to avoid passing of any hazardous current to the skull. In the second stage, an instrumentation amplifier is used for impedance matching. In the third stage, bandpass filters are implemented with the passband frequency range of 0-100 Hz. A 50 Hz notch filter is also designed

Figure 4. International 10-20 system

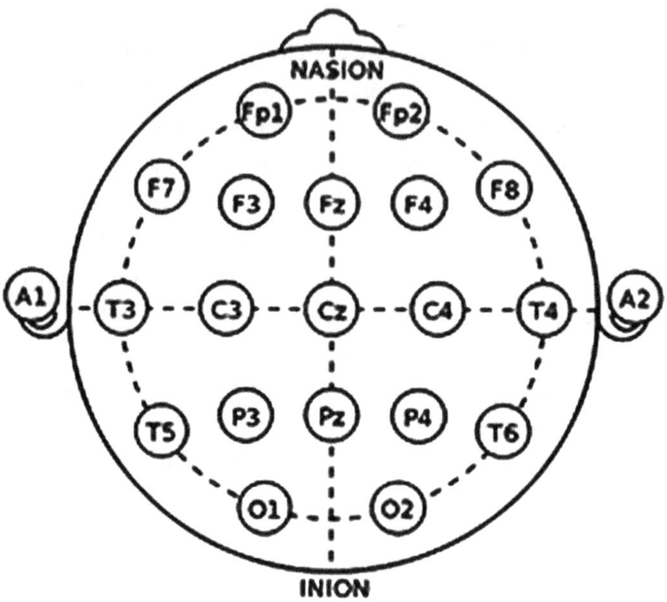

to avoid power line noise. In the last stage, the main amplifiers are connected with adjustable gain. The output signal of the amplifier module is then fed to an analog to digital converter (ADC) for the digitization of the signal. Thus, the output signal is a time-series signal representing brain activities.

Signal Processing

EEG time series is a non- stationary, and random signal, thus its study requires various mathematical and signal analysis tools. It is also highly prone to noises and body artifacts. The types of noises mostly found in acquired EEG are power line 50 Hz noise, environment electromagnetic waves, and thermal noise of the electronic components present in the EEG acquisition device. Most of the noises are rejected by the hardware module of the EEG recorder. Moreover, digital filters are employed at the software level to eliminate the remaining noises. On the other hand, body artifacts are the muscle signals that contaminate the raw EEG data. Some of these body artifacts originate due to the motion of various body parts and can be avoided by instructing the subject not to make any motions while recording EEG. However, artifacts from non-voluntary motions cannot be avoided such as cardiac signal. Blinking and movement of eyes popularly referred as ocular artifacts highly

Table 1. Comparison of Different modalities used for the recoding of the Brain activities

	Year	Portability	Temporal Resolution	Spatial Resolution	Invasive/ Non-Invasive
EEG	1924	Yes	High	Low	Non-invasive
MEG	1968	No	High	Low	Non-invasive
PET	1977	No	Low	High	Non-invasive
fNIRS	1985	Yes	Low	High	Non-invasive
ECoG	early 1950s	No	High	Very high	invasive

affect EEG and subject cannot completely avoid eyeball movements during the acquisition of EEG. For these artifacts signal processing of the contaminated EEG is done. Another need for signal processing is to extract only the useful information from EEG and eliminate redundant data points. In general, there are three types of analysis required to get useful information from the EEG signal namely temporal, spectral and spatial analysis. The temporal resolution of EEG is high and provides good features. However, the frequency and the spatial resolution of EEG are poor. Since EEG signal carries vital information in both frequency and time domain, there is a requirement of signal analysis tools that can extract time and frequency information at the same time. The Fast Fourier Transform (FFT), Short-Time Fourier Transform (STFT), and Wavelet transform have been introduced in most of the studies to analyze EEG (Al-Fahoum & Al-Fraihat, 2014; Easwaramoorthy & Uthayakumar, 2010; Zabidi, Mansor, Lee, & Fadzal, 2012). The FFT represents the spectral component present in the frequency domain but does not provide any time domain information about the signal. On the other hand, STFT overcomes the problem of FFT and provides information from in both time and frequency domain. But the shortcoming of STFT is that it does not provide multi-resolution information of the signal. Wavelet transform shows high multi-resolution properties and is considered as one of the most powerful tools for time-frequency analysis of complex signals like EEG.

Pre-Processing

The brain activities generate EEG in the frequency range of 0.5-30 Hz. As explained earlier noises are the unwanted signals added with the raw brain activities during EEG acquisition and need to be eliminated at the pre-processing stage. Digital band-pass filter designed with a passband frequency between 0.5 and 30 Hz, suppresses the dc values and noises with higher frequency components. Also, a 50 Hz notch filter removes the power line noise. However, the body movement artifacts have the frequency ranges that coincides with that of EEG. For instance, ECG and EMG frequency range is 0-100 Hz, and ocular artifacts frequency range lies between 0 and 10 Hz. Thus, motion artifacts cannot be removed by directly applying the bandpass filtering on the contaminated EEG. To serve this purpose, Independent component analysis (ICA) (Hobson & Hillebrand, 2006), Singular spectrum analysis (Maddirala & Shaik, 2016), wavelet transformation with thresholding (Kumar, Arumuganathan, Sivakumar, & Vimal, n.d.) applied on the decomposed coefficients have been proposed. The authors of this chapter have previously proposed a method in (N. S. Malan & Sharma, 2018), where they decomposed the EEG signal using dual-tree complex wavelet transform (DTCWT) and then applied a quantum adapted threshold on the coefficients of kth scale, i.e., the scale which has a frequency range 0-10 Hz as the strength of ocular artifacts is strong in this range of frequency. Finally, regenerate the artifact-free EEG signal using inverse-DTCWT. The following paragraph explains the details of DTCWT and its application to decompose EEG signal.

Decomposition of EEG Using Dual Tree Complex Wavelet Transform (DTCWT)

DTCWT is an advanced form of discrete wavelet transform (DWT). DTCWT working is based on two-real DWTs arranged in parallel to compute the real and imaginary part of the transform. Figure 5 shows the structure of analysis and synthesis filter banks used by the DTCWT to decompose and reconstruct a given time series. DTCWT is defined as

$$\gamma(t) = \gamma_i(t) + \gamma_j(t) \tag{1}$$

Where $\gamma_i(t)$, and $\gamma_j(t)$ represents the two distinct and real DWTs which are a Hilbert pair.

Feature Extraction

A feature is a quantity that uniquely defines the signals of different classes. The set of different features forms a feature vector. In pattern recognition methods, feature extraction is a technique to identify and highlight the most significant information carried by the signal. In the case of MI EEG feature extraction, selection of appropriate frequency band is a very crucial step as most of the information lies in a particular band of frequency. In (Gert Pfurtscheller & Da Silva, 1999), it has been shown that the motor-related mental tasks generate event-related desynchronization (ERD) and

Figure 5. DTCWT filter banks (a) Analysis (b) Synthesis

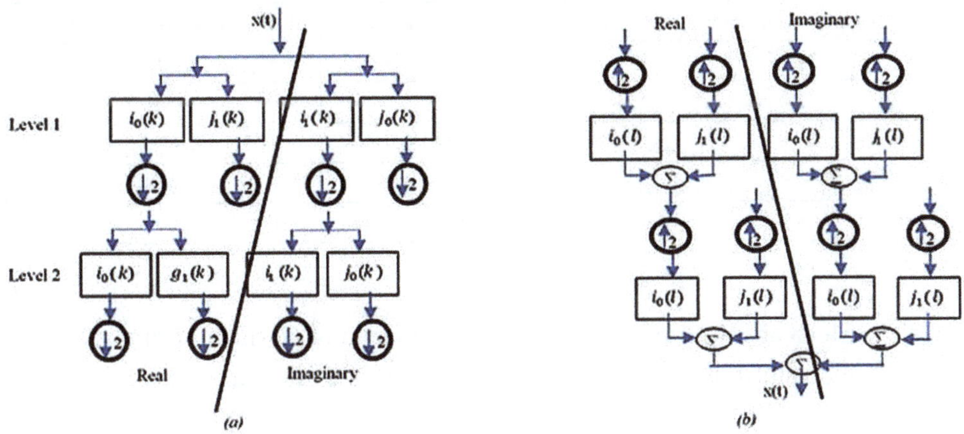

event-related synchronization (ERS) patterns in two frequency bands such as mu (8-13 Hz) and beta (13-30 Hz). It was reported that when the subject thinks about the movement of his limbs, average power in the mu rhythms attenuates and that in the beta rhythms increases. Therefore, for the classification of MI tasks, EEG signal must be bandpass filtered in mu and beta rhythms frequency ranges. Some of the bandpass filters used by researchers are elliptical filter, Butterworth, Chebyshev, and FIR filter (Ang, Chin, Wang, Guan, & Zhang, 2012; Thomas, Guan, Tong, & Prasad, 2008). A few have reported the use of wavelet transform (R. Yang, Song, & Xu, 2010) and wavelet packet decomposition (Hu, Li, & Chen, 2011). The authors of this chapter present a feature extraction method using DTCWT. Firstly, the raw EEG signal is decomposed into different frequency sub-bands as listed in Table 2 using DTCWT to extract the useful features. Secondly, the coefficients of details D3 and D4 are selected for the reconstruction of the EEG time series because these subbands have frequency range same as that of mu and beta rhythms. This will bandpass the original EEG signal into the frequency of interest. Once the EEG signal is filtered, various time, frequency, and phase features are calculated. Some of the features most generally used in MI BCI are explained below.

- **Time Features:** Statistical analysis of EEG in time domain provides the main information exists in the signal that can improve the discrimination scope between the different motor movements related metal tasks (Imran, Talukdar, Sakib, Pathan, & Fattah, 2014). Some of the statistical features are explained below.

Table 2. Frequency Band of each Detail and approximation of DTCWT

Decomposition Level	DTCWT Coefficients	Frequency Band (in Hz)
1	A5	64-128
2	D4	32-64
3	D3	16-32
4	D2	8-16
5	D1	0-8

- Mean absolute value (MAV): It is the mean of all the absolute values of the values in a time series data, $x(n)$. It is defined as

$$MAV = \frac{1}{N}\sum_{i=1}^{N} x(n) \tag{2}$$

Where N is the total number of values in the time series.

- Standard deviation: It calculates the spread of the data about the mean value of the time series. It is defined as

$$S.D. = \sqrt{\frac{\sum_{i=1}^{N}\left[x(n) - \overline{x(n)}\right]^2}{N}} \tag{3}$$

- Variance: It can be defined as the square of the standard deviation. The formula for variance is given by

$$\sigma = \frac{\sum_{i=1}^{N}\left[x(n) - \overline{x(n)}\right]^2}{N} \tag{4}$$

- Sample entropy: It is used to measure the complexity of a given time series using a statistical approach. In this work, authors have used the methodology proposed by [{Citation}] for the calculation of sample entropy.

 - **Frequency Domain Features:** The frequency analysis of EEG provides a lot of information about the signal. Power spectral density is commonly used to extract features from EEG in the frequency domain.
- **Power Spectral Density (PSD):** ERD/ERS is the relative power of the EEG from the channel locations C3 and C4 which provide discriminatory information for two class motor imagery (Gert Pfurtscheller & Da Silva, 1999). To evaluate EEG signal power in the frequency domain, Fourier transform is used. In our work, EEG characteristics are evaluated using the power spectral density (PSD) (Kim et al., 2018) which gives the distribution of signal power over frequency. The PSD of each subband is evaluated for all three channels.
 - **Phase Features:** In order to extract phase features, the phase relation between the EEGs associated with the different task is studied. One such method is phase locking value as defined below.
- **Phase Locking Value:** Phase locking value (PLV) evaluates the phase synchronization between the two signals using the Hilbert transform (Song, Gordon, & Gysels, 2006). The PLV range is [0-1] with value 0 indicating no synchrony between the signals whereas 1 indicates the relative phase between the signals is identical. For feature extraction, the PLV of EEG from channel location C3 and C4 can be evaluated considering Cz as a reference channel.

Feature Selection

Classification of a higher order dimensional feature vector faces the serious problem known as the curse of dimensionality (Lotte, Congedo, Lécuyer, Lamarche, & Arnaldi, 2007). Higher dimensionality of the features makes classification problem a complex exercise and thus causes the classifier to take longer to find true classes. This can be solved by selecting a subset of features from the whole group of features in the feature vector. The selected subset should have the most discrimination properties between the classes to solve the classification problem. Feature selection methods convert the higher m-dimensional feature vector to a lower p-dimensional feature vector by rejecting the irreverent features. The irrelevancy of the feature is measured based on a feature weight numeric value evaluated by the feature selection algorithm. Firstly, the weight of each feature is calculated by the feature selection algorithm. Then, a threshold is chosen and all the weights are compared with it. Features with weights higher than the threshold are selected for classification and rest are rejected. Another advantage of the feature selection procedure is that it reduces the amount of data used for learning the classifier. As a result, the processing time consumed by the classifier reduces. The performance of feature selection method is evaluated

Table 3. Literature review: List of the various state of the art method used by the researchers for the classification of MI data

Name and Year	Subjects/ Public Dataset	Electrodes	Feature Extraction	Feature Selection	Classifier	Results and Remark
(Cantillo-Negrete, Carino-Escobar, Carrillo-Mora, Elias-Vinas, & Gutierrez-Martinez, 2018)	Eight healthy subjects (mean age = 23 years) and 6 stroke patients (Mean age = 55.8 years)	C3, C4, Cz, T3, T4, F3, F4, Fz, P3, P4, and Pz	CSP	PSO	LDA	Stroke patients' average performance was 74.1 ± 11%. And that of healthy users was 76.2 ± 7.6% and 70 ± 6.7,
(Ortega, Asensio-Cubero, Gan, & Ortiz, 2016)	University of Essex BCI data files	15 electrodes placed over sensorimotor cortex area	Multiresolution analysis	Multiobjective optimization in supervised feature selection	linear multiclass SVC or a LDA	Significant reduction in the number of Features is achieved.
(A. Liu et al., 2017)	2008 BCI competition data set 2a	Twenty-two Ag/ AgCl electrodes	Common Spatial Pattern- Local Characteristic-Scale Decomposition (CSP-LCD)	The Firefly Algorithm	Spectral Regression Discriminant Analysis (SRDA)	a real-time brain-computer interface system was designed
	Four subjects, two males and two females, right-handed, aged between 22 and 25	16-channels (Fp1, Fp2, F3, F4, C3, C4, P3, P4, O1, O2, F7, F8, T3, T4, T5, T6)				
(Marchesotti, Bassolino, Serino, Bleuler, & Blanke, 2016)	Twenty-four right-handed subjects (seven females and seventeen males, age between 21–34)	64-channel EEG system (g.tec medical engineering GmbH, Graz, Austria)	CSP		logistic regression	
(Zhang et al., 2018)	BCI Competition III Dataset IIIa, BCI Competition IV Dataset IIb, and BCI Competition IV Dataset IIa	60 channels, 22 channels and three electrodes (C3, Cz, and C4) respectively	Sparse Filter bank CSP (SFBCSP)	multitask learning-based feature multitask learning-based feature	SVM with linear kernel	Averaged accuracies obtained are 88.5%, 83.3%, and 84.3% for the three different MI datasets
(Batula, Kim, & Ayaz, 2017)	Thirteen right-handed subjects (age between18–35),	fNIRS was used to record brain signals, 24 optodes were placed over sensorimotor cortex	correlation-based signal improvement (CBSI), common average referencing (CAR),	recursive feature elimination	LDA	enhancement in accuracy was obtained between the virtual-robot-based BCI and the physical-robot BCI
(Nitesh Singh Malan & Sharma, 2019)	BCI Competition II Dataset III and BCI Competition IV Dataset 2b	C3, CZ, and C4	DTCWT decomposition and Statistical, frquency and phase features	Regularized Neighbourhood component analysis	SVM	average accuracy and kappa coefficient achieved are 80.7% and 0.615. Reduction in feature space is achieved.

using a classifier. If the subset of features chosen by the feature selection method improves the generalization performance of the classifier then only the feature selection is said to be performed adequately. So far, numerous features selection methods have been used in MI- BCI (Ramos, Hernández, & Vellasco, 2016). Based on framework, feature selection methods are categorized into three groups namely the wrapper approach, the filter approach, and the embedded approach. The following paragraph defines the three approaches in detail.

- Wrapper methods use a fitness evaluation model to select feature subsets by assigning a score. The subset with the best score is chosen for the classification task. The score of each subset is evaluated using a learning classifier. Each subset trains the classifier and tested using a hold-out test set. The generalization error of the outcome provides the score for that subset. Due to the separate learning of all the subsets, wrapper methods are time-consuming and computationally expensive, but generally selects the best subset of features and enhance the classification performance for particular classification problem.
- On the contrary, filter methods calculate the best subset of features without using any classification algorithms. There are two stages involved in filter algorithm. In the first stage, features are assigned a rank based on certain performance measuring method. In the second stage, the higher performing features i.e. feature with the ranks above a manually chosen threshold rank are selected for classification. In the recent studies, a numerous performance measuring methods have been proposed such as Fisher score (Gu, Li, & Han, 2012), the mutual information between the features (Ang et al., 2008) and ReliefF and it's advance versions (Kononenko, 1994).
- Filter models are computationally more efficient than the wrapper methods since they evaluate the subset without utilizing the classifier and cross-validation approaches. However, the performance of filter methods is low for some of the applications due to avoidance of the biases of the classifier. For instance, the outcome of ReliefF algorithm would not provide relevant subset of features for Naive-Bayes because it is observed that in most of the problems the generalization performance of Naive-Bayes classifier enhances with the elimination of relevant features (Guyon & Elisseeff, 2003). On the other hand, wrapper model quantifies the features using a predefined classifier and avoids the representational biases of the classifier but takes a longer execution time due to the involvement of cross-validation in its structure that makes it a computationally expensive algorithm. Embedded Models incorporate the advantages of (1) wrapper models - they include the interaction with the classification model and (2) filter models - they are far less computationally intensive than wrapper methods. Examples of embedded methods include Lasso Regularization (Tibshirani, 2017), neighborhood component analysis

(W. Yang, Wang, & Zuo, 2012), recursive feature elimination using support vector machine (SVM) (Lal et al., 2004), ID3 (J. R. Quinlan, 1986), and C4.5 (J. Ross Quinlan, 1993).

Classification

In the last stage of MI BCI system, a decision is made by a classifier to distinguish between the different motor imagery classes correctly. A classifier is an algorithm which learns from the previous data to predict the true class of future data. There are two types of classification methods namely, supervised learning and unsupervised learning. In supervised learning, the previous data also called training data is labeled by its true class. In other words, each training sample is assigned a class label and then used to learn the classifier. When the new data comes, based on previous learning classifier makes a decision. Whereas, in unsupervised learning the training data is unlabeled. In motor imagery classification, supervised learning is most commonly used as the training data is labeled. Numerous studies have experimented the classification of MI data using different classifiers (Fu, Tian, Bao, Meng, & Shi, 2019), but the most commonly used classifier is support vector machine (SVM).

- **Support Vector Machine:** The principal of support vector machine (SVM) is based on statistical learning theory. The framework of SVM is very simple yet effective to solve the problem of classification associated with a small sample size of the dataset, non-linear relationship and multiclass classification (Shawe-Taylor & Sun, 2011). The working of SVM is based on the building of an optimal hyperplane as the decision-making surface to discriminate between the different classes. The SVM model is a representation of the data values as points in space, mapped so that the data values of the different classes are distributed by a clear margin that is globally maximum.

For solving a two class problem using SVM like in MI BCI, the kernel function is implemented in place of the inner product computation, and the dimensions of nonlinear problems are increased to convert them into a linear classification problem. A support vector machine (SVM) classifier with a linear kernel is used to solve the classification problem of two classes. Now, a method to solve a two-class classification problem is explained as follows. Let the sample set is expressed as $\left(x_i, y_i\right), i = 1,2,\ldots,l, x \in \mathbb{R}^N$, where $\in \left\{-1,+1\right\}$ is the class of the data. The discriminant function is expressed as

$$y_i\left[\left(w.x_i\right)+b\right]-1\geq 0, i=1,2,\ldots,l \tag{5}$$

This function can be projected into a dual problem using the Lagrange multiplier. The objective function which is to be optimized is expressed as

$$\min Q\left(a\right)=\frac{1}{2}\sum_{i,j=1}^{l}a_i a_j y_i y_j.K\left(x_i,x_j\right)-\sum_{i=1}^{l}a_j \tag{6}$$

Where $\sum_{i=1}^{l}a_i y_i = 0, 0\leq a_j \leq C$, where a_i is the Lagrange multipliers of M for each constraint and C represents the punishment parameter of the sample. A particular kernel function $K\left(x,xi\right)$ is used to solve the eq. (6). The most popular function used in MI two class problem is a linear kernel. The final optimal objective function of the SVM classifier is obtained as

$$f\left(x\right)=sgn\left(\sum_{i=1}^{l}a_i^* y_i K\left(x,x_i\right)+b^*\right), \tag{7}$$

Where a^* and b^* helps to evaluate the optimal classification surface and are calculated by a support vector.

LITERATURE SURVEY

This section of the chapter presents a brief survey of some of the state-of-the-art signal processing methods used in various studies in tabular form. Table 3 provides information about the signal processing steps followed in some of the recent studies. It also incorporates the results achieved by the researchers.

EXPERIMENTAL STUDY

An Exercise to Classify Two-Class Motor Imagery Data

In this study, authors have presented a signal processing method to extract the time, frequency and phase features using a dual-tree complex wavelet transform

(DTCWT). As explained earlier in this chapter, these features provide most of the discriminatory information for MI task classification. After the feature extraction, classification task is performed using an SVM classifier. A public motor imagery BCI dataset is used to validate the results. To perform this exercise, EEG signal from three channel locations namely C3, Cz and C4 is decomposed using DTCWT into different frequency bands as mentioned in Table 2. The coefficients of details D3 and D4 are used to reconstruct the EEG signal. This will bandpass the EEG in the appropriate frequency range of mu and beta rhythms. After DTCWT filtering, four-time domain features, one frequency domain feature and one phase feature of the EEG are extracted using the methods explained previously in this chapter.

The final feature vector will have features from time, frequency and phase domain. Since there are signals from three channels and two sub-bands the total dimension of the feature vector is

$$3\,channels \times 2\,sub\,bands \times 6\,features = 36\,features\,.$$

The description of the dataset used for this exercise is presented in the following paragraph.

Dataset Description

- **Dataset 1**: For this work, BCI Competition II (Dataset III) (B. Blankertz et al., 2004) dataset acquired from a 25-year-old female while performing a motor imagery task of two classes (left-hand or right-hand movement) is utilized. The sampling frequency of the dataset is 128 Hz and the three channel EEG namely c3,cz, and c4, is prefiltered between 0.5 and 30 Hz. The datset consists of 280 trails, where each trail is of 9 sec under a cue paeced paradigm i.e., a cue is presented at time t=3 and subject was asked to start thinking about the movement of either right hand or left hand.
- **Dataset 2**: This work uses the motor imagery dataset 2b of BCI competition IV (Tangermann et al., 2012). In this dataset, the EEG signals from 9 subjects were recorded while performing a motor imagery task of two classes (i.e., motor imagery of left- hand and right- hand). It comprises of bipolar EEG from 3 channel locations (c3, cz, and c4) mainly associated with the sensory-motor rhythms. The sampling frequency of the acquisition device was 250 Hz, and the data were bandpass filtered between 0.5 Hz and 100 Hz. The data were acquired in five training sessions for each subject, out of which we have selected the data of the third session with smiley feedback. Further, the recorded dataset contains 80 trails for each class.

Performance Measures

The performance measures evaluate how capable a pattern recognition method is to solve a given classification problem. The effectiveness of the different classification algorithms is evaluated using a confusion matrix, which represents the number of times the classifier output was true and how many times the classifier predicted falsely. Based on that classification accuracy is calculated as defined below.

- **Classification Accuracy (CA):** Classification accuracy is defined as "percentage of correct predictions." In other words, in percentage CA is the total number of correct predictions divided by the total number of predictions.
- **Statistical Significance:** Statistical significance is a mathematical approach to investigate that the superior outcome of an experiment or test is not achieved by chance but is instead occurred due to a specific property of the method used. Apart from classification performance, the paired t-test is used for this study to compute the statistical significance of the different feature extraction methods.

RESULTS AND DISCUSSION

This part of the chapter presents the classification results obtained after the feature extraction by the proposed method. A support vector machine (SVM) classifier with a linear kernel is used to perform the classification task. Five-fold cross-validation scheme is chosen to divide the dataset into training and testing sets. To assess the performance of the proposed feature extraction method, classification accuracy (CA) (Schlogl, Kronegg, Huggins, & Mason, 2007) of the SVM classifier is taken as the evaluation criterion.

The proposed feature extraction method was compared in terms of CA with some baseline feature extraction methods such as discrete wavelet transform (DWT), common spatial Patterns (CSP) (Benjamin Blankertz, Dornhege, Krauledat, Muller, & Curio, 2007), Filter Bank CSP (FBCSP) (Ang et al., 2008), Frequency Domain CSP (FDCSP) (Wang, Feng, & Lu, 2017). In all of these studies, SVM classifier was utilized to classify two-class MI EEG. Results of classification performances achieved by the various feature extraction methods are presented in Table 4. The Feature extraction using DWT is done using db5 wavelet with 7 decomposition levels. Only the coefficients of the band 8-32 Hz are extracted to reconstruct the EEG using inverse wavelet transform.

It is notable that the average CA of 82.81% is achieved by the proposed feature extraction method based on DTCWT which is the highest in comparison with the other methods. Also, the proposed feature extraction method gives higher classification results for seven subjects out of a total of nine subjects.

To further evaluate the superiority of the proposed method in comparison with the other methods we performed a paired-sample t-test. It is found that the proposed method is statistically significant ($p<0.05$) than all the other methods. Paired- sample t-test results are shown in table 4.

The proposed scheme utilizes 36 features from time, frequency and phase domain. However, the proposed feature extraction method has achieved better classification performance in comparison to the baseline feature extraction methods, the dimension of the feature vector is very high that degrades the classification performance to some extent. This limits the usability of the proposed scheme to some level. In some of the studies (Boutsidis, Mahoney, & Drineas, 2008; Kannan, Jr, Sharma, & Schoo, 2012; Nitesh Singh Malan & Sharma, 2019) feature selection algorithm such as genetic algorithm (GA), principal component analysis (PCA), and Neighborhood Component Analysis (NCA) are used to reduce the high feature dimensions of EEG. This work can be investigated using feature selection approaches to further improve the classification performance.

FUTURE RESEARCH DIRECTIONS

In the context of MI BCI, the brain response to MI task is different for different subjects. In other words, BCI performance is subject specific since the neural response of brain to MI events varies between subjects. Therefore it is very important to evaluate the start time of the motor imagery to further improve the classification performance. In some studies, researchers have used time-shifted windows of EEG and evaluated the classification performance (Feng et al., 2018; Y. Zhang et al., 2018). However, this adds more dimensions to the data and makes the structure of the data more complex. The study of complex relationship in feature space has been investigated using subspace regularization-based algorithms in applications including brain disease diagnosis, imaging processing, and so on (Lei, Yang, Wang, Chen, & Ni, 2017; Liu & Zhang, 2016; Nie et al., 2019). Also, tensor-based decomposition and multiway learning applied on different biomedical dataset show promising potential in preserving the structural relationship and analysis of the data (Yu Zhang et al., 2017; Zhou et al., 2016). For future studies above mentioned methods can investigated for motor imagery classification.

CONCLUSION

This chapter described the designing aspects of a motor imagery (MI) based brain-computer interface (BCI) system including its applications in various research fields. Also, a feature extraction exercise is performed for two-class motor imagery EEG based on DTCWT. In the conducted study, the first step involves the decomposition of MI EEG into different frequency bands using DTCWT. Then, the frequency bands associated with mu and beta rhythms are used to reconstruct the EEG time series. This applied filtering on the raw EEG data employing the superior properties of DTCWT. Thereby, time, frequency and phase features are extracted and used to train the SVM classifier with a linear kernel. Classification accuracy is measured and compared with other popular methods shows that our proposed scheme outperforms the other feature extraction methods. Further, paired-sample t-test was performed and results verified that the proposed method was statistically significant in comparison with CSP, FBCSP, and FDCSPP. The average classification accuracy achieved by our method is 82.81%. Hence, this feature extraction method can be employed to enhance the classification performance of two class motor imagery EEG. For future work, this feature extraction method can be applied for multi-class motor imagery classification. Also, the feature dimensions of the generated feature vector can be reduced using feature selection algorithms.

Table 4. Comparison of Classification Accuracy between four feature extraction methods: CSP, FBCSP, FDCSP, and proposed method. Values in boldness indicates the largest values. Also, results of paired-sample t-test is are listed.

Subject ID	Feature Extraction Methods with classifier				
	DWT (db5) +SVM	CSP + SVM	FBCSP + SVM	FDCSP + SVM	Proposed Method + SVM
Dataset 1	72.3	73.12	76.45	79.81	**82.1**
B0103T	70.6	76.56	77.50	78.13	**87.50**
B0203T	61.9	55.56	55.94	69.03	**78.10**
B0303T	**67.5**	52.62	53.75	58.19	57.5
B0403T	95.6	98.06	98.87	99.38	**99.4**
B0503T	77.5	88.19	90.44	86.88	**91.3**
B0603T	66.3	69.37	78.06	79.37	**81.9**
B0703T	75.6	83.44	86.50	**90.63**	88.9
B0803T	85.0	86.56	88.75	88.12	**94.4**
B0903T	77.5	81.75	83.88	81.87	**87.5**
Mean Value	74.98	76.523	79.014	81.141	**84.86**
p Value	$p<0.05$	$p<0.05$	$p<0.05$	$p<0.05$	--

REFERENCES

Abiyev, R. H., Akkaya, N., Aytac, E., Günsel, I., & Çağman, A. (2016). Brain-Computer Interface for Control of Wheelchair Using Fuzzy Neural Networks. *BioMed Research International*, *2016*, 1–9. doi:10.1155/2016/9359868 PMID:27777953

Al-Fahoum, A. S., & Al-Fraihat, A. A. (2014). Methods of EEG Signal Features Extraction Using Linear Analysis in Frequency and Time-Frequency Domains. *ISRN Neuroscience*, *2014*, 1–7. doi:10.1155/2014/730218 PMID:24967316

Ang, K. K., Chin, Z. Y., Wang, C., Guan, C., & Zhang, H. (2012). Filter Bank Common Spatial Pattern Algorithm on BCI Competition IV Datasets 2a and 2b. *Frontiers in Neuroscience*, *6*. doi:10.3389/fnins.2012.00039 PMID:22479236

Ang, K. K., Chin, Z. Y., Zhang, H., & Guan, C. (2008). Filter bank common spatial pattern (FBCSP) in brain-computer interface. In *IEEE International Joint Conference On Neural Networks. (IEEE World Congress on Computational Intelligence)*, 2390–2397. Piscataway, NJ: IEEE.

Bashar, S. K., Hassan, A. R., & Bhuiyan, M. I. H. (2015). Identification of motor imagery movements from EEG signals using Dual Tree Complex Wavelet Transform. *2015 International Conference on Advances in Computing, Communications and Informatics (ICACCI)*, 290–296. 10.1109/ICACCI.2015.7275623

Bi, L., Fan, X., & Liu, Y. (2013). EEG-Based Brain-Controlled Mobile Robots: A Survey. *IEEE Transactions on Human-Machine Systems*, *43*(2), 161–176. doi:10.1109/TSMCC.2012.2219046

Blankertz, B., Dornhege, G., Krauledat, M., Müller, K.-R., & Curio, G. (2007). The non-invasive Berlin Brain-Computer Interface: Fast acquisition of effective performance in untrained subjects. *NeuroImage*, *37*(2), 539–550. doi:10.1016/j.neuroimage.2007.01.051 PMID:17475513

Blankertz, B., Muller, K., Curio, G., Vaughan, T. M., Schalk, G., Wolpaw, J. R., ... Birbaumer, N. (2004). The BCI competition 2003: Progress and perspectives in detection and discrimination of EEG single trials. *IEEE Transactions on Biomedical Engineering*, *51*(6), 1044–1051. doi:10.1109/TBME.2004.826692 PMID:15188876

Boutsidis, C., Mahoney, M. W., & Drineas, P. (2008). Unsupervised feature selection for principal components analysis. *Proceedings of the 14th ACM SIGKDD International Conference on Knowledge Discovery and Data Mining*, 61–69. New York, NY: ACM. 10.1145/1401890.1401903

Cantillo-Negrete, J., Carino-Escobar, R. I., Carrillo-Mora, P., Elias-Vinas, D., & Gutierrez-Martinez, J. (2018). Motor Imagery-Based Brain-Computer Interface Coupled to a Robotic Hand Orthosis Aimed for Neurorehabilitation of Stroke Patients. *Journal of Healthcare Engineering*, *2018*, 1–10. doi:10.1155/2018/1624637 PMID:29849992

Chaudhary, U., Birbaumer, N., & Ramos-Murguialday, A. (2016). Brain-computer interfaces for communication and rehabilitation. *Nature Reviews. Neurology*, *12*(9), 513–525. doi:10.1038/nrneurol.2016.113 PMID:27539560

Chaudhury, K. N., & Unser, M. (2010). On the shiftability of dual-tree complex wavelet transforms. *IEEE Transactions on Signal Processing*, *58*(1), 221–232. doi:10.1109/TSP.2009.2028962

Easwaramoorthy, D. & Uthayakumar, R. (2010). Analysis of biomedical EEG signals using Wavelet Transforms and Multifractal Analysis. *2010 International Conference on Communication Control and Computing Technologies*, 544–549. doi:10.1109/ICCCCT.2010.5670780

Feng, J., Yin, E., Jin, J., Saab, R., Daly, I., Wang, X., ... Cichocki, A. (2018). Towards correlation-based time window selection method for motor imagery BCIs. *Neural Networks*, *102*, 87–95. doi:10.1016/j.neunet.2018.02.011 PMID:29558654

Fu, R., Tian, Y., Bao, T., Meng, Z., & Shi, P. (2019). Improvement Motor Imagery EEG Classification Based on Regularized Linear Discriminant Analysis. *Journal of Medical Systems*, *43*(6), 169. doi:10.100710916-019-1270-0 PMID:31062175

Grosse-Wentrup, M., Liefhold, C., Gramann, K., & Buss, M. (2009). Beamforming in noninvasive brain–computer interfaces. *IEEE Transactions on Biomedical Engineering*, *56*(4), 1209–1219. doi:10.1109/TBME.2008.2009768 PMID:19423426

Gu, Q., Li, Z., & Han, J. (2012). Generalized Fisher Score for Feature Selection. *ArXiv:1202.3725 [Cs, Stat]*. Retrieved from http://arxiv.org/abs/1202.3725

Guyon, I., & Elisseeff, A. (2003). An Introduction to Variable and Feature Selection. *Journal of Machine Learning Research*, *3*(Mar), 1157–1182.

Hobson, A. R., & Hillebrand, A. (2006). Independent component analysis of the EEG: Is this the way forward for understanding abnormalities of brain-gut signalling? *Gut*, *55*(5), 597–600. doi:10.1136/gut.2005.081703 PMID:16609130

Hsu, W.-Y. (2013). Wavelet-coherence features for motor imagery EEG analysis posterior to EOG noise elimination. *International Journal of Innovative Computing, Information, & Control*, *9*, 465–475.

Hu, D., Li, W., & Chen, X. (2011). Feature extraction of motor imagery EEG signals based on wavelet packet decomposition. *The 2011 IEEE/ICME International Conference on Complex Medical Engineering*, 694–697. doi:10.1109/ICCME.2011.5876829

Imran, S. M., Talukdar, M. T. F., Sakib, S. K., Pathan, N. S., & Fattah, S. A. (2014). Motor imagery EEG signal classification scheme based on wavelet domain statistical features. *2014 International Conference on Electrical Engineering and Information Communication Technology*, 1–4. 10.1109/ICEEICT.2014.6919172

Kamousi, B., Liu, Z., & He, B. (2005). Classification of motor imagery tasks for brain-computer interface applications by means of two equivalent dipoles analysis. *IEEE Transactions on Neural Systems and Rehabilitation Engineering*, *13*(2), 166–171. doi:10.1109/TNSRE.2005.847386 PMID:16003895

Kannan, A. G. Q. M., Jr., Sharma, A., & Schoo, P. (2012). Genetic Algorithm Based Feature Selection Algorithm for Effective Intrusion Detection in Cloud Networks. *2012 IEEE 12th International Conference on Data Mining Workshops*, 416–423. doi:10.1109/ICDMW.2012.56

Kawasaki, T. (2017). *Clinical Application of Motor Imagery Training*. Neurological Physical Therapy. doi:10.5772/67518

Kim, C., Sun, J., Liu, D., Wang, Q., & Paek, S. (2018). An effective feature extraction method by power spectral density of EEG signal for 2-class motor imagery-based BCI. *Medical & Biological Engineering & Computing*, 1–14. PMID:29497931

Kononenko, I. (1994). Estimating attributes: Analysis and extensions of RELIEF. *European Conference on Machine Learning*, 171–182. Berlin, Germany: Springer. 10.1007/3-540-57868-4_57

Kumar, P. S., Arumuganathan, R., Sivakumar, K., & Vimal, C. (n.d.). Removal of ocular artifacts in the EEG through wavelet transform without using an EOG reference channel. *Int. J. Open Probl. Comput. Math*, 188–200.

LaFleur, K., Cassady, K., Doud, A., Shades, K., Rogin, E., & He, B. (2013). Quadcopter control in three-dimensional space using a noninvasive motor imagery-based brain–computer interface. *Journal of Neural Engineering*, *10*(4), 046003. doi:10.1088/1741-2560/10/4/046003 PMID:23735712

Lal, T. N., Schroder, M., Hinterberger, T., Weston, J., Bogdan, M., Birbaumer, N., & Scholkopf, B. (2004). Support vector channel selection in BCI. *IEEE Transactions on Biomedical Engineering*, *51*(6), 1003–1010. doi:10.1109/TBME.2004.827827 PMID:15188871

Lei, B., Yang, P., Wang, T., Chen, S., & Ni, D. (2017). Relational-Regularized Discriminative Sparse Learning for Alzheimer's Disease Diagnosis. *IEEE Transactions on Cybernetics*, *47*(4), 1102–1113. doi:10.1109/TCYB.2016.2644718 PMID:28092591

Li, T., Zhang, J., Xue, T., & Wang, B. (2017). *Development of a Novel Motor Imagery Control Technique and Application in a Gaming Environment*. Comp. Int. and Neurosc. doi:10.1155/2017/5863512

Liu, M., & Zhang, D. (2016). Pairwise Constraint-Guided Sparse Learning for Feature Selection. *IEEE Transactions on Cybernetics*, *46*(1), 298–310. doi:10.1109/TCYB.2015.2401733 PMID:26151948

Lotte, F., Congedo, M., Lécuyer, A., Lamarche, F., & Arnaldi, B. (2007). A review of classification algorithms for EEG-based brain–computer interfaces. *Journal of Neural Engineering*, *4*(2), R1–R13. doi:10.1088/1741-2560/4/2/R01 PMID:17409472

Maddirala, A. K., & Shaik, R. A. (2016). Removal of EOG Artifacts From Single Channel EEG Signals Using Combined Singular Spectrum Analysis and Adaptive Noise Canceler. *IEEE Sensors Journal*, *16*(23), 8279–8287. doi:10.1109/JSEN.2016.2560219

Malan, N. S. & Sharma, S. (2018). Removal of Ocular Atrifacts from Single Channel EEG Signal Using DTCWT with Quantum Inspired Adaptive Threshold. *2018 2nd International Conference on Biomedical Engineering (IBIOMED)*, 94–99. doi:10.1109/IBIOMED.2018.8534915

Malan, N. S., & Sharma, S. (2019). Feature selection using regularized neighbourhood component analysis to enhance the classification performance of motor imagery signals. *Computers in Biology and Medicine*, *107*, 118–126. doi:10.1016/j.compbiomed.2019.02.009 PMID:30802693

Mellinger, J., Schalk, G., Braun, C., Preissl, H., Rosenstiel, W., Birbaumer, N., & Kübler, A. (2007). An MEG-based brain-computer interface (BCI). *NeuroImage*, *36*(3), 581–593. doi:10.1016/j.neuroimage.2007.03.019 PMID:17475511

Ming, M., Shaona, L., Haitao, M., Yuliang, M., & Yunyuan, G. (2015). Feature extraction method of motor imagery EEG based on DTCWT sample entropy. *2015 34th Chinese Control Conference (CCC)*, 3964–3968. doi:10.1109/ChiCC.2015.7260250

Mishchenko, Y., Kaya, M., Ozbay, E., & Yanar, H. (2017). Developing a 3- to 6-state EEG-based brain-computer interface for a robotic manipulator control. *bioRxiv*. doi:10.1101/171025

Naseer, N., & Hong, K.-S. (2015). fNIRS-based brain-computer interfaces: A review. *Frontiers in Human Neuroscience, 9*. doi:10.3389/fnhum.2015.00003

Navarro, A. A., Ceccaroni, L., Velickovski, F., Torrellas, S., Miralles, F., Allison, B. Z. … Faller, J. (2011). Context-Awareness as an Enhancement of Brain-Computer Interfaces. *IWAAL*. doi:10.1007/978-3-642-21303-8_30

Nie, D., Wang, L., Adeli, E., Lao, C., Lin, W., & Shen, D. (2019). 3-D Fully Convolutional Networks for Multimodal Isointense Infant Brain Image Segmentation. *IEEE Transactions on Cybernetics, 49*(3), 1123–1136. doi:10.1109/TCYB.2018.2797905 PMID:29994385

Norcia, A. M., Appelbaum, L. G., Ales, J. M., Cottereau, B. R., & Rossion, B. (2015). The steady-state visual evoked potential in vision research: A review. *Journal of Vision (Charlottesville, Va.), 15*(6), 4–4. doi:10.1167/15.6.4 PMID:26024451

Novi, Q., Guan, C., Dat, T. H., & Xue, P. (2007). Sub-band common spatial pattern (SBCSP) for brain-computer interface. In *3rd International IEEE/EMBS Conference On Neural Engineering, 2007. CNE'07*, 204–207. Piscataway, NJ: IEEE.

Peng, Z. K., Jackson, M. R., Rongong, J. A., Chu, F. L., & Parkin, R. M. (2009). On the energy leakage of discrete wavelet transform. *Mechanical Systems and Signal Processing, 23*(2), 330–343. doi:10.1016/j.ymssp.2008.05.014

Penn, A. A., & Shatz, C. J. (1999). Brain waves and brain wiring: The role of endogenous and sensory-driven neural activity in development. *Pediatric Research, 45*(4 Pt 1), 447–458. doi:10.1203/00006450-199904010-00001 PMID:10203134

Pfurtscheller, G. & Neuper, C. (2001). Motor imagery and direct brain-computer communication. *Proceedings of the IEEE, 89*(7), 1123–1134.

Pfurtscheller, G., Flotzinger, D., Pregenzer, M., Wolpaw, J. R., & McFarland, D. (1995). EEG-based brain computer interface (BCI). Search for optimal electrode positions and frequency components. *Medical Progress Through Technology, 21*(3), 111–121. PMID:8776708

Pfurtscheller, G., & Lopes da Silva, F. H. (1999). Event-related EEG/MEG synchronization and desynchronization: Basic principles. *Clinical Neurophysiology, 110*(11), 1842–1857. doi:10.1016/S1388-2457(99)00141-8 PMID:10576479

Quinlan, J. R. (1986). Induction of Decision Trees. *Machine Learning, 1*(1), 81–106. doi:10.1007/BF00116251

Quinlan, J. R. (1993). *C4.5: Programs for Machine Learning*. San Francisco, CA: Morgan Kaufmann Publishers.

Ramos, A. C., Hernández, R. G., & Vellasco, M. (2016). Feature selection methods applied to motor imagery task classification. In *2016 IEEE Latin American Conference On Computational Intelligence (LA-CCI)*, 1–6. Piscataway, NJ: IEEE.

Ramoser, H., Muller-Gerking, J., & Pfurtscheller, G. (2000). Optimal spatial filtering of single trial EEG during imagined hand movement. *IEEE Transactions on Rehabilitation Engineering*, *8*(4), 441–446. doi:10.1109/86.895946 PMID:11204034

Rao, R. P. N., & Scherer, R. (2010). Brain-Computer Interfacing [In the Spotlight]. *IEEE Signal Processing Magazine*, *27*(4), 152–150. doi:10.1109/MSP.2010.936774

Schalk, G., & Leuthardt, E. C. (2011). Brain-computer interfaces using electrocorticographic signals. *IEEE Reviews in Biomedical Engineering*, *4*, 140–154. doi:10.1109/RBME.2011.2172408 PMID:22273796

Schlogl, A., Kronegg, J., Huggins, J., & Mason, S. (2007). *19 evaluation criteria for bci research*. Toward Brain-Computer Interfacing.

Sharanreddy, P. K. K. (2013, March). Detection of primary brain tumor present in eeg signal using wavelet transform and neural network [Journal (Paginated)]. Retrieved from https://www.biomedscidirect.com/990/detection_of_primary_brain_tumor_present_in_eeg_signal_using_wavelet_transform_and_neural_network/articlescategories

Shawe-Taylor, J., & Sun, S. (2011). A review of optimization methodologies in support vector machines. *Neurocomputing*, *74*(17), 3609–3618. doi:10.1016/j.neucom.2011.06.026

Song, L. & Gordon, E. (n.d.). *Phase Synchrony Rate for the Recognition of Motor Imagery in BCI*. 8.

Song, L., Gordon, E., & Gysels, E. (2006). Phase Synchrony Rate for the Recognition of Motor Imagery in Brain-Computer Interface. In Y. Weiss, B. Schölkopf, & J. C. Platt (Eds.), Advances in Neural Information Processing Systems Vol. 18, pp. 1265–1272. Retrieved from http://papers.nips.cc/paper/2849-phase-synchrony-rate-for-the-recognition-of-motor-imagery-in-brain-computer-interface.pdf

Sur, S., & Sinha, V. K. (2009). Event-related potential: An overview. *Industrial Psychiatry Journal*, *18*(1), 70–73. doi:10.4103/0972-6748.57865 PMID:21234168

Tangermann, M., Müller, K.-R., Aertsen, A., Birbaumer, N., Braun, C., Brunner, C., ... Mueller-Putz, G. (2012). Review of the BCI competition IV. *Frontiers in Neuroscience*, *6*, 55. doi:10.3389/fnins.2012.00055 PMID:22811657

Thomas, K. P., Guan, C., Tong, L. C., & Prasad, V. A. (2008). An adaptive filter bank for motor imagery based Brain Computer Interface. In *Proceedings of Annual International Conference of the IEEE Engineering in Medicine and Biology Society.* 1104–1107. 10.1109/IEMBS.2008.4649353

Tibshirani, R. (2017). Regression shrinkage and selection via the lasso: A retrospective. *Journal of the Royal Statistical Society. Series B, Statistical Methodology*, 273–282. doi:10.1111/j.1467-9868.2011.00771.x@10.1111/(ISSN)1467-9868.TOP_SERIES_B_RESEARCH

Wang, J., Feng, Z., & Lu, N. (2017). Feature extraction by common spatial pattern in frequency domain for motor imagery tasks classification. *2017 29th Chinese Control and Decision Conference (CCDC),* 5883–5888. Piscataway, NJ: IEEE. 10.1109/CCDC.2017.7978220

Xu, B., & Song, A. (2008). Pattern recognition of motor imagery EEG using wavelet transform. *Journal of Biomedical Science and Engineering, 1*(01), 64–67. doi:10.4236/jbise.2008.11010

Yang, R., Song, A., & Xu, B. (2010). Feature extraction of motor imagery eeg based on wavelet transform and higher-order statistics. *International Journal of Wavelets, Multresolution, and Information Processing*, *8*(3), 373–384. doi:10.1142/S0219691310003535

Yang, W., Wang, K., & Zuo, W. (2012). Neighborhood Component Feature Selection for High-Dimensional Data. *JCP*, *7*(1), 161–168.

Yu, Y., Zhou, Z., Yin, E., Jiang, J., Tang, J., Liu, Y., & Hu, D. (2016). Toward brain-actuated car applications: Self-paced control with a motor imagery-based brain-computer interface. *Computers in Biology and Medicine*, *77*, 148–155. doi:10.1016/j.compbiomed.2016.08.010 PMID:27544071

Yuan, H., & He, B. (2014). Brain-computer interfaces using sensorimotor rhythms: Current state and future perspectives. *IEEE Transactions on Biomedical Engineering*, *61*(5), 1425–1435. doi:10.1109/TBME.2014.2312397 PMID:24759276

Zabidi, A., Mansor, W., Lee, Y. K., & Fadzal, C. C. W. (2012). Short-time Fourier Transform analysis of EEG signal generated during imagined writing. *2012 International Conference on System Engineering and Technology (ICSET)*, 1–4. 10.1109/ICSEngT.2012.6339284

Zhang, Y., Nam, C. S., Zhou, G., Jin, J., Wang, X., & Cichocki, A. (2018). Temporally Constrained Sparse Group Spatial Patterns for Motor Imagery BCI. *IEEE Transactions on Cybernetics*, 1–11. doi:10.1109/TCYB.2018.2841847 PMID:29994667

Zhang, Yu., Zhou, G., Jin, J., Zhang, Y., Wang, X., & Cichocki, A. (2017). Sparse Bayesian multiway canonical correlation analysis for EEG pattern recognition. *Neurocomputing*, *225*, 103–110. doi:10.1016/j.neucom.2016.11.008

Zhou, G., Zhao, Q., Zhang, Y., Adalı, T., Xie, S., & Cichocki, A. (2016). Linked Component Analysis From Matrices to High-Order Tensors: Applications to Biomedical Data. *Proceedings of the IEEE, 104*(2), 310–331. doi:10.1109/JPROC.2015.2474704

Zhu, Y., Xu, K., Xu, C., Zhang, J., Ji, J., Zheng, X., ... Tian, M. (2016). PET Mapping for Brain-Computer Interface Stimulation of the Ventroposterior Medial Nucleus of the Thalamus in Rats with Implanted Electrodes. *Journal of Nuclear Medicine: Official Publication, Society of Nuclear Medicine*, *57*(7), 1141–1145. doi:10.2967/jnumed.115.171868 PMID:26917709

Chapter 10
A Study on the Examination of RGB Scale Retinal Pictures Using Recent Methodologies

A. Swarnalatha
St. Joseph's College of Engineering, India

K. Palani Thanaraj
https://orcid.org/0000-0003-3897-4460
St. Joseph's College of Engineering, India

A. Sheryl Oliver
St. Joseph's College of Engineering, India

M. Esther Hannah
St. Joseph's College of Engineering, India

ABSTRACT

Retinal disease/condition examination is one of the significant areas of the medical field. A variety of retinal abnormality assessments based on fundus image-assisted trials are widely proposed by the researchers to examine the parts of the retina. Recently, traditional and soft computing-based approaches are executed to inspect the optic disc and the blood vessels of the retina to discover disease/damages. This work implements (i) A two-phase methodology based on Jaya Algorithm (JA) and Kapur's Entropy (KE) thresholding and level-set segmentation for the optic disc evaluation and (ii) JA-based Multi-scale Matched Filter (MMF) for the blood vessel assessment. During this analysis, various benchmark datasets such as RIM-ONE, DRIVE, and STARE are considered. The experimental study substantiates that JA-assisted retinal picture examination offers better results than other related existing methodologies.

DOI: 10.4018/978-1-7998-0326-3.ch010

INTRODUCTION

Eyes are the vital organs in human body which play a crucial role in human sensory arrangement. It translates the light signals into understandable picture and transmits it to the brain through optic-nerve in the form of electro-chemical pulses. A shortcoming or injury in eyes may affects translation of light signals into pictures, which may cause momentary or permanent loss of vision. Hence, a pre-screening procedure is always suggested by the ophthalmologist to ensure the safe functioning of eyes. During this screening practice, various regions of eyes are examined using a visual check and also using the imaging procedures (Rabbani et al., 2015; Mahmudi et al., 2014; Golabbakhsh & Rabbani, 2013).

Retina is an inmost deposit in eye and automatic assessment of fundamental retinal parts are very significant to discover a range of retinal diseases (Mahmudi et al., 2013). If the cause and the nature of retinal-infection is discovered, then the doctor will suggest a well-organized treatment to cure or minimize the infection. In literature, retinal pictures recorded with ocular fundus image (Golabbakhsh & Rabbani, 2013), fluorescein angiography (Rabbani et al., 2015), and optical coherence tomography (Mahmudi et al., 2014) are extensively used to examine different elements in retina.

Earlier works confirms that, retinal examination is essential in identification and handling of Ocular-Hypertension (OHT), Diabetic-Retinopathy, Macular-Edema, glaucoma, Retinal-Vasculature (RV), Optic-Nerve Disorder (OND), malaria, papilloedema and Cardiovascular-Diseases (CD) (Jahromi et al., 2014; Wilkinson et al., 2003; Hajeb et al., 2012; 2014; Esmaeili et al., 2012; Sivakamasundari et al., 2015; Raja et al., 2012). These works also confirms the need of assessing the geometrical and physical disparity in Retinal-Optic-Disc (ROD) and Retinal-Blood-Vessel (RBV) to identify a range of illnesses.

This paper proposes two semi-automated procedures to examine the Fundus-Retinal-Pictures (FRP). Initially, the examination of Optic-Disc (OD) is implemented using the Jaya Algorithm (Rao, 2016; Rao & More, 2017) and Kapur's Entropy (Anitha et al., 2017) (JA+KE) based pre-processing and the Level-Set Segmentation (LSS) as the post-processing section. This technique is implemented to extract the OD from the RGB scale FRP obtained from normal (255 pictures) and Glaucoma (200 pictures) cases existing in RIM-ONE database. This work also examines the OD of other images, such as Normal (118 pictures), Early (12 pictures), Moderate (14 pictures), Deep (14 pictures) and OHT (11) available in the RIM-ONE database. The above said pictures are associated with five numbers of the expert's annotations called the Ground-Truth (GT). A relative assessment among the extracted OD and GT is executed to confirm the superiority of proposed procedure based on the computed values of picture likeliness measure (PLM). The higher values of PLM confirm the better superiority. Further, the superiority of Kapur's thresholding is confirmed against the Otsu's (Sudhan et al., 2017) and Shannon's (Shree et al., 2018) techniques.

Finally, JA assisted Multiscale-Matched-Filter (MMF) is designed to trace and extract the blood vessels from the complete FRP and the superiority of the proposed tool is confirmed with a relative examination against the ground truths. The outcome is also confirmed against other related approaches. During the blood-vessel examination, FRP datasets, such as DRIVE, STARE and Fluorescein Angiography Retinal Image (FARI) are considered and the experimental outcome confirms the superiority of the proposed procedure.

BACKGROUND

Due to its importance, a large number of traditional, semi-automated and computerized methodologies are proposed and employed by the researchers to evaluate various retinal diseases.

Sree et al. (2018) proposed a Jaya-Algorithm assisted image processing scheme for the optic-disc extraction approach and they implemented as experimental investigation using the Shannon's approach and level-set segmentation (LSS). In this work, they considered the RIM-ONE dataset (Fumero et al., 2011) and obtained better picture similarity values on the chosen test pictures. Sudhan et al. (2017) discussed about the Otsu's thresholding and LSS approach to extract the optic-disc on a chosen test pictures of the RIM-ONE dataset. Sivakamasundari et al. (2015) presented content based retinal image retrieval using papamarkos thresholding scheme. Raja et al (2012) implemented an analysis for vasculature detection in retinal pictures based on the PSO and Tsallis thresholding. Jahromi et al. (2014) proposed an automated segmentation of borders of corneal layers in OCT pictures with gaussian mixture models and obtained better results. Fumero et al. (2011) contributed the RIM-ONE benchmark dataset to test the OD extraction approaches. Sofka and Stewart (2006) developed the Multiscale-Matched-Filters (MMF) to extract the Blood-Vessels from the FRPs. The work of Sreejini and Govindan (2015) implemented the PSO assisted MMF to extract the BV. This work presented an enhanced result compared with the other related procedures existing in the literature. Recently, Keerthana et al. (2017) proposed a MMF procedure to enhance the outcome during BV extraction from the DRIVE benchmark pictures are achieved a better result compared to other related existing methods.

The recent works also confirms the participation of heuristic-algorithm based approaches to investigate the medical pictures to measure the harshness of infections. These facilities also substantiate that, heuristic-algorithm supported scheme also tender improved exactness compared with traditional approaches considered in early days. Hence, in the proposed work, the recently developed heuristic procedure called Jaya-Algorithm is implemented to enhance the outcome of the OD and BV extraction from the benchmark FRP datasets.

MAIN FOCUS OF THIS CHAPTER

Recent works confirms the accessibility of considerable amount of medical picture examination practices proposed and implemented to assist the doctors in identifying the infection rate and also to plan for a possible treatment procedures (Ashour et al., 2015; Balan et al., 2016; Dey et al., 2018; Fernandes et al., 2017; Lakshmi et al., 2016). The FRP examination procedures based on traditional and soft-computing methodologies are also available to examine various retinal parts (Niemeijer et al., 2004; Staal et al., 2004; Hoover et al., 2000; Hoover and Goldbaum, 2003). Compared to the conventional methodologies, soft-computing based procedures will help to achieve better result and it also helps to implement the semi-automated and automated tools to enhance the outcome during the FRP assessment. The main aim of this chapter is to propose semi-automated assessment tool for (i) Optic-Disc examination and (ii) Blood-Vessel examination. This work implements a recent optimization algorithm called the Jaya-Algorithm (JA) to enhance the outcome during the FRP evaluation. The OD assessment is done with a hybrid procedure based on JA+KE and LSS using both the normal and Glaucoma case FRPs with an image count of 624 (255 normal and 369 abnormal case). The difficulty in these FRPs is, all are in RGB scale, hence the investigation requires more computation time. The experimental outcome obtained with Matlab7 confirms that, proposed technique requires lesser computation effort compared to Otsu's and Shannon's approaches. Additionally, an examination scheme is also developed to extract BV from the FRPs with an image count of 507 pictures (40 from DRIVE, 397 from STARE and 70 from FARI). This procedure is also implemented in Matlab7 and better results are obtained. Other details regarding the construction and implementation of proposed approaches are presented below.

Examination of Retinal Optic-Disc

Figure 1 presents different stages involved in Optic-Disc examination method. Initially, the chosen test-picture (normal/abnormal case) experience a three-level thresholding process based on the JA and KE. The thresholding task will enhance the OD section by eliminating the other unwanted sections in the chosen FRP (Sudhan et al., 2017; Sree et al., 2018). The OD in thresholded picture is then mined using the LSS, which

Figure 1. Block diagram of the Optic-Disc mining procedure

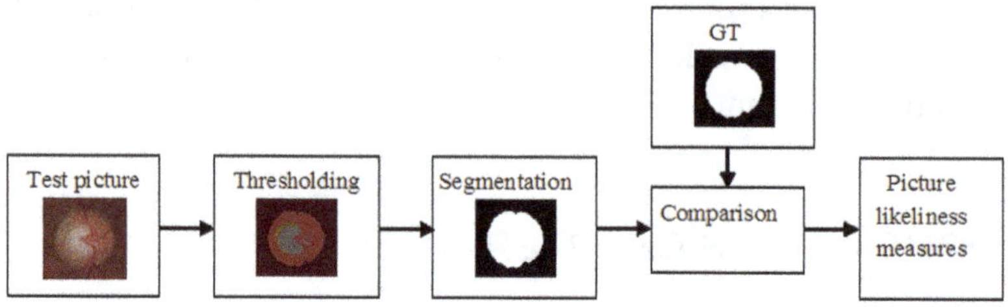

works with the help of a manually assigned bounding-box. When the iteration of LSS increase, the box will shrink towards the interior of the OD and extracts the section with greater accuracy. Later, the extracted OD is then compared with the GTs, and the necessary picture likeliness measures are then computed to validate the superiority of the proposed tool. During this procedure, the FRP is processed in its RGB scale, which offers a better result compared to the gray scale FRPs.

Jaya Algorithm

JA is a recently projected population supported optimization methodology by Rao (2016). The advantage of the JA contrast to other related procedure is, it requires nominal preliminary constraints to be allocated.

Let $G(x)_{min}$ is the preferred objective function, $\Re 1 = \Re 2$ are the subjective number of choice [0,1], N is the population size (ie. $n=1,2,...,N$) and i and D denotes the number of iterations and dimensions (ie. $j=1,2,...,D$) respectively. At some instance, $G(x)_{best}$ and $G(x)_{worst}$ signifies the best & worst answers attained via the candidate of the population.

The chief equation of JA is accessible below (Rajinikanth et al., 2019; Manic et al., 2019; Satapathy & Rajinikanth, 2018)

$$X^{1}_{j,n,i} = X_{j,n,i} + \Re 1_{j,i}\left(X_{jbest,i} - \left|X_{j,n,i}\right|\right) - \Re 2_{j,i}\left(X_{jworst,i} - \left|X_{j,n,i}\right|\right) \tag{1}$$

where, $X_{j,n,i}$ represents the jth variable of nth candidate at i^{th} iteration and $X^{1}_{j,n,i}$ denoted the updated value. More details regarding the JA can be found in (Rao and More, 2017; Wang et al., 2017).

Kapur's Based Threshoding

This division presents a capable entropy utility called Kapur's function, initially discussed in 1985 (Kapur et al., 1985). Kapur's approach was firstly implemented to split gray-level pictures based on its histogram. This approach determines the optimal threshold (T) by exploiting the overall image's entropy.

Let, T = $[T_1, T_2, ..., T_{k-1}]$, the vector for image thresholds. Then, Kapur's function will be;

$$J_{\max} = f_{Kapur}(T) = \sum_{j=1}^{k} H_j^C \; for \, C \{1,2,3\} \tag{2}$$

Entropy for IR_{GB} is calculated for Red, Green and Blue segment based on the assigned T value. For multi- threshold case, this process can be expressed as;

$$\begin{aligned} H_1^C &= \sum_{j=1}^{T_1} \frac{Ph_j^C}{\omega_0^C} \ln\left(\frac{Ph_j^C}{\omega_0^C}\right), \\ H_2^C &= \sum_{j=T_1+1}^{T_2} \frac{Ph_j^C}{\omega_1^C} \ln\left(\frac{Ph_j^C}{\omega_1^C}\right), \\ &\vdots \\ H_k^C & \sum_{j=T_k+1}^{L} \frac{Ph_j^C}{\omega_{k-1}^C} \ln\left(\frac{Ph_j^C}{\omega_{K-1}^C}\right) \end{aligned} \tag{3}$$

where Ph_j^C is the probability allocation of intensity regions and $\omega_0^C, \omega_1^C, ...\omega_{k-1}^C$ are probability incidence for k stages. Complete description of Kapur's approach is available in (Shriranjani et al., 2018; Anitha et al., 2017; Lakshmi et al., 2016).

Level-Set-Segmentation

From the year 1990's (Caselles et al., 1993; Malladi et al., 1995) Level-Set-Segmentation (LSS) has been largely used to examine traditional and medical images. The chief advantage of the LSS technique contrast to other approach is, it can create contours with multifaceted procedure to carry dividing and merging maneuver during the picture outline exploration.

This chapter employs modern edition of LSS called the Distance-Regularized-LS (DRLS) proposed by Li et al., (2010) in order to extract the OD from FRP of RIM-ONE database. The DRLS technique has the following formula;

$$\text{The arc development is} = \frac{\partial C'(s,t)}{\partial t} = FW \tag{4}$$

where, C' - arc vector with spatial (s) and temporal (t) parameter, F - swiftness variable and W - deepest usual vector of arc C.

The arc progress of Eqn. (4) can be formed as DRLS by inserting $C'(s,t)$ as zero LS of a time exciting LS utility ϕ (x,y,t). The variable ϕ presents negative standards inside the zero-stage curve and positive value exterior.

The vector N is expressed as;

$$N = \frac{-\nabla\varphi}{\nabla\varphi} \tag{5}$$

where ∇ is the slope variable.

The LS development is;

$$\frac{\partial\varphi}{\partial t} = F\left|\nabla\varphi\right| \tag{6}$$

Related details on DRLS available in (Vaishnavi et al., 2014).

Examination of Retinal Blood-Vessel

Figure 2 shows various phases existing in Blood-Vessel examination using FRPs. Initially, the RGB scale DRIVE database picture is chosen as the test-picture and is then processed with the JA assisted MMF. When the RGB FRP is passed through the tool, MMF helps to extract the traces made by the BV of FRP. Later, the extracted BV is then evaluated along with the GT, and the essential picture similarity values are then calculated to authenticate the superiority of the proposed tool. During this procedure, the RGB scale and the gray scale FRP are examined and the experimental outcome confirms that, this tool helps to extract the BV with greater accuracy.

Figure 2. Block diagram of Blood-Vessel mining procedure

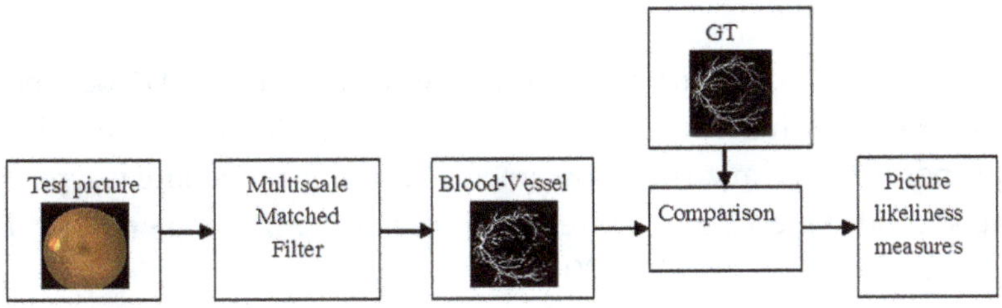

Multiscale Matched Filter

The idea of Matched Filter (MF) is based on the template corresponding procedure and is generally considered to resolve the retinal blood vessel segmentation difficulty (Sofka & Stewart, 2006; Sreejini & Govindan, 2015; Keerthana et al., 2017).

It works based on the following statement:

Let, the Gaussian MF is defined as;

$$K(a,b) = -\exp(-a^2 / 2\sigma^2)\forall |b| \leq L / 2 \tag{7}$$

where σ is the filter scale, L is the one directional of the vessel segmentation, and K(a,b) is image parameter.

Throughout this procedure, *K(a,b)* is rotated in diverse directions arbitrarily to recognize the vessel traces. The number of kernels, *K(a,b)* depends regularly on the angle of rotation.

The related vicinity values can be expressed as;

$$NH = \left\{(u,v), |u| \leq G, |v| \leq L / 2\right\} \tag{8}$$

where G is the location where the Gaussian arc should be cut and this value is chosen as $3*\sigma$.

When, the initial kernel *K(a,b)* is rotated, then a new neighborhood, p_i is attained.

$$p_i = \begin{bmatrix} u & v \end{bmatrix} = \begin{bmatrix} a & b \end{bmatrix} \begin{bmatrix} \cos\theta & -\sin\theta \\ \sin\theta & \cos\theta \end{bmatrix} \tag{9}$$

where θ is the angle of rotation and [u v] the new coordinates.

The updated weights of the new kernel are then expressed as;

$$K_i(a,b) = -\exp(-a^2 / 2\sigma^2)\forall p_i \in NH \tag{10}$$

From Eqn. (7) and (8), it can be noted that, the accuracy of the MF depends mainly on the parameters, such as L, σ and G. In this paper, JA based three-dimensional search is proposed to optimize these parameters, and this procedure is repeated twice to have the second stage values. More details regarding the implemented filter can be found in (Sreejini & Govindan, 2015).

Evaluation of ROI With GT

The aim of this chapter is to extract OD/BV from FRP and to calculate the picture likeliness measures for supplementary assessment. This work considers a benchmark FRPs (RIM-ONE and DRIVE), in which test pictures are associated with GTs. After extracting OD/BV from FRP, a relative examination among the OD and GT as well as BV and GT is to be performed and the values, like True-Positive-Rate (TPR), True-Negative-Rate (TNR), False-Positive-Rate (FPR), False-Negative-Rate (FNR), Jaccard-Index (JI), Dice-Coefficient (DC), Sensitivity (SE), Specificity (SP), Accuracy (AC) and Precision (PR) are computed as discussed in (Chaddad & Tanougast, 2016; Rajinikanth et al., 2017).

The equations for these parameters are presented below:

$$FPR(I_{gt}, I_t) = \left(I_{gt}/I_t\right)/(I_{gt} \cup I_t) \tag{11}$$

$$FNR(I_{gt}, I_t) = \left(I_t/I_{gt}\right)/(I_{gt} \cup I_t) \tag{12}$$

$$JI(I_{gt}, I_t) = I_{gt} \cap I_t / I_{gt} \cup I_t \tag{13}$$

$$DC(I_{gt}, I_t) = 2\left(I_{gt} \cap I_t\right)/\left|I_{gt}\right| \cup \left|I_t\right| \tag{14}$$

where, I_{gt} signify the GT and I_t symbolize mined section.

$$SE = T_P/(T_P + F_N) \tag{15}$$

$$SP = T_N/(T_N + F_P) \tag{16}$$

$$AC = (T_P + T_N)/(T_P + T_N + F_P + F_N) \tag{17}$$

$$PR = T_P/(T_P + F_P) \tag{18}$$

where, I_{GT} is ground truth, I_S is mined region, T_N, T_P, F_N and F_P signifies true-negative, true-positive, false-negative and false-positive; correspondingly. If these values are better, then it can be assumed that, proposed image examination tool works well.

(during the comparison, if GT and OD/BV are high, then it is called T_P, when GT is high and OD/BV is low, then it is known as F_P, when GT is low and OD/BV section is high, then it is F_N, when GT and OD/BV image are low, then it is T_N. where low and high represents the pixel size of images)

SOLUTIONS AND RECOMMENDATIONS

This work considers a variety of FRPs for the examination available in various datasets. Initial examination is executed using the RGB scale version of RIM-ONE pictures (normal/abnormal cases) based on a semi-automated tool implemented using Matlab7. Later, the extraction and evaluation of the BV is executed using the RGB and the gray scale test pictures of DRIVE, STARE and FARI. Proposed testing is performed using the computer; AMD C70 Dual Core 1 GHz CPU with 4 GB of RAM. In both the cases, the JA parameters are assigned as; number of agents = 30, search dimension = 3, iteration size = 1000 and the stopping criteria = maximized objective-function.

Initially, the OD examination procedure is executed using the RIM-ONE database. This database consist of RGB scaled Retinal-Optic-Disc (ROD) pictures of varied dimension (562 x 524 pixels, …, etc). The earlier research works with the RGB scale picture confirms that, examination of RGB is more complex compared with the gray scale picture due to its complex histogram pattern (Red, Green & Blue). The initial part of the OD evaluation tool employs a three-level threshold process to enhance the disc section of FRP using the JA+KE. When, JA+KE is executed, the JA algorithm continuously explores the three-dimensional search space to identify the optimized threshold for the test picture which maximizes Kapur's entropy value.

After implementing possible pre-processing scheme, a post-processing based on the LSS is employed to mine the OD from the threshold picture.

This scheme works as follows:

Step 1: Initialize the JA algorithm with the chosen algorithm parameters

Step 2: Apply a three-level thresholding (*T=3*) using the JA assisted Kapur's entropy in order to group the similar pixel levels (this procedure will remove the major portion of the retinal blood vessel from the RGB test image and will enhance the optic disc region).

Step 3: Apply LSS to divide the threshold image

Step 4: Consider the segmented optic disc section; apply RGB to gray scale conversion and record the black & white (BW) image.

Step 5: Apply the image feature extraction and performance metric procedures to record the necessary data from the segmented OD.

Figure 3 presents the sample pictures initially considered to test the OD examination tool. Here, a sum of 455 (255 normal case and 200 glaucoma case) RGB scaled FRPs are initially examined. Later, the specific FRPs available along with the GT (5 numbers for each image) is considered for the examination and its samples are shown in Figure 4. These pictures are categorized into five groups based on the severity of OD infection as shown in figure. During this examination, around 169 RGB scale pictures are examined separately and its results are recorded for further investigation. The quality of the OD segmented using LSS based on JA+KE is also compared with the related approaches like Otsu and Shannon existing in the previous research works. Finally, a relative study between mined OD and GTs are performed and the average results are then considered to confirm the superiority of the JA+KE technique. The average experimental result also confirms that, KE procedure takes minimal computation time (138.26 sec) compared to Otsu (152.19 sec) and Shannon (167.33 sec). This confirms that, JA+KE approach will offer better throughput compared with other existing procedures.

Figure 5 presents the chosen normal FRP available with the GTs. Table 1 presents computed picture similarity values obtained with the image considered in Figure 5. Similar procedure is implemented for other images (169 pictures) and the average value of the similarity values are shown in Figure 6. This figure confirms that, Kapur's function offers better result (Red coloured values) compared with Otsu (Gray colour) and Shannon's (Green colour) procedure. This result confirms that, proposed OD evaluation scheme offers better outcome. Further, proposed approach is compared against the results obtained by Mohamed et al. (2014) as shown in Table 2. Expert 1 to Expert 4 also exists in Mohamed et al. (2014). This result also confirms that, proposed procedure provides better result. JA+Otsu can be found in

Figure 3. Sample images of RIM-ONE database. (a1) - (a4) Normal OD and (b1) - (b4) Abnormal OD

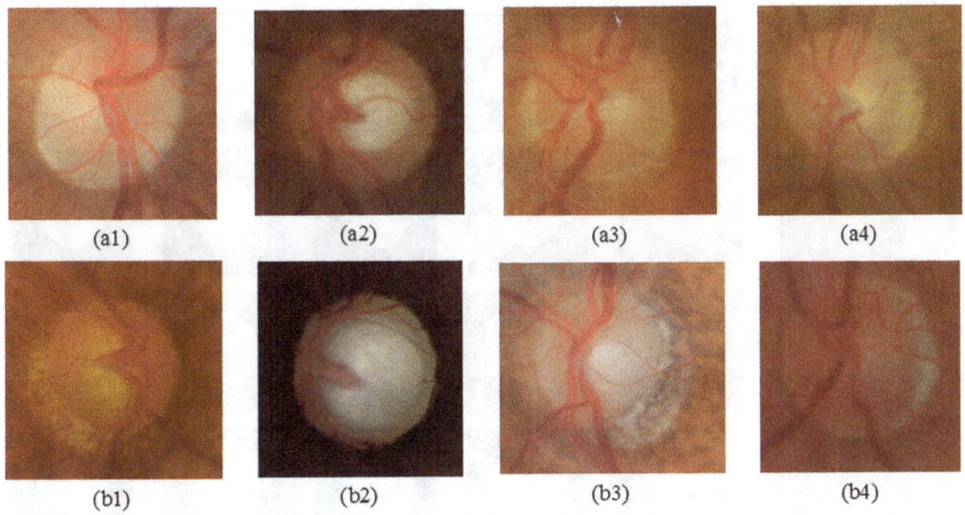

and JA+Shannon is available in Shree et al. (2018). This table also verifies that, proposed JA+KE and LSS offers better results compared to other methodologies considered in this study.

The BV extraction based on JA+MMF is then implemented to extract the Blood-Vessels from FRPs of chosen database.

Segmentation procedure for RGB fundus images:

Step 1: Initialise the JA algorithm with the chosen algorithm parameters
Step 2: Extract the green channel image and implement the FA based matched filter.
Step 3: Store the extracted blood vessel.
Step 4: Apply the image performance metric procedures to record the necessary data in order to validate the segmented image with the GT.

The JA with a three dimension search and the following values are arrived for MMF constraints L, σ and G: (2, 2, 78) and (2, 3, 7).

The FRPs of DRIVE dataset is considered for the initial evaluation process. This database consist 40 RGB scale pictures along with two GTs. This database has 20 test images and 20 train images with the ground truth (GT) provided by the experts. The proposed experimental work is implemented on the DRIVE dataset and the extracted vessel is validated against the GT. All the necessary picture likeliness values are then computed as in Table 1 and the specific values like SE, SP and AC are considered to compare the obtained result with the previous results. The outcome

Figure 4. Various cases of test pictures considered to assess the OD extraction tool. (a) Category, (b) Sample test picture, (c) – (f) GT1 – GT5.

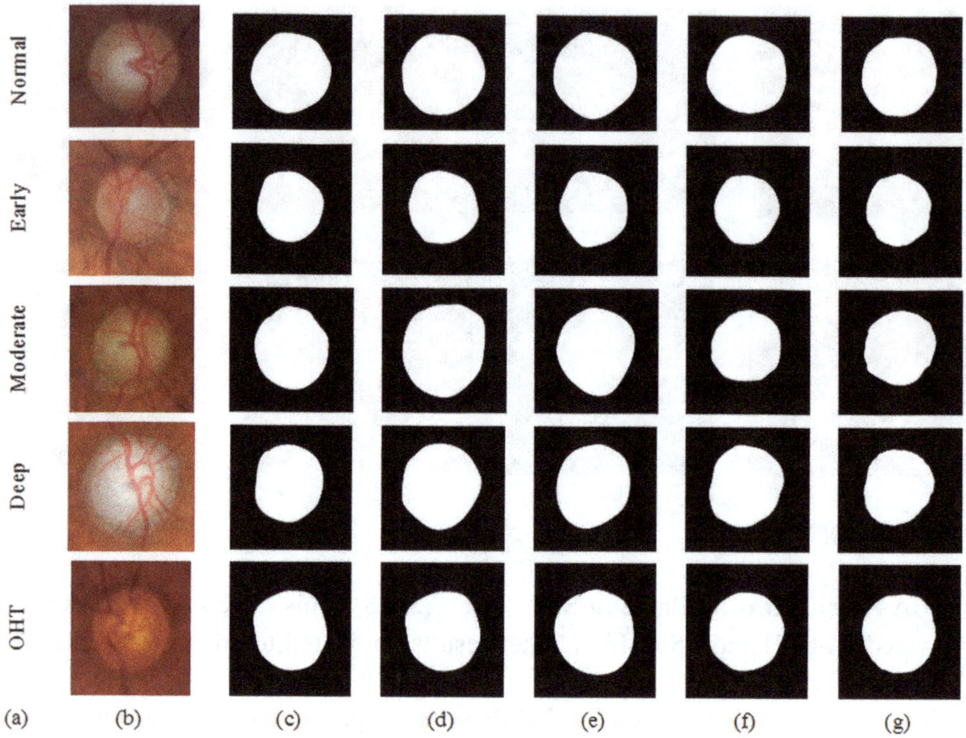

of this work confirm that, proposed method is efficient in extracting the vessel from the retinal images and provides better sensitivity and specificity compared to other methods existing in the literature.

The MMF designed based on JA is then executed on the considered FRPs. Figure 7 shows the outcome obtained for sample test pictures. Fig 7 (a) presents the pseudo image name, Fig 7 (b) shows the test picture, Fig 7 (c) & (d) presents the GTs and Fig 7 (e) shows the extracted vessel. The average result is then compared against other related approaches and found that, JA+MMF offers satisfactory results for the considered DRIVE pictures.

Alike procedure is then executed for the STARE and FARI images and the corresponding results are presented in Figure 8 and Figure 9 respectively. The STARE is a well-known database to analyze the retinal BV. Similarly, the FARI is also a noted image database widely adopted to examine the BV from the disease infected retinal section. The result of Figure 8 confirms that, proposed procedure is very efficient in extracting the BV from the normal and the infected retinal section. Similar procedure is then implemented on the FARU pictures and the result obtained

Figure 5. Results of OD examination scheme. (a1) Kapur's thresholding, (b1) Otsu's thresholding, (c1) Shannon's thresholding, (a2) OD of Kapur's + LSS, (b2) OD of Otsu's + LSS, (c2) Shannon's + LSS

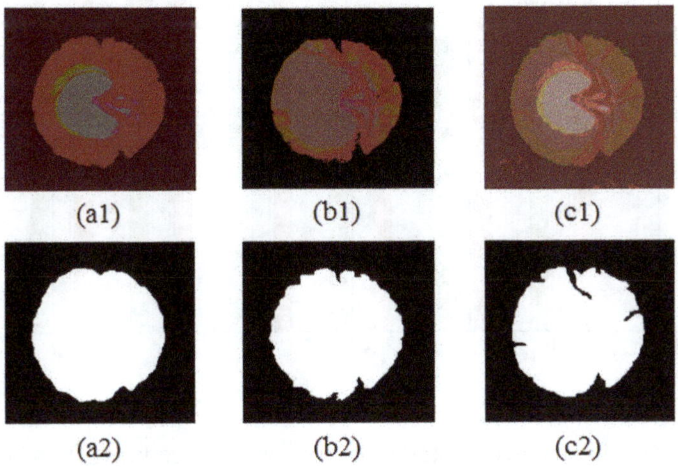

for this picture is depicted in Figure 9. The BV section of this picture is also extracted as discussed in DRIVE picture.

Table 1. PLM obtained with RIM-ONE dataset

Method	GT	TPR	FNR	TNR	FPR	JI	DC	SE	SP	AC	PR
Kapur	1	0.9971	0.0029	0.9440	0.0560	0.9077	0.9516	0.9971	0.9440	0.9632	0.9101
	2	0.9893	0.0107	0.9727	0.0273	0.9479	0.9732	0.9893	0.9727	0.9791	0.9577
	3	0.9738	0.0262	0.9812	0.0188	0.9466	0.9726	0.9738	0.9812	0.9783	0.9714
	4	0.9954	0.0046	0.9245	0.0755	0.8729	0.9321	0.9954	0.9245	0.9493	0.8764
	5	0.9959	0.0041	0.9099	0.0901	0.8471	0.9172	0.9959	0.9099	0.9391	0.8501
Otsu	1	0.9832	0.0168	0.9716	0.0284	0.9363	0.9671	0.9832	0.9716	0.9758	0.9516
	2	0.9597	0.0403	0.9909	0.0091	0.9460	0.9722	0.9597	0.9909	0.9789	0.9851
	3	0.9362	0.0638	0.9940	0.0060	0.9277	0.9625	0.9362	0.9940	0.9711	0.9903
	4	0.9859	0.0141	0.9542	0.0458	0.9085	0.9521	0.9859	0.9542	0.9653	0.9205
	5	0.9825	0.0175	0.9373	0.0627	0.8755	0.9336	0.9825	0.9373	0.9526	0.8894
Shannon	1	0.9608	0.0392	0.9587	0.0413	0.8957	0.9450	0.9608	0.9587	0.9595	0.9297
	2	0.9464	0.0536	0.9824	0.0176	0.9204	0.9586	0.9464	0.9824	0.9685	0.9711
	3	0.9239	0.0761	0.9857	0.0143	0.9042	0.9497	0.9239	0.9857	0.9612	0.9769
	4	0.9615	0.0385	0.9409	0.0591	0.8663	0.9284	0.9615	0.9409	0.9481	0.8974
	5	0.9587	0.0413	0.9249	0.0751	0.8363	0.9109	0.9587	0.9249	0.9364	0.8675

Figure 6. Average results obtained for the RIM-ONE dataset

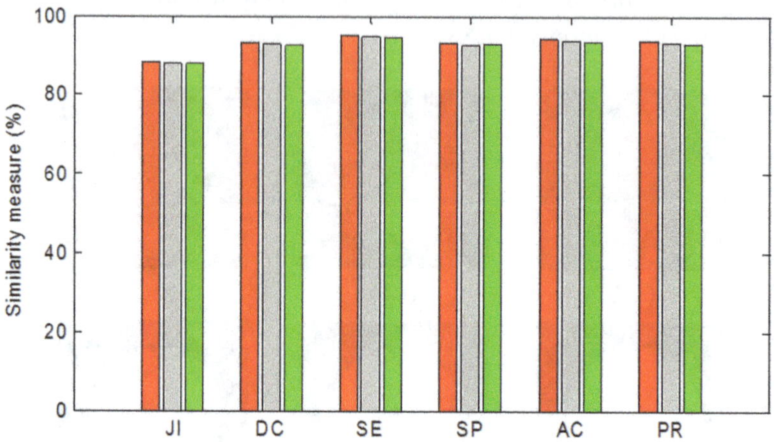

From these results, it can be noted that, proposed procedure offers better result of the other existing FRPs. The above results confirm that, the JA + MMF procedure is efficient in extracting the BV region from the RGB scale and Gray scale pictures. Hence, in future, this procedure can be used to examine the real time picture obtained from the eye testing centers.

FUTURE RESEARCH DIRECTIONS

In order to recognize the infection harshness and also to plan for the supplementary handling task, it is necessary to investigate the FRP with the help of doctors. Recently, most of the eye testing clinics has the ability to record digital fundus

Table 2. Performance metrics for RIM-ONE FRPs

Procedures	Sensitivity (%)	Specificity (%)	Accuracy (%)
Expert 1	81.9867	97.1064	95.8758
Expert 2	87.6188	97.2064	94.7085
Expert 3	91.3886	97.1895	94.6889
Expert 4	90.4135	96.1164	95.2057
Mohamed et al. (2014)	91.38	97.03	-
JA+Kapur	93.2706	97.4927	96.2632
JA+Otsu	93.1074	96.8297	95.5917
JA+Shannon	92.8122	97.1615	95.7406

Table 3. Performance metrics for DRIVE FRPs

Approaches	Sensitivity (%)	Specificity (%)	Accuracy (%)
Frederic and Klein (2001)	69.71	93.77	89.84
Moazam et al. (2012)	71.52	97.69	94.30
Bob et al. (2010)	71.20	97.24	93.82
Perez et al. (2007)	66.00	96.12	92.20
Martinez-Perez et al. (1999)	72.46	96.55	93.44
Saleh and Ali (2011)	73.52	97.95	94.58
Sreejini and Govindan (2015)	71.32	98.66	96.33
Keerthana et al. (2017)	79.16	98.03	87.19
Proposed JA+MMF	76.38	98.57	95.26

images of retina. In order to have a pre-opinion concerning the retinal irregularity in medical level, it is necessary to use an appropriate image evaluation scheme to assess the FRPs. The aim of the research work offered in this chapter is to develop a Jaya Algorithm (JA) supported semi-automated image examination to scrutinize the irregular retinal sections. In this work, image processing system based on the JA assisted Kapur's entropy and LSS is proposed to examine OD region of FRP and JA + MMF scheme to mine the BV from the chosen FRPs. This chapter focuses on extracting and analyzing the abnormal section of the retinal pictures.

Figure 7. Extracted BV for sample DRIVE FRP. (a) Pseudo name, (b) Test picture, (c) GT1, (d) GT2, (e) Mined BV using JA+MMF

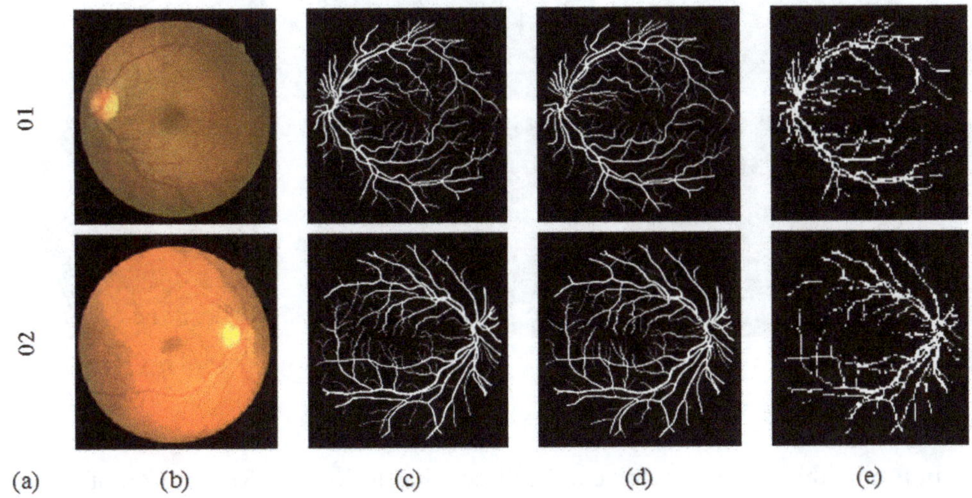

Figure 8. Mined BV for sample STARE FRP. (a) Disease condition, (b) Test picture, (e) Extracted BV

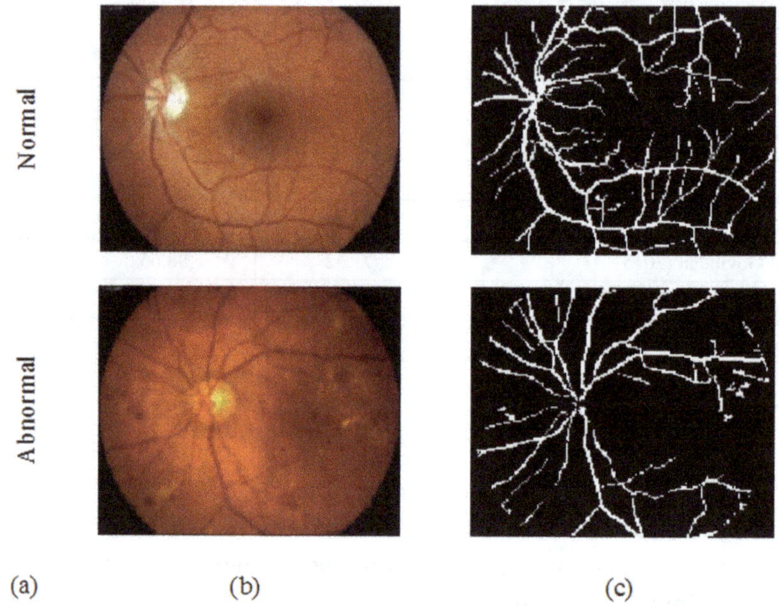

Figure 9. Testing of FARI picture. (a) Disease condition, (b) Test picture, (c) Extracted BV, (d) Complement picture

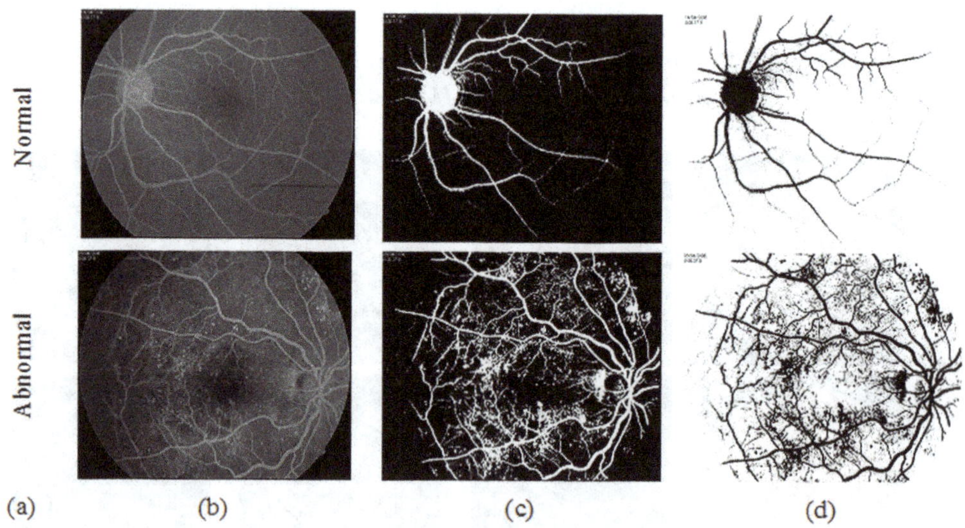

In future, this research work can be directed as follows: i) Realization of recent heuristic procedures to improve the accuracy of proposed tool, ii) Enhancing the results of OD extraction procedures by employing other thresholding procedures, such as water-shed, seed-based region-growing, principle-component-analysis, and active-contour, iii) Implementing the well-known segmentation approaches, like principal component analysis to improve the picture likeness measures, iv) Extracting texture features of the OD/BV and implementing a suitable classifier unit for the automated detection and diagnose of retinal irregularities.

CONCLUSION

The anticipated practice executes an image analyzing tool for the RGB and gray scale Retinal-Fundus-Picture (RFP) by implementing a separate scheme for Optic-Disc and Blood-Vessel using Jaya Algorithm assisted tool. The first examination approach is created based on the JA + KE based thresholding and LSS based extraction and the second tool is realized with JA + MMF to extract the BV from the RGB and gray scale FRPs. This work considers four well known retinal image datasets, like RIM-ONE, DRIVE, STARE and FARI. Initially, the proposed procedure is tested using FRPs of RIM-ONE dataset and its performance is appraised with the well known image quality measures existing in the literature. Later, the proposed approach is tested using the benchmark DRIVE, STARE and FARI dataset. The outcome of this experimental work confirms that, proposed scheme is very efficient in extracting the OD/BV from the considered FRPs with improved accuracy compared with other related existing procedures. Hence, in future, he proposed schemes can be used to inspect the real clinical retinal images.

REFERENCES

Anitha, P., Bindhiya, S., Abinaya, A., Satapathy, S. C., Dey, N., & Rajinikanth, V. (2017). RGB image multi-thresholding based on Kapur's entropy—A study with heuristic algorithms. In *Proceedings of Second International Conference on Electrical, Computer and Communication Technologies (ICECCT)*. 10.1109/ICECCT.2017.8117823

Ashour, A. S., Samanta, S., Dey, N., Kausar, N., Abdessalemkaraa, W. B., & Hassanien, A. E. (2015). Computed tomography image enhancement using cuckoo search: A log transform based approach. *Journal of Signal and Information Processing*, *6*(3), 244–257. doi:10.4236/jsip.2015.63023

Balan, N. S., Kumar, A. S., Raja, N. S. M., & Rajinikanth, V. (2016). Optimal multilevel image thresholding to improve the visibility of plasmodium sp. in blood smear images. *Advances in Intelligent Systems and Computing*, *397*, 563–571. doi:10.1007/978-81-322-2671-0_54

Bob, Z., Lin, Z., Lei, Z., & Fakhri, K. (2010). Retinal vessel extraction by matched filter with first order derivative of Gaussian. *Computers in Biology and Medicine*, *40*(4), 438–445. doi:10.1016/j.compbiomed.2010.02.008 PMID:20202631

Caselles, V., Catte, F., Coll, T., & Dibos, F. (1993). A geometric model for active contours in image processing. *Numerische Mathematik*, *66*(1), 1–31. doi:10.1007/BF01385685

Chaddad, A., & Tanougast, C. (2016). Quantitative evaluation of robust skull stripping and tumor detection applied to axial MR images. *Brain Informatics*, *3*(1), 53–61. doi:10.100740708-016-0033-7 PMID:27747598

Dey, N., Rajinikanth, V., Amira, S., Ashour, A. S., & Tavares, J. M. R. S. (2018). Social Group Optimization Supported Segmentation and Evaluation of Skin Melanoma Images. *Symmetry*, *10*(2), 51. doi:10.3390ym10020051

Esmaeili, M., Rabbani, H., Dehnavi, A. M., & Dehghani, A. (2012). Automatic detection of exudates and optic disk in retinal images using curvelet transform. *IET Image Processing*, *6*(7), 1005–1013. doi:10.1049/iet-ipr.2011.0333

Fernandes, S. L., Gurupur, V. P., Lin, H., & Martis, R. J. (2017). A novel fusion approach for early lung cancer detection using computer aided diagnosis techniques. *Journal of Medical Imaging and Health Informatics*, *7*(8), 1841–1850. doi:10.1166/jmihi.2017.2280

Frederic, Z., & Klein, J. C. (2001). Segmentation of vessel-like patterns using mathematical morphology and curvature evaluation. *IEEE Transactions on Image Processing*, *10*(7), 1010–1019. doi:10.1109/83.931095 PMID:18249674

Fumero, F., Alayon, S., Sanchez, J. L., Sigut, J., & Gonzalez-Hernandez, M. (2011). RIM-ONE: An open retinal image database for optic nerve evaluation. In *2011 24th International Symposium on Computer-Based Medical Systems (CBMS),* 1–6.

Golabbakhsh, M., & Rabbani, H. (2013). Vessel-based registration of fundus and optical coherence tomography projection images of retina using a quadratic registration model. *IET Image Processing*, *7*(8), 768–776. doi:10.1049/iet-ipr.2013.0116

Hajeb, S. H., Rabbani, H., & Akhlaghi, M. R. (2012). Diabetic retinopathy grading by digital curvelet transform. Computational and Mathematical Methods in Medicine, 1607-1614.

Hajeb, S. H., Rabbani, H., & Akhlaghi, M. R. (2014). A new combined method based on curvelet transform and morphological operators for automatic detection of foveal avascular zone. *Signal, Image and Video Processing*, *8*(2), 205–222. doi:10.100711760-013-0530-6

Hoover, A., & Goldbaum, M. (2003). Locating the optic nerve in a retinal image using the fuzzy convergence of the blood vessels. *IEEE Transactions on Medical Imaging*, *22*(8), 951–958. doi:10.1109/TMI.2003.815900 PMID:12906249

Hoover, A., Kouznetsova, V., & Goldbaum, M. (2000). Locating blood vessels in retinal images by piece-wise threhsold probing of a matched filter response. *IEEE Transactions on Medical Imaging*, *19*(3), 203–210. doi:10.1109/42.845178 PMID:10875704

Jahromi, M. K., Kafieh, R., Rabbani, H., & .... (2014). An automatic algorithm for segmentation of the boundaries of corneal layers in optical coherence tomography images using gaussian mixture model. *Journal of Medical Signals and Sensors*, *4*(3), 171–180. PMID:25298926

Kapur, J. N., Sahoo, P. K., & Wong, A. K. C. (1985). A new method for gray-level picture thresholding using the entropy of the histogram. *Computer Vision Graphics and Image Processing*, *29*(3), 273–285. doi:10.1016/0734-189X(85)90125-2

Keerthana, K., Jayasuriya, T. J., Raja, N. S. M., & Rajinikanth, V. (2017). Retinal vessel extraction based on firefly algorithm guided multi-scale matched filter. *Int J Mod Sci Technol*, *2*(2), 74–80.

Lakshmi, V. S., Tebby, S. G., Shriranjani, D., & Rajinikanth, V. (2016). Chaotic cuckoo search and Kapur/Tsallis approach in segmentation of T.cruzi from blood smear images. *Int. J. Comp. Sci. Infor. Sec. (IJCSIS)*, 14, 51-56.

Li, C., Xu, C., Gui, C., & Fox, M. D. (2010). Distance regularized level set evolution and its application to image segmentation. *IEEE Transactions on Image Processing*, *19*(12), 3243–3254. doi:10.1109/TIP.2010.2069690 PMID:20801742

Mahmudi, T., Kafieh, R., & Rabbani, H. (2014, Feb. 15-20). Comparison of macular OCTs in right and left eyes of normal people. In *Proc. SPIE 9038, Medical Imaging 2014: Biomedical Applications in Molecular, Structural, and Functional Imaging, 90381K*, San Diego, CA. doi:10.1117/12.2044046

Malladi, R., Sethian, J. A., & Vemuri, B. C. (1995). Shape modeling with front propagation: A level set approach. *IEEE T. Pattern Anal. Mac. Int.*, *17*(2), 158–175. doi:10.1109/34.368173

Manic, K. S., Naimi, I. S. I., Hasoon, F. N., & Rajinikanth, V. (2019). Jaya algorithm-assisted evaluation of tooth elements using digital bitewing radiography images. *Computational Techniques for Dental Image Analysis,* 107-128. doi:. doi:10.4018/978-1-5225-6243-6.ch005

Martínez-Pérez, M. E., Hughes, A. D., Stanton, A. V., Thom, S. A., Bharath, A. A., & Parker, K. H. (1999, September). Retinal blood vessel segmentation by means of scale-space analysis and region growing. In International Conference on Medical Image Computing and Computer-Assisted Intervention (pp. 90-97). Springer, Berlin, Germany.

Moazam, F. M., Barman, S. A., Paolo, R., Andreas, H., Abdul, B., Bunyarit, U., ... Christopher, O. G. (2012). An approach to localize the retinal blood vessels using bit planes and centerline detection. *Computer Methods and Programs in Biomedicine*, *108*(2), 600–616. doi:10.1016/j.cmpb.2011.08.009 PMID:21963241

Mohamed, N. A., Zulkifley, M. A., & Hussain, A. (2014). Local binary patterns for optic disc segmentation. In *Proceedings of International Conference on Applied Computer and Applied Computational Science*, 149–153. doi:10.1109/ISCAIE.2015.7298324

Niemeijer, M., Staal, J. J., Ginneken, B. V., Loog, M., & Abramoff, M. D. (2004). Comparative study of retinal vessel segmentation methods on a new publicly available database. In *J. M. Fitzpatrick & M. Sonka (Eds.), S.* P. I. E. Medical Imaging, 5370, pp. 648–656. doi:10.1117/12.535349

Perez, M., Alun, H. D., Thorn, S. A., & Kim, P. H. (2007). Improvement of a retinal blood vessel segmentation method using the insight segmentation and registration toolkit (ITK). In *29th Annual International Conference of the Engineering in Medicine and Biology Society, EMBS 2007.* Piscataway, NJ: IEEE. 892-895.

Rabbani, H., Allingham, M. J., Mettu, P. S., Cousins, S. W., & Farsiu, S. (2015). Fully automatic segmentation of fluorescein leakage in subjects with diabetic macular edema. *Investigative Ophthalmology & Visual Science*, *56*(3), 1482–1492. doi:10.1167/iovs.14-15457 PMID:25634978

Raja, N. S. M., Kavitha, G., & Ramakrishnan, S. (2012). Analysis of vasculature in human retinal images using particle swarm optimization based Tsallis multi-level thresholding and similarity measures. *Lecture Notes in Computer Science*, *7677*, 380–387. doi:10.1007/978-3-642-35380-2_45

Rajinikanth, V., Dey, N., Kumar, R., Panneerselvam, J., & Raja, N. S. M. (2019). Fetal head periphery extraction from ultrasound image using Jaya algorithm and Chan-Vese segmentation. *Procedia Computer Science*, *152*, 66–73. doi:10.1016/j.procs.2019.05.028

Rajinikanth, V., Raja, N. S. M., Satapathy, S. C., & Fernandes, S. L. (2017). Otsu's multi-thresholding and active contour snake model to segment dermoscopy images. *Journal of Medical Imaging and Health Informatics*, *7*(8), 1837–1840. doi:10.1166/jmihi.2017.2265

Rao, R. V. (2016). Jaya: A simple and new optimization algorithm for solving constrained and unconstrained optimization problems. *International Journal of Industrial Engineering Computations*, *7*, 19–34.

Rao, R. V., & More, K. C. (2017). Design optimization and analysis of selected thermal devices using self-adaptive Jaya algorithm. *Energy Conversion and Management*, *140*, 24–35. doi:10.1016/j.enconman.2017.02.068

Saleh, M. M., & Ali, M. (2011). Retinal image analysis using curvelet transform and multistructure elements morphology by reconstruction. *IEEE Transactions on Biomedical Engineering*, *58*(5), 1183–1192. doi:10.1109/TBME.2010.2097599 PMID:21147592

Satapathy, S. C. & Rajinikanth, V. (2018). Jaya algorithm guided procedure to segment tumor from brain MRI. *Journal of Optimization*. doi:10.1155/2018/3738049

Shree, V. T. D., Revanth, K., Raja, N. S. M., & Rajinikanth, V. (2018). A hybrid image processing approach to examine abnormality in retinal optic disc. *Procedia Computer Science*, *125*, 157–164. doi:10.1016/j.procs.2017.12.022

Shriranjani, D., Tebby, S. G., Satapathy, S. C., Dey, N., & Rajinikanth, V. (2018). Kapur's entropy and active contour-based segmentation and analysis of retinal optic disc. *Lecture Notes in Electrical Engineering*, *490*, 287–295. doi:10.1007/978-981-10-8354-9_26

Sivakamasundari, J., Kavitha, G., Natarajan, V., & Ramakrishnan, S. (2015). An approach to content based retinal image retrieval using papamarkos multilevel thresholding method. *J. Med. Imaging Health Inf.*, *5*(3), 527–532. doi:10.1166/jmihi.2015.1419

Sofka, M., & Stewart, C. V. (2006). Retinal vessel centerline extraction using multiscale matched filters, confidence and edge measures. *IEEE Transactions on Medical Imaging*, *25*(12), 1531–1546. doi:10.1109/TMI.2006.884190 PMID:17167990

Sreejini, K. S., & Govindan, V. K. (2015). Improved multiscale matched filter for retina vessel segmentation using PSO algorithm. *Egyptian Informatics Journal, 16*(3), 253–260. doi:10.1016/j.eij.2015.06.004

Staal, J. J., Abramoff, M. D., Niemeijer, M., Viergever, M. A., & Ginneken, B. V. (2004). Ridge based vessel segmentation in color images of the retina. *IEEE Transactions on Medical Imaging, 23*(4), 501–509. doi:10.1109/TMI.2004.825627 PMID:15084075

Sudhan, G. H. H., Aravind, R. G., Gowri, K., & Rajinikanth, V. (2017). Optic disc segmentation based on Otsu's thresholding and level set. In *International Conference on Computer Communication and Informatics (ICCCI)*. 10.1109/ICCCI.2017.8117688

Vaishnavi, G. K., Jeevananthan, K., Begum, S. R., & Kamalanand, K. (2014). Geometrical analysis of schistosome egg images using distance regularized level set method for automated species identification. *J. Bioinformatics Intell. Cont, 3*(2), 147–152. doi:10.1166/jbic.2014.1080

Wang, S., Rao, R. V., Chen, P., Zhang, Y., Liu, A., & Wei, L. (2017). Abnormal breast detection in mammogram images by feed-forward neural network trained by Jaya algorithm. *Fundamenta Informaticae, 151*(1-4), 191–211. doi:10.3233/FI-2017-1487

Wilkinson, C. P., Ferris, F. L. III, Klein, R. E., Lee, P. P., Agardh, C. D., Davis, M., ... Verdaguer, J. T. (2003). Proposed international clinical diabetic retinopathy and diabetic macular edema disease severity scales. *Ophthalmology, 110*(9), 1677–1682. doi:10.1016/S0161-6420(03)00475-5 PMID:13129861

ADDITIONAL READING

Admin. (n.d.). Algorithm Validation. Retrieved from http://medimrg.webs.ull.es/research/retinal-imaging/rim-one/

DRIVE. Digital Retinal Images for Vessel Extraction. (n.d.). Retrieved from https://www.isi.uu.nl/Research/Databases/DRIVE/The Stare Project. (n.d.). STructured Analysis of the Retina. Retrieved from http://cecas.clemson.edu/~ahoover/stare/ Available Datasets. (n.d.). Available Datasets - Dr Hossein Rabbani. Retrieved from https://sites.google.com/site/hosseinrabbanikhorasgani/datasets-1

Chapter 11
Classification of Skin Lesion Using (Segmentation) Shape Feature Detection

Satheesha T.Y.
Department of Electrical and Computer Engineering, School of Engineering and Technology, CMR University, Bangalore, India

ABSTRACT

Malignant melanoma has caused countless deaths in recent years. Many calculation methods have been created for automatic melanoma detection. In this chapter, based on the traditional concept of shape signature and convex hull, an improved boundary description shape signature is developed. The convex defect-based signature (CDBS) proposed in this paper scans contour irregularities and is applied to skin lesion classification in macroscopic images. Border irregularities of skin lesions are the predominant criteria for ABCD (asymmetry, border, color, and diameter) to distinguish between melanoma and nonmelanoma. The performance of the CDBS is compared with popular shape descriptors: shape signature, indentation depth function, invariant elliptic Fourier descriptor (IEFD), and rotation invariant wavelet descriptor (RIWD), where the proposed descriptor shows better results. Multilayer perceptron neural network is used as a classifier in this work. Experimental results show that the proposed approach achieves significant performance with mean accuracy of 90.49%.

DOI: 10.4018/978-1-7998-0326-3.ch011

INTRODUCTION

Skin cancer is known as one of the most usual forms of cancer in different countries (Oliveira et al., 2016). There are three commonly known types of skin cancers including basal cell carcinoma (BCC), squamous cell carcinomas (SCC), and melanoma. However, malignant melanoma is considered as the deadliest type of skin cancers and is the cause of majority of deaths (75%) related to skin cancer (Jerant et al., 2000). The American Cancer Society estimated that there will be about 87110 new cases (52170 in men and 34940 in women) and about 9730 deaths (6380 in men and 3350 in women) related to melanoma in the United States in 2017 ("American Cancer Society", 2017).

Early detection of melanoma can help dermatologists find appropriate treatment and survive patient (Jerant et al., 2000). The clinical methods for diagnosing skin lesions are established on visual examination. Several approaches were suggested by dermatologists, such as ABCD(E) (asymmetry, border, color, diameter, and evolution) (Blum et al., 2003; Nachbar et al., 1994), seven-point check list (MacKie & Doherty, 1991), and Menzies method (Menzies et al., 1996).

Rapidly growth of melanoma incidence rate and also possibility of misdiagnosis encouraged the development of computational methods for melanoma detection. Principal steps of computer aided diagnosis (CAD) systems for identifying skin lesions include image acquisition, preprocessing, segmentation, feature extraction, and classification (Wighton et al., 2011).

Macroscopy and dermoscopy are common non-invasive imaging techniques of skin lesions (Smith & MacNeil, 2011). Whereas dermoscopic images are captured by a proper device to provide a magnified visualization of the skin surface, macroscopic images are ac- quired by standard camera, a more accessible device (Engasser & Warshaw, 2010).

The rest of this paper is organized as follows. Section II presents the newly suggested descriptor, its feature set, and also a shape and textural feature set. Section III discusses the experimental results of the proposed feature set. Finally, Section IV provides the summary and conclusion.

PROPOSED METHOD

In this section, we represent our extension to the shape sig- nature and show it can be more helpful in describing a concave contour in comparison with the conventional shape signature. The new signature is created based on a known concept: convex hull. Hence, we firstly give the definition of conventional signature and convex hull and then define the new signature. Finally, a dozen of shape and textural feature set will be presented to link with new signature attributes to improve melanoma prognosis.

Conventional Shape Signature

Shape signature is a common method for one-dimensional description of shape contour.

Shape signature is a common method for one-dimensional description of shape contour. For a closed contour $C(t) = (x(t), y(t))$: $[1, T] \rightarrow \mathbb{N}2$, (Gon^zalez & Woods, 2008).

For example, signature curve of a melanoma lesion is depicted in Figure 1(c). While for an arbitrary θ melanoma lesion (Figure 1(a)) has three intersection points, its equivalent signature curve only considers the first centroid distance. Also, shaded region in Figure 1(a) shows the region that is not properly de- scribed by shape signature.

Convex Deficiency Based Signature

The convex hull of a region is the smallest convex region containing it. Convex hull is a useful tool for shape description, particularly when the shape boundary includes significant con- cavities (Gonzalez & Woods, 2008).

As an example, Figure 1(a) demonstrates contour of a melanoma lesion and its convex hull. The CDBS curves of melanoma lesion is plotted in Figure 1(d). It is comprehended from CDBS diagram that shapes with abrupt boundaries have more significant peaks on their CDBS curves, and also shape with smooth boundaries tend to have more zero-incidence points. Therefore, concavities of non-convex contours can be exhibited accurately by CDBS curve is plotted in Figure 1(c).

EXPERIMENTAL RESULTS

Dataset Description

The datasets used in this paper comprise 206 macroscopic images which were extracted from online databases Dermatology Information System ("Dermatology Information System", 2012) and DermQuest (2012). These images categorized into two types: malignant melanoma (119 images) and nevi or non-melanoma (87 images).

Figure 1. Illustrations of shape signature and proposed CDBS curves of a melanoma lesion

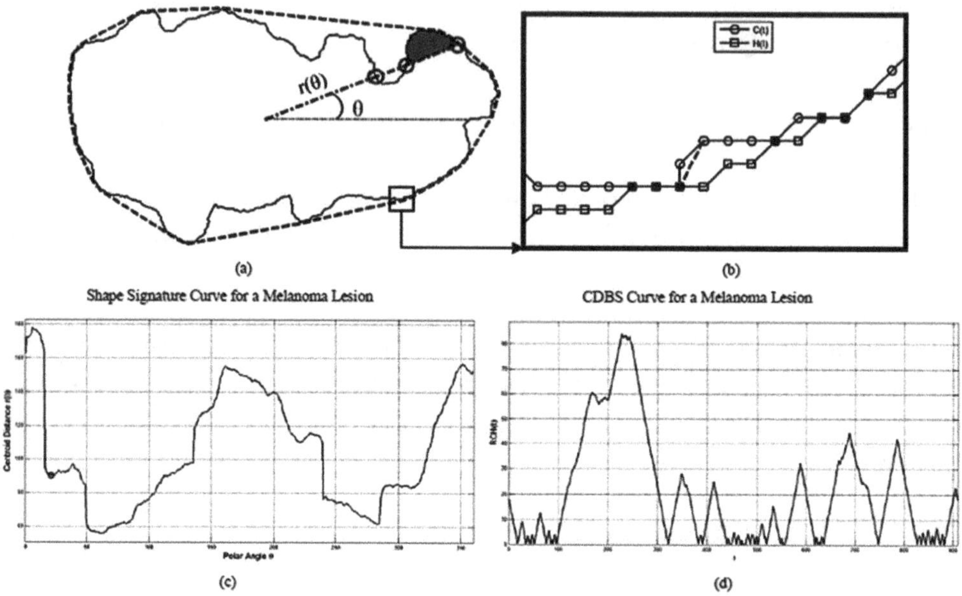

Preprocessing

In this step, in order to preserve rotation-invariant of images, first each image was rotated until major axis of lesion that passes through its center was aligned with the horizontal axis. Then, shading attenuation model of healthy skin (Cavalcanti and Scharcanski, 2011) was per- formed to attenuate illumination artifacts of input macroscopic images. An example of applying this method on a melanoma lesion is illustrated in Figure 2.

Figure 2. Example of applying shading attenuation method. (a) Original melanoma image; (b) Result of applying shading attenuation method on (a).

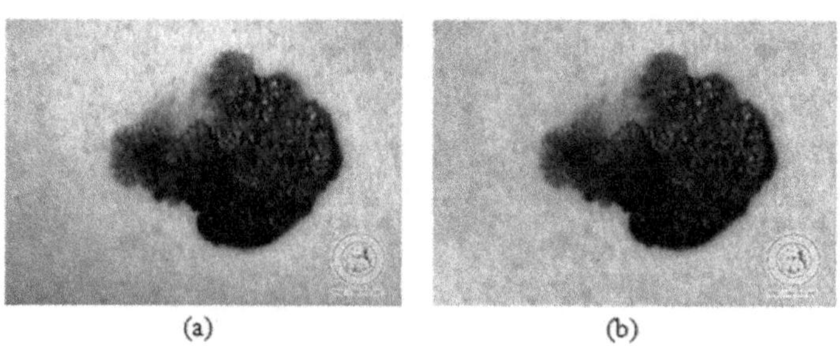

Classification

Classification step was evaluated by measuring average performance of the procedure across 10 individual trials. In each trial, 5-fold cross-validation was employed to randomly split samples into 5 folds. Then, training and testing phases were repeated 5 times with different train and test subsamples to obtain classification performance. Therefore, each time 4 folds (80% of samples) were used for training process and one remaining fold (20% of samples) was used for testing process. Finally, outcomes of this process were computed using statistical measures accuracy, sensitivity, specificity, and precision, which are defined in (1) to (4).

$$\text{Accuracy} = (TP+TN) / (TP+FP+FN+TN) \tag{1}$$

$$\text{Sensitivity} = (TP) / (TP+FN) \tag{2}$$

$$\text{Specificity} = (TN) / (TN+FP) \tag{3}$$

$$\text{Precision} = (TP) / (TP+FP) \tag{4}$$

where, TP (true positive) and TN (true negative) respectively are number of correct melanoma and non melanoma estimations, and FP (false positive) and FN (false negative) respectively are number of incorrect melanoma and non-melanoma estimations.

RESULTS AND DISCUSSION

In experiments, Fourier descriptor (Gonzalez & Woods, 2008) is computed separately for the proposed CDBS and four mentioned boundary descriptors. The Fourier coefficients are normalized with first one. The first 20 coefficients of Fourier descriptor (except the first one which is always "1") were employed for evaluation.

Also, RIWD coefficients are calculated in four levels using approximation coefficients of "Daubechies" wavelet, and coefficients of each level are evaluated separately. The first 20 coefficients of IEFD, and RIWD in the first 3 levels (except the first one) were utilized. Also, for the 4th level of RIWD, only the first 10 coefficients (except the first one) were used. Feature extraction is a part of recognition procedure, so its run-time can be considered as a complexity measure of the algorithm in skin

Table 1. Comparision of classification results and feature extraction run-time among proposed cdbs in this work and common boundary descriptors (shape signature, indentation depth function, iefds, and riwds)

Feature set	*NOFs.	*Acc. (%)	*Sen. (%)	*Spe. (%)	*Pre. (%)	*FERT. (sec)
Signature (Fourier descriptor)	19	55.91	63.35	**45.75**	61.07	16.40
Indentation depth function (Fourier descriptor)	19	36.63	40.20	31.87	45.74	31.20
IEFDs	19	49.98	66.06	27.78	55.97	251.82
RIWDs (1st level)	19	54.31	70.91	31.67	60.91	13.77
RIWDs (2nd level)	19	55.85	70.57	35.95	60.52	13.91
RIWDs (3rd level)	19	56.21	72.29	34.19	60.30	14.11
RIWDs (4th level)	9	55.29	72.33	31.89	59.10	14.44
Proposed CDBS (Fourier descriptor)	19	**59.71**	**73.15**	41.37	**63.49**	**12.91**

*NOFs: Number of features, Acc: Accuracy, Sen: Sensitivity, Spe: Specificity, Pre: Precision, FERT: Feature Extraction Run-Time.

Best result of each measure and lowest feature extraction run-time are marked in boldface.

lesion diagnosis problem. Feature extraction run-time (FERT) is computed as time spent (in seconds) to compute entire features of the set for all samples. The computed FERTs for acquiring Fourier coefficients of the CDBS and four mentioned boundary descriptors are represented in the last column of Table I.

CONCLUSION

In this paper, a new boundary descriptor was introduced in order to improve the performance of melanoma detection. Shape signature and convex hull models were used to create the proposed descriptor that was called CDBS. A consistent feature set was designed for CDBS to describe border irregularity and shape concavity of skin lesions. Result analysis indicated that the proposed feature vector has robust features for an automatic melanoma diagnosis framework, since it has highest classification outcomes and less feature dimension in comparison with previous works on Dermatology Information System and DermQuest datasets.

REFERENCES

(2017, March 1). American Cancer Society. (2017). *Cancer facts & figures 2017*. Available at https://www.cancer.org/research/cancer-factsstatistics.Html

Blum, A., Rassner, G., & Garbe, C. (2003). Modified ABC-point list of dermoscopy: A simplified and highly accurate dermoscopic algorithm for the diagnosis of cutaneous melanocytic lesions. *Journal of the American Academy of Dermatology*, *48*(5), 672–678. doi:10.1067/mjd.2003.282 PMID:12734495

Cavalcanti, P. G., & Scharcanski, J. (2011). Automated prescreening of pigmented skin lesions using standard cameras. *Computerized Medical Imaging and Graphics*, *35*(6), 481–491. doi:10.1016/j.compmedimag.2011.02.007 PMID:21489751

Dermatology Information System. (2012). Available at http://www.dermis.net

DermQuest. (2012). Available at http://www.dermquest.com

Engasser, H. C. & Warshaw, E. M. (2010). Dermatoscopy use by US dermatologists: a cross-sectional survey. *Journal of the American Academy of Dermatology, 63,* pp. 412-419. e2.

Gonzalez, R. C. & Woods, R. E. (2008). Digital image processing. Upper Saddle River, NJ: Prentice Hall.

Jerant, A. F., Johnson, J. T., Sheridan, C., & Caffrey, T. J. (2000). Early detection and treatment of skin cancer. *American Family Physician*, *62*, 357–386. PMID:10929700

MacKie, R., & Doherty, V. (1991). Seven-point checklist for melanoma. *Clinical and Experimental Dermatology*, *16*(2), 151–152. doi:10.1111/j.1365-2230.1991.tb00329.x PMID:1867692

Menzies, S. W., Ingvar, C., Crotty, K. A., & McCarthy, W. H. (1996). Frequency and morphologic characteristics of invasive melanomas lacking specific surface microscopic features. *Archives of Dermatology*, *132*(10), 1178–1182. doi:10.1001/archderm.1996.03890340038007 PMID:8859028

Nachbar, F., Stolz, W., Merkle, T., Cognetta, A. B., Vogt, T., Landthaler, M., ... Plewig, G. (1994). The ABCD rule of dermatoscopy: High prospective value in the diagnosis of doubtful melanocytic skin lesions. *Journal of the American Academy of Dermatology*, *30*(4), 551–559. doi:10.1016/S0190-9622(94)70061-3 PMID:8157780

Oliveira, R. B., Papa, J. P., Pereira, A. S., & Tavares, J. M. R. (2016). Computational methods for pigmented skin lesion classification in images: Review and future trends. *Neural Computing & Applications*, 1–24.

Smith, L., & MacNeil, S. (2011). State of the art in non-invasive imaging of cutaneous melanoma. *Skin Research and Technology*, *17*(3), 257–269. doi:10.1111/j.1600-0846.2011.00503.x PMID:21342292

Wighton, P., Lee, T. K., Lui, H., McLean, D. I., & Atkins, M. S. (2011). Generalizing common tasks in automated skin lesion diagnosis. *IEEE Transactions on Information Technology in Biomedicine*, *15*(4), 622–629. doi:10.1109/TITB.2011.2150758 PMID:21550892

Compilation of References

(2017, March 1). American Cancer Society. (2017). *Cancer facts & figures 2017*. Available at https://www.cancer.org/research/cancer-factsstatistics.Html

Abdelnabi, M. H. (2019). Cardiovascular clinical implications of heart rate variability. *International Journal of the Cardiovascular Academy*, *5*(2), 37. doi:10.4103/IJCA.IJCA_36_18

Abiyev, R. H., Akkaya, N., Aytac, E., Günsel, I., & Çağman, A. (2016). Brain-Computer Interface for Control of Wheelchair Using Fuzzy Neural Networks. *BioMed Research International*, *2016*, 1–9. doi:10.1155/2016/9359868 PMID:27777953

Abou-Abbas, L., Tadj, C., & Fersaie, H. A. (2017). A fully automated approach for baby cry signal segmentation and boundary detection of expiratory and inspiratory episodes. *The Journal of the Acoustical Society of America*, *142*(3), 1318–1331. doi:10.1121/1.5001491 PMID:28964073

Acharya, R. U., Lim, C. M., & Joseph, P. (2002). Heart rate variability analysis using correlation dimension and detrended fluctuation analysis. *ITBM-RBM*, *23*(6), 333–339. doi:10.1016/S1297-9562(02)90002-1

Acharya, R., Kannathal, N., Sing, O. W., Ping, L. Y., & Chua, T. (2004). Heart rate analysis in normal subjects of various age groups. *Biomedical Engineering Online*, *3*(1), 24. doi:10.1186/1475-925X-3-24 PMID:15260880

Acharya, U. R., Joseph, K. P., Kannathal, N., Lim, C. M., & Suri, J. S. (2006). Heart rate variability: A review. *Medical & Biological Engineering & Computing*, *44*(12), 1031–1051. doi:10.100711517-006-0119-0 PMID:17111118

Agelink, M. W., Malessa, R., Baumann, B., Majewski, T., Akila, F., Zeit, T., & Ziegler, D. (2001). Standardized tests of heart rate variability: Normal ranges obtained from 309 healthy humans, and effects of age, gender, and heart rate. *Clinical Autonomic Research*, *11*(2), 99–108. doi:10.1007/BF02322053 PMID:11570610

Aggarwal, Y., Singh, N., Ghosh, S., & Sinha, R. K. (2014). Eye Gaze–Induced Mental Stress Alters the Heart Rate Variability Analysis. *Journal of Clinical Engineering*, *39*(2), 79–89. doi:10.1097/JCE.0000000000000023

Akbulut, F. P., & Akan, A. (2018). A smart wearable system for short term cardiovascular risk assessment with emotional dynamics. *Measurement*, *128*, 237–246. doi:10.1016/j.measurement.2018.06.050

Alesanco, A., & Garcıa, J. (2010). Clinical Assessment of Wireless ECG Transmission in Real-Time Cardiac Telemonitoring. *IEEE Transactions on Information Technology in Biomedicine*, *14*(5), 1144–1152. doi:10.1109/TITB.2010.2047650 PMID:20378476

Al-Fahoum, A. S., & Al-Fraihat, A. A. (2014). Methods of EEG Signal Features Extraction Using Linear Analysis in Frequency and Time-Frequency Domains. *ISRN Neuroscience*, *2014*, 1–7. doi:10.1155/2014/730218 PMID:24967316

Ang, K. K., Chin, Z. Y., Zhang, H., & Guan, C. (2008). Filter bank common spatial pattern (FBCSP) in brain-computer interface. In *IEEE International Joint Conference On Neural Networks. (IEEE World Congress on Computational Intelligence)*, 2390–2397. Piscataway, NJ: IEEE.

Ang, K. K., Chin, Z. Y., Wang, C., Guan, C., & Zhang, H. (2012). Filter Bank Common Spatial Pattern Algorithm on BCI Competition IV Datasets 2a and 2b. *Frontiers in Neuroscience*, *6*. doi:10.3389/fnins.2012.00039 PMID:22479236

Anitha, P., Bindhiya, S., Abinaya, A., Satapathy, S. C., Dey, N., & Rajinikanth, V. (2017). RGB image multi-thresholding based on Kapur's entropy—A study with heuristic algorithms. In *Proceedings of Second International Conference on Electrical, Computer and Communication Technologies (ICECCT)*. 10.1109/ICECCT.2017.8117823

Ansari, S. (2017). Novel developments and trends of analytical methods for drug analysis in biological and environmental samples by molecularly imprinted polymers. *TrAC Trends in Analytical Chemistry*, *89*, 146–162.

Anthea, M., Hopkins, J., McLaughlin, C. W., Johnson, S., Warner, M. Q., LaHart, D., & Wright, J. D. (1993). *Human biology and health. 1993*. Englewood Cliffs, NJ: Prentice Hall.

Antoch, G., Stattaus, J., Nemat, A. T., Marnitz, S., Beyer, T., Kuehl, H., ... Freudenberg, L. S. (2003). Non–small cell lung cancer: Dual-modality PET/CT in preoperative staging. *Radiology*, *229*(2), 526–533. doi:10.1148/radiol.2292021598 PMID:14512512

Arcaute, K., Mann, B. K., & Wicker, R. B. (2006). Stereolithography of three-dimensional bioactive poly (ethylene glycol) constructs with encapsulated cells. *Annals of Biomedical Engineering*, *34*(9), 1429–1441.

Arole, V. M. (2014). Fabrication of nanomaterials by top-down and bottom-up approaches-an overview. JAAST:Material Science, 89-93.

Arun, U., Sriraam, N., & Avvaru, S. (2016, October). Study and investigation of continuous cardiac monitoring using vernier EKG with myRIO processor. In 2016 International Conference on Circuits, Controls, Communications and Computing (I4C) (pp. 1-4). IEEE.

Ashour, A. S., Samanta, S., Dey, N., Kausar, N., Abdessalemkaraa, W. B., & Hassanien, A. E. (2015). Computed tomography image enhancement using cuckoo search: A log transform based approach. *Journal of Signal and Information Processing*, *6*(3), 244–257. doi:10.4236/jsip.2015.63023

Ávila, H. M., Schwarz, S., Rotter, N., & Gatenholm, P. (2016). 3D bioprinting of human chondrocyte-laden nanocellulose hydrogels for patient-specific auricular cartilage regeneration. *Bioprinting*, *1*, 22–35.

Azar, A. T., & El-Said, S. A. (2014). Performance analysis of support vector machines classifiers in breast cancer mammography recognition. *Neural Computing & Applications*, *24*(5), 1163–1177. doi:10.100700521-012-1324-4

Baars, B. J. (2005). Global workspace theory of consciousness: Toward a cognitive neuroscience of human experience. *Progress in Brain Research*, *150*, 45–53. doi:10.1016/S0079-6123(05)50004-9 PMID:16186014

Bajura, M., & Fuchs, H. (1992). Merging virtual objects with the real world: seeing ultrasound imagery within the patient. In *proceedings of the 19th annual conference on computer graphics and interactive techniques.* (pp. 203-210), New York, NY. 10.1145/133994.134061

Balan, N. S., Kumar, A. S., Raja, N. S. M., & Rajinikanth, V. (2016). Optimal multilevel image thresholding to improve the visibility of plasmodium sp. in blood smear images. *Advances in Intelligent Systems and Computing*, *397*, 563–571. doi:10.1007/978-81-322-2671-0_54

Barton, A. J., Sagers, R. D., & Pitt, W. G. (1996). Bacterial adhesion to orthopedic implant polymers. *Journal of Biomedical Materials Research: An Official Journal of The Society for Biomaterials and The Japanese Society for Biomaterials*, *30*(3), 403–410.

Bashar, S. K., Hassan, A. R., & Bhuiyan, M. I. H. (2015). Identification of motor imagery movements from EEG signals using Dual Tree Complex Wavelet Transform. *2015 International Conference on Advances in Computing, Communications and Informatics (ICACCI)*, 290–296. 10.1109/ICACCI.2015.7275623

Ben Ali, M., Ondarcuhu, T., Brust, M., & Joachim, C. (2002). Atomic force microscope tip nanoprinting of gold nanoclusters. *Langmuir*, *18*(3), 872–876.

Berry, D. A., Cronin, K. A., Plevritis, S. K., Fryback, D. G., Clarke, L., Zelen, M., & Feuer, E. J. (2005). Effect of screening and adjuvant therapy on mortality from breast cancer. *The New England Journal of Medicine*, *353*(17), 1784–1792. doi:10.1056/NEJMoa050518 PMID:16251534

Bettermann, H., Kröz, M., Girke, M., & Heckmann, C. (2001). Heart rate dynamics and cardiorespiratory coordination in diabetic and breast cancer patients. *Clinical Physiology and Functional Imaging*, *21*(4), 411–420. PMID:11442574

Bhatia, S. (2016). Nanoparticles types, classification, characterization, fabrication methods and drug delivery applications. In *Natural polymer drug delivery systems* (pp. 33–93). Cham: Springer.

Bi, L., Fan, X., & Liu, Y. (2013). EEG-Based Brain-Controlled Mobile Robots: A Survey. *IEEE Transactions on Human-Machine Systems*, *43*(2), 161–176. doi:10.1109/TSMCC.2012.2219046

Billiet, T., Gevaert, E., De Schryver, T., Cornelissen, M., & Dubruel, P. (2014). The 3D printing of gelatin methacrylamide cell-laden tissue-engineered constructs with high cell viability. *Biomaterials*, *35*(1), 49–62.

Blagden, S. P., Charman, S. C., Sharples, L. D., Magee, L. R. A., & Gilligan, D. (2003). Performance status score: Do patients and their oncologists agree? *British Journal of Cancer*, *89*(6), 1022–1027. doi:10.1038j.bjc.6601231 PMID:12966419

Blankertz, B., Dornhege, G., Krauledat, M., Müller, K.-R., & Curio, G. (2007). The non-invasive Berlin Brain-Computer Interface: Fast acquisition of effective performance in untrained subjects. *NeuroImage*, *37*(2), 539–550. doi:10.1016/j.neuroimage.2007.01.051 PMID:17475513

Blankertz, B., Muller, K., Curio, G., Vaughan, T. M., Schalk, G., Wolpaw, J. R., ... Birbaumer, N. (2004). The BCI competition 2003: Progress and perspectives in detection and discrimination of EEG single trials. *IEEE Transactions on Biomedical Engineering*, *51*(6), 1044–1051. doi:10.1109/TBME.2004.826692 PMID:15188876

Blum, A., Rassner, G., & Garbe, C. (2003). Modified ABC-point list of dermoscopy: A simplified and highly accurate dermoscopic algorithm for the diagnosis of cutaneous melanocytic lesions. *Journal of the American Academy of Dermatology*, *48*(5), 672–678. doi:10.1067/mjd.2003.282 PMID:12734495

Bob, Z., Lin, Z., Lei, Z., & Fakhri, K. (2010). Retinal vessel extraction by matched filter with first order derivative of Gaussian. *Computers in Biology and Medicine*, *40*(4), 438–445. doi:10.1016/j.compbiomed.2010.02.008 PMID:20202631

Bonnemeier, H., Wiegand, U. K., Brandes, A., Kluge, N., Katus, H. A., Richardt, G., & Potratz, J. (2003). Circadian profile of cardiac autonomic nervous modulation in healthy subjects. *Journal of Cardiovascular Electrophysiology*, *14*(8), 791–799. doi:10.1046/j.1540-8167.2003.03078.x PMID:12890036

Boonnithi, S., & Phongsuphap, S. (2011, September). Comparison of heart rate variability measures for mental stress detection. IEEE. *Computers in Cardiology*, *2011*, 85–88.

Boutsidis, C., Mahoney, M. W., & Drineas, P. (2008). Unsupervised feature selection for principal components analysis. *Proceedings of the 14th ACM SIGKDD International Conference on Knowledge Discovery and Data Mining*, 61–69. New York, NY: ACM. 10.1145/1401890.1401903

Breiman, L. (2001). Random forests. *Machine Learning*, *45*(1), 5–32. doi:10.1023/A:1010933404324

Brennan, M., Palaniswami, M., & Kamen, P. (2001). Do existing measures of Poincare plot geometry reflect nonlinear features of heart rate variability? *IEEE Transactions on Biomedical Engineering*, *48*(11), 1342–1347. doi:10.1109/10.959330 PMID:11686633

Breslow, L. A., & Aha, D. W. (1997). *Simplifying Decision Trees: A Survey*. Washington, DC: Navy Center for Applied Research in Artificial Intelligence, Naval Research Laboratory.

Brøgger, A. L., Kwasny, D., Bosco, F. G., Silahtaroglu, A., Tümer, Z., Boisen, A., & Svendsen, W. E. (2012). Centrifugally driven microfluidic disc for detection of chromosomal translocations. *Lab on a Chip*, *12*(22), 4628–4634.

Çakir, P. C. (2013). Protein-Size Molecularly Imprinted Polymer Nanogels as Synthetic Antibodies, by Localized Polymerization with Multi-initiators. *Advanced Materials*, *25*(7), 1048–1051.

Cantillo-Negrete, J., Carino-Escobar, R. I., Carrillo-Mora, P., Elias-Vinas, D., & Gutierrez-Martinez, J. (2018). Motor Imagery-Based Brain-Computer Interface Coupled to a Robotic Hand Orthosis Aimed for Neurorehabilitation of Stroke Patients. *Journal of Healthcare Engineering*, *2018*, 1–10. doi:10.1155/2018/1624637 PMID:29849992

Casali, A. G., Gosseries, O., Rosanova, M., Boly, M., Sarasso, S., Casali, K. R. ... Massimini, M. (2013). A theoretically based index of consciousness independent of sensory processing and behavior. *Science translational medicine*, *5*(198).

Caselles, V., Catte, F., Coll, T., & Dibos, F. (1993). A geometric model for active contours in image processing. *Numerische Mathematik*, *66*(1), 1–31. doi:10.1007/BF01385685

Castelletti, S., Dagradi, F., Goulene, K., Danza, A. I., Baldi, E., Stramba-Badiale, M., & Schwartz, P. J. (2018). A wearable remote monitoring system for the identification of subjects with a prolonged QT interval or at risk for drug-induced longQT syndrome. *International Journal of Cardiology*, *266*, 89–94. doi:10.1016/j.ijcard.2018.03.097 PMID:29887480

Cavalcanti, P. G., & Scharcanski, J. (2011). Automated prescreening of pigmented skin lesions using standard cameras. *Computerized Medical Imaging and Graphics*, *35*(6), 481–491. doi:10.1016/j.compmedimag.2011.02.007 PMID:21489751

Chaddad, A., & Tanougast, C. (2016). Quantitative evaluation of robust skull stripping and tumor detection applied to axial MR images. *Brain Informatics*, *3*(1), 53–61. doi:10.100740708-016-0033-7 PMID:27747598

Chalmers, D. J. (1996). The conscious mind: In search of a fundamental theory. Oxford, UK: Oxford University Press.

Chalmers, D. J. (1995). Facing up to the problem of consciousness. *Journal of Consciousness Studies*, *2*(3), 200–219.

Chandra, P. (2018) *Eigenvalue decomposition based analysis and classification of electromyogram signals.* (Master's thesis), Indian Institute of Technology, Indore, India.

Chatterjee, K. S. (2014). Core/shell nanoparticles in biomedical applications. *Advances in Colloid and Interface Science*, *209*, 8–39.

Chaudhary, U., Birbaumer, N., & Ramos-Murguialday, A. (2016). Brain-computer interfaces for communication and rehabilitation. *Nature Reviews. Neurology*, *12*(9), 513–525. doi:10.1038/nrneurol.2016.113 PMID:27539560

Chaudhury, K. N., & Unser, M. (2010). On the shiftability of dual-tree complex wavelet transforms. *IEEE Transactions on Signal Processing*, *58*(1), 221–232. doi:10.1109/TSP.2009.2028962

Chen, M., Li, Y. F., & Besenbacher, F. (2014). Electrospun Nanofibers-Mediated On-Demand Drug Release. *Advanced Healthcare Materials*, *3*(11), 1721–1732.

Chen, S., Li, R., Li, X., & Xie, J. (2018). Electrospinning: An enabling nanotechnology platform for drug delivery and regenerative medicine. *Advanced Drug Delivery Reviews*, *132*, 188–213.

Christodoulou, C. I., & Pattichis, C. S. (1999). Unsupervised pattern recognition for the classification of EMG signals. *IEEE Transactions on Biomedical Engineering*, *46*(2), 169–178. doi:10.1109/10.740879 PMID:9932338

ChuDuc, H., Stein, P. K., & PhamManh, H. (2013). Effect of calculation algorithm on heart rate variability by chaos theory. *International Journal of Electronics and Electrical Engineering*, *1*(3), 145–148. doi:10.12720/ijeee.1.3.145-148

Chuto, G. R. (2010). Les nanoparticules. *Médecine Nucléaire (Paris)*, ▪▪▪, 370–376.

Collier, J. H. (2010). Multi-component extracellular matrices based on peptide self-assembly. *Chemical Society Reviews*, *39*(9), 3413–342.

Collister, D., Ferguson, T., Komenda, P., & Tangri, N. (2016). The Patterns, Risk Factors, and Prediction of Progression in Chronic Kidney Disease: A Narrative Review. *Seminars in Nephrology*, *36*(4), 273–282. doi:10.1016/j.semnephrol.2016.05.004 PMID:27475658

Constant, J. (1997). *Essentials of Learning Electrocardiography: A Complete Course for the Non-Cardiologist*. New York, NY: Parthenon Pub Group.

Cysarz, D., Bettermann, H., & van Leeuwen, P. (2000). Entropies of short binary sequences in heart period dynamics. *American Journal of Physiology. Heart and Circulatory Physiology*, *278*(6), H2163–H2172. doi:10.1152/ajpheart.2000.278.6.H2163 PMID:10843917

Da Motta, G. D. C. P., Schardosim, J. M., & Da Cunha, M. L. C. (2015). Neonatal infant pain scale: Cross-cultural adaptation and validation in Brazil. *Journal of Pain and Symptom Management*, *50*(3), 394–401. doi:10.1016/j.jpainsymman.2015.03.019 PMID:26025270

Daraee, H. E. (2016). Application of liposomes in medicine and drug delivery. *Artificial Cells, Nanomedicine, and Biotechnology*, *44*(1), 381–391.

De Couck, M., & Gidron, Y. (2013). Norms of vagal nerve activity, indexed by Heart Rate Variability, in cancer patients. *Cancer Epidemiology*, *37*(5), 737–741. doi:10.1016/j.canep.2013.04.016 PMID:23725879

de la Rochefordière, A., Abner, A. L., Silver, B., Vicini, F., Recht, A., & Harris, J. R. (1992). Are cosmetic results following conservative surgery and radiation therapy for early breast cancer dependent on technique?. *International Journal of Radiation Oncology* Biology* Physics*, *23*(5), 925-931.

Derakhshanfar, S., Mbeleck, R., Xu, K., Zhang, X., Zhong, W., & Xing, M. (2018). 3D bioprinting for biomedical devices and tissue engineering: A review of recent trends and advances. Bioactive materials, 3(2), 144-156.

Dermatology Information System. (2012). Available at http://www.dermis.net

DermQuest. (2012). Available at http://www.dermquest.com

DeVita, V. T., Lawrence, T. S., & Rosenberg, S. A. (2015). *Cancer of the Skin: Cancer: Principles & Practice of Oncology*. Philadelphia, PA: Lippincott Williams & Wilkins.

Dey, N., Rajinikanth, V., Amira, S., Ashour, A. S., & Tavares, J. M. R. S. (2018). Social Group Optimization Supported Segmentation and Evaluation of Skin Melanoma Images. *Symmetry*, *10*(2), 51. doi:10.3390ym10020051

Di Rienzo, M., Vaini, E., & Lombardi, P. (2018). Development of a smart garment for the assessment of cardiac mechanical performance and other vital signs during sleep in microgravity. *Sensors and Actuators. A, Physical*, *274*, 19–27. doi:10.1016/j.sna.2018.02.034

Doulah, A. B. M. S. U. & Fattah, S. A. (2014, April). Neuromuscular disease classification based on mel-frequency cepstrum of motor unit action potential. In *2014 International Conference on Electrical Engineering and Information & Communication Technology (ICEEICT),* (pp. 1-4). 10.1109/ICEEICT.2014.6919167

Doulah, A. B. M. S. U. & Jumana, M. A. (2012, May). ALS disease detection in EMG using time-frequency method. In *2012 International Conference on Informatics, Electronics & Vision (ICIEV),* (pp. 648-651).

Dua, D. & Graff, C. (2019). UCI Machine Learning Repository. Retrieved from http://archive.ics.uci.edu/ml. Irvine, CA: University of California, School of Information and Computer Science.

Duan, B. (2017). State-of-the-art review of 3D bioprinting for cardiovascular tissue engineering. *Annals of Biomedical Engineering*, *45*(1), 195–209.

Dunham, M. H. (2006). *Data Mining: Introductory and Advanced Topics. Pearson Education India* (p. 315). Pearson Education India. Retrieved from http://www.amazon.com/Data-Mining-Introductory-Advanced-Topics/dp/0130888923

Easwaramoorthy, D. & Uthayakumar, R. (2010). Analysis of biomedical EEG signals using Wavelet Transforms and Multifractal Analysis. *2010 International Conference on Communication Control and Computing Technologies*, 544–549. doi:10.1109/ICCCCT.2010.5670780

Eckmann, J. P., Kamphorst, S. O., & Ruelle, D. (1987). Recurrence plots of dynamical systems. *Europhysics Letters*, *4*(9), 973–977. doi:10.1209/0295-5075/4/9/004

Edwards, P. J. & Gleeson, M. (2004). Clinical experience and perception in stereo augmented reality surgical navigation. *Medical imaging and augmented reality lecture notes in computer science, 3150*, 369-376.

Egervari, K., Szollosi, Z., & Nemes, Z. (2007). Tissue microarray technology in breast cancer HER2 diagnostics. *Pathology, Research and Practice*, *203*(3), 169–177.

Eglash, R. (2011). Nanotechnology and Traditional Knowledge Systems. In Nanotechnology and Global Sustainability (pp. 74-97). CRC Press.

Eigler, D. M. (1990). Positioning single atoms with a scanning tunnelling microscope. *Nature*, *344*(6266), 524–526.

El Nahas, M. (2005). The global challenge of chronic kidney disease. *Kidney International*, *68*(6), 2918–2929. Retrieved from http://www.ncbi.nlm.nih.gov/pubmed/21212690. doi:10.1111/j.1523-1755.2005.00774.x PMID:16316385

Emam, A. N., Loutfy, S. A., Mostafa, A. A., Awad, H., & Mohamed, M. B. (2017). Cytotoxicity, biocompatibility and cellular response of carbon dots–plasmonic based nano-hybrids for bioimaging. *RSC Advances*, *7*(38), 23502–23514.

Engasser, H. C. & Warshaw, E. M. (2010). Dermatoscopy use by US dermatologists: a cross-sectional survey. *Journal of the American Academy of Dermatology, 63,* pp. 412-419. e2.

Esmaeili, M., Rabbani, H., Dehnavi, A. M., & Dehghani, A. (2012). Automatic detection of exudates and optic disk in retinal images using curvelet transform. *IET Image Processing*, *6*(7), 1005–1013. doi:10.1049/iet-ipr.2011.0333

Fakhrullin, R. (2014). *Cell surface engineering: fabrication of functional nanoshells*. Royal Society of Chemistry.

Fattah, S. A., Iqbal, M. A., Jumana, M. A., & Doulah, A. S. U. (2012). Identifying the motor neuron disease in EMG signal using time and frequency domain features with comparison. *Signal and Image Processing: an International Journal*, *3*(2), 99–114. doi:10.5121ipij.2012.3207

Feng, J., Yin, E., Jin, J., Saab, R., Daly, I., Wang, X., ... Cichocki, A. (2018). Towards correlation-based time window selection method for motor imagery BCIs. *Neural Networks*, *102*, 87–95. doi:10.1016/j.neunet.2018.02.011 PMID:29558654

Fernandes, S. L., Gurupur, V. P., Lin, H., & Martis, R. J. (2017). A novel fusion approach for early lung cancer detection using computer aided diagnosis techniques. *Journal of Medical Imaging and Health Informatics*, *7*(8), 1841–1850. doi:10.1166/jmihi.2017.2280

Feynman, R. P. (1960). There's plenty of room at the bottom. *Engineering and Science*, *23*(5), 22–36.

Filipponi, L. (2013). *Nanotechnologies: principles, applications, implications and hands-on activities*. Luxembourg: Publications Office of the European Union.

Francesco, B., Maria Grazia, B., Emanuele, G., Valentina, F., Sara, C., Chiara, F., & Francesco, F. (2012). Linear and nonlinear heart rate variability indexes in clinical practice. *Computational and Mathematical Methods in Medicine*. PMID:22400047

Frederic, Z., & Klein, J. C. (2001). Segmentation of vessel-like patterns using mathematical morphology and curvature evaluation. *IEEE Transactions on Image Processing*, *10*(7), 1010–1019. doi:10.1109/83.931095 PMID:18249674

Fuglsang-Frederiksen, A. (2000). The utility of interference pattern analysis. *Muscle & Nerve: Official Journal of the American Association of Electrodiagnostic Medicine*, *23*(1), 18–36. doi:10.1002/(SICI)1097-4598(200001)23:1<18::AID-MUS4>3.0.CO;2-B PMID:10590403

Fuhrhop, S., Lamparth, S., & Heuer, S. A. (2009). Textile Integrated Long-Term ECG Monitor with Capacitively Coupled Electrodes. *Proc. of the IEEE BioCAS* (pp. 21–24). 10.1109/BIOCAS.2009.5372095

Fullum, T., & Gunnarsson, C. (2009). Comparison of the clinical and economic outcomes between open and minimally invasive appendectomy and colectomy: Evidence from a large commercial payer database. *Surgical Endoscopy*, *24*(4), 845–853. doi:10.100700464-009-0675-0 PMID:19730950

Fumero, F., Alayon, S., Sanchez, J. L., Sigut, J., & Gonzalez-Hernandez, M. (2011). RIM-ONE: An open retinal image database for optic nerve evaluation. In *2011 24th International Symposium on Computer-Based Medical Systems (CBMS),* 1–6.

Fung, E., Järvelin, M. R., Doshi, R. N., Shinbane, J. S., Carlson, S. K., Grazette, L. P. ... Peters, N. S. (2015). Electrocardiographic Patch Devices and Contemporary Wireless Cardiac Monitoring. *Frontiers in Physics*, *6*, 149. doi:10.3389/fphys.2015.00149 PMID:26074823

Fu, R., Tian, Y., Bao, T., Meng, Z., & Shi, P. (2019). Improvement Motor Imagery EEG Classification Based on Regularized Linear Discriminant Analysis. *Journal of Medical Systems*, *43*(6), 169. doi:10.100710916-019-1270-0 PMID:31062175

Fu, X., Cai, J., Zhang, X., Li, W. D., Ge, H., & Hu, Y. (2018). Top-down fabrication of shape-controlled, monodisperse nanoparticles for biomedical applications. *Advanced Drug Delivery Reviews*.

Galeev, A. R., Igisheva, L. N., & Kazin, E. M. (2002). Heart rate variability in healthy six-to sixteen-year-old children. *Human Physiology*, *28*(4), 428–432. doi:10.1023/A:1016529931519 PMID:12187882

Gazit, E. (2013). *Plenty of room for biology at the bottom: An introduction to bionanotechnology*. World Scientific.

Gazzoni, M., Farina, D., & Merletti, R. (2004). A new method for the extraction and classification of single motor unit action potentials from surface EMG signals. *Journal of Neuroscience Methods*, *136*(2), 165–177. doi:10.1016/j.jneumeth.2004.01.002 PMID:15183268

Ghosh, D., Debnath, D. S., & Bose, S. (2012). A Comparative Study of Performance of Fpgabased Melfilter Bank & Bark Filter Bank. *International Journal of Artificial Intelligence & Applications*, *3*(3), 37–54. doi:10.5121/ijaia.2012.3304

Giannatsis, J., & Dedoussis, V. (2009). Additive fabrication technologies applied to medicine and health care: A review. *International Journal of Advanced Manufacturing Technology*, *40*(1-2), 116–127.

Ginger, D. S., Zhang, H., & Mirkin, C. A. (2004). The evolution of dip-pen nanolithography. *Angewandte Chemie International Edition*, *43*(1), 30–45.

Gittard, S. D., & Narayan, R. J. (2010). Laser direct writing of micro-and nano-scale medical devices. *Expert Review of Medical Devices*, *7*(3), 343–356.

Giuliano, A. E., Connolly, J. L., Edge, S. B., Mittendorf, E. A., Rugo, H. S., Solin, L. J., & Hortobagyi, G. N. (2017). Breast cancer—major changes in the American Joint Committee on Cancer eighth edition cancer staging manual. CA: A Cancer Journal for Clinicians, 67(4), 290-303.

Gjoreski, H., Rashkovska, A., Kozina, S., Lustrek, M., & Gams, M. (2014). Telehealth using ECG sensor and accelerometer. In *Proceedings of the 2014 37th International Convention on Information and Communication Technology, Electronics and Microelectronics (MIPRO)*. doi:10.1109/mipro.2014.6859575

Golabbakhsh, M., & Rabbani, H. (2013). Vessel-based registration of fundus and optical coherence tomography projection images of retina using a quadratic registration model. *IET Image Processing*, *7*(8), 768–776. doi:10.1049/iet-ipr.2013.0116

Gonzalez, R. C. & Woods, R. E. (2008). Digital image processing. Upper Saddle River, NJ: Prentice Hall.

Goodman, A. M., Neumann, O., Nørregaard, K., Henderson, L., Choi, M. R., Clare, S. E., & Halas, N. J. (2017). Near-infrared remotely triggered drug-release strategies for cancer treatment. *Proceedings of the National Academy of Sciences of the United States of America*, *114*(47), 12419–12424.

Goodsell, D. S. (2004). *Bionanotechnology: lessons from nature*. John Wiley & Sons.

Greiser, K. H., Kluttig, A., Schumann, B., Swenne, C. A., Kors, J. A., Kuss, O., & Werdan, K. (2009). Cardiovascular diseases, risk factors and short-term heart rate variability in an elderly general population: The CARLA study 2002–2006. *European Journal of Epidemiology*, *24*(3), 123–142. doi:10.100710654-009-9317-z PMID:19199053

Grimnes, S., & Martinsen, G. (2008). *Bioimpedance and Bioelectricity Basics*. London, UK: Academic Press.

Grosse-Wentrup, M., Liefhold, C., Gramann, K., & Buss, M. (2009). Beamforming in noninvasive brain–computer interfaces. *IEEE Transactions on Biomedical Engineering*, *56*(4), 1209–1219. doi:10.1109/TBME.2008.2009768 PMID:19423426

Gu, Q., Li, Z., & Han, J. (2012). Generalized Fisher Score for Feature Selection. *ArXiv:1202.3725 [Cs, Stat]*. Retrieved from http://arxiv.org/abs/1202.3725

Güler, N. F., & Koçer, S. (2005). Classification of EMG signals using PCA and FFT. *Journal of Medical Systems*, *29*(3), 241–250. doi:10.100710916-005-5184-7 PMID:16050079

Gulzar, T., Singh, A., & Sharma, S. (2014). Comparative Analysis of LPCC, MFCC and BFCC for the Recognition of Hindi Words Using Artificial Neural Networks. *International Journal of Computers and Applications*, *101*(12), 22–27.

Guyon, I., & Elisseeff, A. (2003). An Introduction to Variable and Feature Selection. *Journal of Machine Learning Research*, *3*(Mar), 1157–1182.

Hadizadeh, E., Rabbani, R., Azizi, Z., Barekatain, M., Hakhamaneshi, K., Khoram, E., & Fotowat-Ahmady, A. (2019). Ultra Low-Power System for Remote ECG Monitoring.

Hadjiiski, L., Sahiner, B., Helvie, M. A., Chan, H. P., Roubidoux, M. A., Paramagul, C., ... Foster, M. (2006). Breast masses: Computer-aided diagnosis with serial mammograms. *Radiology*, *240*(2), 343–356. doi:10.1148/radiol.2401042099 PMID:16801362

Hajeb, S. H., Rabbani, H., & Akhlaghi, M. R. (2012). Diabetic retinopathy grading by digital curvelet transform. Computational and Mathematical Methods in Medicine, 1607-1614.

Hajeb, S. H., Rabbani, H., & Akhlaghi, M. R. (2014). A new combined method based on curvelet transform and morphological operators for automatic detection of foveal avascular zone. *Signal, Image and Video Processing*, *8*(2), 205–222. doi:10.100711760-013-0530-6

Hall, M., Frank, E., Holmes, G., Pfahringer, B., Reutemann, P., & Witten, I. H. (2009). The WEKA data mining software: an update. *ACM SIGKDD explorations newsletter, 11*(1), 10-18.

Hall, J. M., Lee, M. K., Newman, B., Morrow, J. E., Anderson, L. A., Huey, B., & King, M. C. (1990). Linkage of early-onset familial breast cancer to chromosome 17q21. *Science*, *250*(4988), 1684–1689. doi:10.1126cience.2270482 PMID:2270482

Hanahan, D. & Weinberg, R. A. (2000). The hallmarks of cancer. *cell, 100*(1), 57-70.

Han, F., Jia, X., Dai, D., Yang, X., Zhao, J., Zhao, Y., & Yuan, X. (2013). Performance of a multilayered small-diameter vascular scaffold dual-loaded with VEGF and PDGF. *Biomaterials*, *34*(30), 7302–7313.

Henry, B., Lovell, N., & Camacho, F. (2001). Nonlinear dynamics time series analysis. In Nonlinear Biomedical Signal Processing: Dynamic Analysis and Modeling (pp. 1–39). New York, NY: IEEE.

Herrera, A., & Del Rio, F. (2010). Frequency bark cepstral coefficients extraction for speech analysis by synthesis. *The Journal of the Acoustical Society of America*, *128*(4), 2290. doi:10.1121/1.3508042 PMID:20370010

Herry, C. L., Burns, P., Desrochers, A., Fecteau, G., Durosier, L. D., Cao, M. . . . Frasch, M. G. (2019). Decoding vagal contributions to fetal heart rate variability. *arXiv*:1901.06431.

Hervault, A. D. (2016). Doxorubicin loaded dual pH-and thermo-responsive magnetic nanocarrier for combined magnetic hyperthermia and targeted controlled drug delivery applications. *Nanoscale*, *8*(24), 12152–12161.

Hobson, A. R., & Hillebrand, A. (2006). Independent component analysis of the EEG: Is this the way forward for understanding abnormalities of brain-gut signalling? *Gut*, *55*(5), 597–600. doi:10.1136/gut.2005.081703 PMID:16609130

Hoover, A., & Goldbaum, M. (2003). Locating the optic nerve in a retinal image using the fuzzy convergence of the blood vessels. *IEEE Transactions on Medical Imaging*, *22*(8), 951–958. doi:10.1109/TMI.2003.815900 PMID:12906249

Hoover, A., Kouznetsova, V., & Goldbaum, M. (2000). Locating blood vessels in retinal images by piece-wise threhsold probing of a matched filter response. *IEEE Transactions on Medical Imaging*, *19*(3), 203–210. doi:10.1109/42.845178 PMID:10875704

Hopkins, A. M., DeSimone, E., Chwalek, K., & Kaplan, D. L. (2015). 3D in vitro modeling of the central nervous system. *Progress in Neurobiology*, *125*, 1–25.

Housa, R., Munib, Q., & Moussa, A. (2005). Breast cancer diagnosis system based on wavelet analysis and fuzzy-neural. *Expert Systems with Applications*, *28*(4), 713–723. doi:10.1016/j.eswa.2004.12.028

Hsieh, F. Y., & Hsu, S. H. (2015). 3D bioprinting: A new insight into the therapeutic strategy of neural tissue regeneration. *Organogenesis*, *11*(4), 153–158.

Hsu, W.-Y. (2013). Wavelet-coherence features for motor imagery EEG analysis posterior to EOG noise elimination. *International Journal of Innovative Computing, Information, & Control*, *9*, 465–475.

Hu, D., Li, W., & Chen, X. (2011). Feature extraction of motor imagery EEG signals based on wavelet packet decomposition. *The 2011 IEEE/ICME International Conference on Complex Medical Engineering*, 694–697. doi:10.1109/ICCME.2011.5876829

Huang, N. E., Shen, Z., Long, S. R., Wu, M. C., Shih, H. H., Zheng, Q. . . . Liu, H. H. (1998, March). The empirical mode decomposition and the Hilbert spectrum for nonlinear and non-stationary time series analysis. In *Proceedings of the Royal Society of London A: mathematical, physical and engineering sciences* (Vol. 454, No. 1971, pp. 903-995). 10.1098/rspa.1998.0193

Huang, H. C., Huang, S. Y., Lin, C. I., & Lee, Y. D. (2007). A multi-array sensor via the integration of acrylic molecularly imprinted photoresists and ultramicroelectrodes on a glass chip. *Analytica Chimica Acta*, *582*(1), 137–146.

Huang, H. C., Lin, C. I., Joseph, A. K., & Der Lee, Y. (2004). Photo-lithographically impregnated and molecularly imprinted polymer thin film for biosensor applications. *Journal of Chromatography. A*, *1027*(1-2), 263–268.

HuiáShin, H. a. (2012). A facile and sensitive detection of pathogenic bacteria using magnetic nanoparticles and optical nanocrystal probes. *Analyst (London)*, *137*(16), 3609–3612.

Hull, C. W. (1986). U.S. Patent No. 4,575,330. Washington, DC: U.S. Patent and Trademark Office.

Hundsberger, T., Omlin, A., Haegele-Link, S., Vehoff, J., & Strasser, F. (2014). Autonomic dysfunction in cancer cachexia coincides with large fiber polyneuropathy. *Journal of Pain and Symptom Management*, *48*(4), 611–618. doi:10.1016/j.jpainsymman.2013.11.018 PMID:24709363

Hutchins, G., & Grabsch, H. I. (2018). How to make tissue microarrays. *Diagnostic Histopathology*, *24*(4), 127–135.

Illingworth, R. S. (1972). The Normal Child and Some Problems of the Early Years and Their Treatment (10th ed.). Philadelphia, PA: W. B. Saunders Co.

Imran, S. M., Talukdar, M. T. F., Sakib, S. K., Pathan, N. S., & Fattah, S. A. (2014). Motor imagery EEG signal classification scheme based on wavelet domain statistical features. *2014 International Conference on Electrical Engineering and Information Communication Technology*, 1–4. 10.1109/ICEEICT.2014.6919172

Jahromi, M. K., Kafieh, R., Rabbani, H., & … . (2014). An automatic algorithm for segmentation of the boundaries of corneal layers in optical coherence tomography images using gaussian mixture model. *Journal of Medical Signals and Sensors*, *4*(3), 171–180. PMID:25298926

Jerant, A. F., Johnson, J. T., Sheridan, C., & Caffrey, T. J. (2000). Early detection and treatment of skin cancer. *American Family Physician*, *62*, 357–386. PMID:10929700

Jessop, Z. M., Al-Sabah, A., Gardiner, M. D., Combellack, E., Hawkins, K., & Whitaker, I. S. (2017). 3D bioprinting for reconstructive surgery: Principles, applications and challenges. *Journal of Plastic, Reconstructive & Aesthetic Surgery; JPRAS*, *70*(9), 1155–1170.

Jiang, X., Shao, N., Jing, W., Tao, S., Liu, S., & Sui, G. (2014). Microfluidic chip integrating high throughput continuous-flow PCR and DNA hybridization for bacteria analysis. *Talanta*, *122*, 246–250.

Jojoa, J. A., Rivera, C. E., Delgado, E. M., Casas, H. M., Rosas, G. M., Rosero, C. Y., & Montenegro, F. A. (2017). (2017). New ABC Chronic Kidney Disease Classification. *Int J Nephrol Kidney Failure*, *3*(2). doi:10.16966/2380-5498.144

Jones, S. W. (2005). Introduction to integrated circuit technology. IC Knowlegde LLC, Georgetown, MA Revision, Nov.

Josephson, B. D. (1996). First-Person Experience and the Scientific Exploration of Consciousness. In Biomedical and Life Physics (pp. 383-389). Vieweg+ Teubner Verlag. doi:10.1007/978-3-322-85017-1_38

Joshi, D., Tripathi, A., Sharma, R., & Pachori, R. B. (2017, February). Computer aided detection of abnormal EMG signals based on tunable-Q wavelet transform. In *2017 4th International Conference on Signal Processing and Integrated Networks (SPIN),* (pp. 544-549). 10.1109/SPIN.2017.8050010

Kamińska, D., Sapiński, T., & Pelikant, A. (2013). *Comparison of Perceptual Features Efficiency for Automatic Identification of Emotional States from Speech* (pp. 210–213). doi:10.1109/HSI.2013.6577824

Kamousi, B., Liu, Z., & He, B. (2005). Classification of motor imagery tasks for brain-computer interface applications by means of two equivalent dipoles analysis. *IEEE Transactions on Neural Systems and Rehabilitation Engineering, 13*(2), 166–171. doi:10.1109/TNSRE.2005.847386 PMID:16003895

Kandel, E. R., Schwartz, J. H., Jessell, T. M., Jessell, M. B. T., Siegelbaum, S., & Hudspeth, A. (2000). Principles of neural science, 4. New York, NY: McGraw-Hill.

Kannaian, T., Neelaveni, R., & Thilagavathi, G. (2013). Design and development of embroidered textile electrodes for continuous measurement of electrocardiogram signals. *Journal of Industrial Textiles, 42*(3), 303–318. doi:10.1177/1528083712438069

Kannan, A. G. Q. M., Jr., Sharma, A., & Schoo, P. (2012). Genetic Algorithm Based Feature Selection Algorithm for Effective Intrusion Detection in Cloud Networks. *2012 IEEE 12th International Conference on Data Mining Workshops*, 416–423. doi:10.1109/ICDMW.2012.56

Kaplan, D. T., Furman, M. I., Pincus, S. M., Ryan, S. M., Lipsitz, L. A., & Goldberger, A. L. (1991). Aging and the complexity of cardiovascular dynamics. *Biophysical Journal, 59*(4), 945–949. doi:10.1016/S0006-3495(91)82309-8 PMID:2065195

Kapur, J. N., Sahoo, P. K., & Wong, A. K. C. (1985). A new method for gray-level picture thresholding using the entropy of the histogram. *Computer Vision Graphics and Image Processing, 29*(3), 273–285. doi:10.1016/0734-189X(85)90125-2

Karpati, G., Carpenter, S., & Nelson, R. F. (1970). Type I muscle fibre atrophy and central nuclei: A rare familial neuromuscular disease. *Journal of the Neurological Sciences, 10*(5), 489–500. doi:10.1016/0022-510X(70)90027-4 PMID:4910660

Karp, J. M., Yeh, J., Eng, G., Fukuda, J., Blumling, J., Suh, K. Y., ... Khademhosseini, A. (2007). Controlling size, shape and homogeneity of embryoid bodies using poly (ethylene glycol) microwells. *Lab on a Chip, 7*(6), 786–794.

Katsis, C. D., Exarchos, T. P., Papaloukas, C., Goletsis, Y., Fotiadis, D. I., & Sarmas, I. (2007). A two-stage method for MUAP classification based on EMG decomposition. *Computers in Biology and Medicine, 37*(9), 1232–1240. doi:10.1016/j.compbiomed.2006.11.010 PMID:17208215

Kawasaki, T. (2017). *Clinical Application of Motor Imagery Training*. Neurological Physical Therapy. doi:10.5772/67518

Keerthana, K., Jayasuriya, T. J., Raja, N. S. M., & Rajinikanth, V. (2017). Retinal vessel extraction based on firefly algorithm guided multi-scale matched filter. *Int J Mod Sci Technol, 2*(2), 74–80.

Khandoker, A. H., Lai, D. T., Begg, R. K., & Palaniswami, M. (2007). Wavelet-based feature extraction for support vector machines for screening balance impairments in the elderly. *IEEE Transactions on Neural Systems and Rehabilitation Engineering*, *15*(4), 587–597. doi:10.1109/TNSRE.2007.906961 PMID:18198717

Khor, W. S., Baker, B., Amin, K., Patel, K., & Wong, J. (2016). Augmented and virtual reality in surgery- the digital surgical environment: Application, limitations and legal pitfalls. *Annals of Translational Medicine*, *4*(23), 454. doi:10.21037/atm.2016.12.23 PMID:28090510

Kim, J., Ko, I., Seol, Y., Atala, A., Yoo, J. J., & Lee, S. (2016, December). 3D Bioprinting of Functional Skeletal Muscle Tissue for Volumetric Muscle Tissue Loss. In Tissue Engineering Part A, (Vol. 22, pp. S5-S5). 140 HUGUENOT STREET, 3RD FL, NEW ROCHELLE, NY 10801 USA: MARY ANN LIEBERT, INC.

Kim, C., Sun, J., Liu, D., Wang, Q., & Paek, S. (2018). An effective feature extraction method by power spectral density of EEG signal for 2-class motor imagery-based BCI. *Medical & Biological Engineering & Computing*, 1–14. PMID:29497931

Kim, D. H., Rozhkova, E. A., Ulasov, I. V., Bader, S. D., Rajh, T., Lesniak, M. S., & Novosad, V. (2010). Biofunctionalized magnetic-vortex microdiscs for targeted cancer-cell destruction. *Nature Materials*, *9*(2), 165.

Kim, J., Elsnab, J., Gehrke, C., Li, J., & Gale, B. K. (2013). Microfluidic integrated multi-walled carbon nanotube (MWCNT) sensor for electrochemical nucleic acid concentration measurement. *Sensors and Actuators. B, Chemical*, *185*, 370–376.

King, T. A., Muhsen, S., Patil, S., Koslow, S., Oskar, S., Park, A., & Morrow, M. (2013). Is there a role for routine screening MRI in women with LCIS? *Breast Cancer Research and Treatment*, *142*(2), 445–453. doi:10.100710549-013-2725-5 PMID:24141896

Kirstein, T., Cottet, D., Grzyb, J., & Tröster, G. (2002, October). Textiles for signal transmission in wearables. In *Proc. ACM of First Workshop on Electronic Textiles (MAMSET 2002)*, San Jose, CA.

Kohavi, R. (1995) A study of cross-validation and bootstrap for accuracy estimation and model selection. *In proceedings of the 14th International Joint Conference on Artificial Intelligence*, Morgan Kaufmann Publishers, San Francisco, CA, pp. 1137-1143.

Kononen, J., Bubendorf, L., Kallionimeni, A., Bärlund, M., Schraml, P., Leighton, S., & Kallionimeni, O. P. (1998). Tissue microarrays for high-throughput molecular profiling of tumor specimens. *Nature Medicine*, *4*(7), 844.

Kononenko, I. (1994). Estimating attributes: Analysis and extensions of RELIEF. *European Conference on Machine Learning*, 171–182. Berlin, Germany: Springer. 10.1007/3-540-57868-4_57

Kouchaki, S., Boostani, R., & Parsaei, H. (2012, May). A new feature selection method for classification of EMG signals. In *2012 16th CSI International Symposium on Artificial Intelligence and Signal Processing (AISP),* (pp. 585-590). 10.1109/AISP.2012.6313814

Krummel, T. M., Yock, P. G., Zenios, S. A., Brinton, T. J., Kumar, U. N., Watkins, F. T., & Makower, J. (2017). *Biodesign: The process of innovating medical technologies*. Cambridge, UK: Cambridge University Press.

Kumar, C., ur Rehman, F., Kumar, S., Mehmood, A. & Shabir, G. (2018). Analysis of MFCC and BFCC in a speaker identification system. In *Proceedings of 2018 International Conference on Computing, Mathematics and Engineering Technologies (iCoMET)*, Sukkur, Pakistan, pp. 1-5. doi:10.1109/ICOMET.2018.8346330

Kumar, M. (2016). Prediction of Chronic Kidney Disease Using Random Forest Machine Learning Algorithm. *Journal of Computer Science and Mobile Computing*, *5*(2), 24–33.

Kumar, P. S., Arumuganathan, R., Sivakumar, K., & Vimal, C. (n.d.). Removal of ocular artifacts in the EEG through wavelet transform without using an EOG reference channel. *Int. J. Open Probl. Comput. Math*, 188–200.

Kumar, M., Pachori, R. B., & Acharya, U. R. (2016). An efficient automated technique for CAD diagnosis using flexible analytic wavelet transform and entropy features extracted from HRV signals. *Expert Systems with Applications*, *63*, 165–172. doi:10.1016/j.eswa.2016.06.038

Kumar, M., Pachori, R. B., & Acharya, U. R. (2017). Characterization of coronary artery disease using flexible analytic wavelet transform applied on ECG signals. *Biomedical Signal Processing and Control*, *31*, 301–308. doi:10.1016/j.bspc.2016.08.018

Kumar, M., Pachori, R. B., & Acharya, U. R. (2017a). Automated diagnosis of myocardial infarction ECG signals using sample entropy in flexible analytic wavelet transform framework. *Entropy (Basel, Switzerland)*, *19*(9), 488. doi:10.3390/e19090488

Kumar, M., Pachori, R. B., & Acharya, U. R. (2018). Automated diagnosis of atrial fibrillation ECG signals using entropy features extracted from flexible analytic wavelet transform. *Biocybernetics and Biomedical Engineering*, *38*(3), 564–573. doi:10.1016/j.bbe.2018.04.004

Kusiak, A. (2003). Data mining based decision-making approach for predicting survival of kidney dialysis patients. In IFAC Proceedings Volumes (IFAC-Papers Online)(Vol. 36, pp. 35–39). IFAC Secretariat. 10.1016/S1474-6670(17)33468-7

Kusiak, A. (2001). Feature transformation methods in data mining. *IEEE Transactions on Electronics Packaging Manufacturing*, *24*(3), 214–221. doi:10.1109/6104.956807

LaFleur, K., Cassady, K., Doud, A., Shades, K., Rogin, E., & He, B. (2013). Quadcopter control in three-dimensional space using a noninvasive motor imagery-based brain–computer interface. *Journal of Neural Engineering*, *10*(4), 046003. doi:10.1088/1741-2560/10/4/046003 PMID:23735712

Lake, D. E., Richman, J. S., Griffin, M. P., & Moorman, J. R. (2002). Sample entropy analysis of neonatal heart rate variability. *American Journal of Physiology. Regulatory, Integrative and Comparative Physiology*, *283*(3), R789–R797. doi:10.1152/ajpregu.00069.2002 PMID:12185014

Lakshmi, V. S., Tebby, S. G., Shriranjani, D., & Rajinikanth, V. (2016). Chaotic cuckoo search and Kapur/Tsallis approach in segmentation of T.cruzi from blood smear images. *Int. J. Comp. Sci. Infor. Sec. (IJCSIS)*, 14, 51-56.

Lal, T. N., Schroder, M., Hinterberger, T., Weston, J., Bogdan, M., Birbaumer, N., & Scholkopf, B. (2004). Support vector channel selection in BCI. *IEEE Transactions on Biomedical Engineering*, *51*(6), 1003–1010. doi:10.1109/TBME.2004.827827 PMID:15188871

Langer, R. (2000). Biomaterials in drug delivery and tissue engineering: One laboratory's experience. *Accounts of Chemical Research*, *33*, 94–101.

Lange, S. A., Benes, V., Kern, D. P., Hörber, J. H., & Bernard, A. (2004). Microcontact printing of DNA molecules. *Analytical Chemistry*, *76*(6), 1641–1647.

Lasisi, T. J., Raji, Y. R., & Salako, B. L. (2016). Salivary creatinine and urea analysis in patients with chronic kidney disease: A case control study. *BMC Nephrology*, *17*(1), 10. doi:10.118612882-016-0222-x PMID:26775026

Laurent, S. F. (2008). Magnetic iron oxide nanoparticles: Synthesis, stabilization, vectorization, physicochemical characterizations, and biological applications. *Chemical Reviews*, *108*(6), 2064–2110.

Lee, K. B., Kim, E. Y., Mirkin, C. A., & Wolinsky, S. M. (2004). The use of nanoarrays for highly sensitive and selective detection of human immunodeficiency virus type 1 in plasma. *Nano Letters*, *4*(10), 1869–1872.

Lee, K. B., Park, S. J., Mirkin, C. A., Smith, J. C., & Mrksich, M. (2002). Protein nanoarrays generated by dip-pen nanolithography. *Science*, *295*(5560), 1702–1705.

Lee, M., Kang, D. K., Yang, H. K., Park, K. H., Choe, S. Y., Kang, C., & Kang, I. C. (2006). Protein nanoarray on Prolinker™ surface constructed by atomic force microscopy dip-pen nanolithography for analysis of protein interaction. *Proteomics*, *6*(4), 1094–1103.

Lee, S. S., Hsu, E. L., Mendoza, M., Ghodasra, J., Nickoli, M. S., Ashtekar, A., & Nelson, D. (2015). Gel scaffolds of BMP-2-binding peptide amphiphile nanofibers for spinal arthrodesis. *Advanced Healthcare Materials*, *4*(1), 131–141.

Lee, T. T., García, J. R., Paez, J. I., Singh, A., Phelps, E. A., Weis, S., & García, A. J. (2015). Light-triggered in vivo activation of adhesive peptides regulates cell adhesion, inflammation and vascularization of biomaterials. *Nature Materials*, *14*(3), 352.

Lei, B., Yang, P., Wang, T., Chen, S., & Ni, D. (2017). Relational-Regularized Discriminative Sparse Learning for Alzheimer's Disease Diagnosis. *IEEE Transactions on Cybernetics*, *47*(4), 1102–1113. doi:10.1109/TCYB.2016.2644718 PMID:28092591

Lempel, A., & Ziv, J. (1976). On the complexity of finite sequences. *IEEE Transactions on Information Theory*, *22*(1), 75–81. doi:10.1109/TIT.1976.1055501

Levey, A. S., Eckardt, K. U., Tsukamoto, Y., Levin, A., Coresh, J., Rossert, J., ... Eknoyan, G. (2005). Definition and classification of chronic kidney disease: A position statement from Kidney Disease: Improving Global Outcomes (KDIGO). *Kidney International*, *67*(6), 2089–2100. doi:10.1111/j.1523-1755.2005.00365.x PMID:15882252

Levine, J. (1983). Materialism and qualia: The explanatory gap. *Pacific philosophical quarterly*, *64*(4), 354-361.

Liaw, C. Y., & Guvendiren, M. (2017). Current and emerging applications of 3D printing in medicine. *Biofabrication*, *9*(2), 024102.

Li, C., Xu, C., Gui, C., & Fox, M. D. (2010). Distance regularized level set evolution and its application to image segmentation. *IEEE Transactions on Image Processing*, *19*(12), 3243–3254. doi:10.1109/TIP.2010.2069690 PMID:20801742

Lichman, M. (2013). *UCI Machine Learning Repository. Retrieved from* http://archive.ics.uci.edu/ml. Irvine, CA: University of California, School of Information and Computer Science.

Linares, A. V., Falcimaigne-Cordin, A., Gheber, L. A., & Haupt, K. (2011). Patterning nanostructured, synthetic, polymeric receptors by simultaneous projection photolithography, nanomolding, and molecular imprinting. *Small*, *7*(16), 2318–2325.

Lippmann, R. (1987). An introduction to computing with neuralnets. *IEEE ASSP Magazine*, *4*(2), 4–22. doi:10.1109/MASSP.1987.1165576

Li, S.-H., Lin, B.-S., Wang, C.-A., & Yang, C.-T. (2017). Design of wearable and wireless multi-parameter monitoring system for evaluating cardiopulmonary function. *Medical Engineering & Physics*, *47*, 144–150. doi:10.1016/j.medengphy.2017.06.009 PMID:28684215

Li, T., Zhang, J., Xue, T., & Wang, B. (2017). *Development of a Novel Motor Imagery Control Technique and Application in a Gaming Environment.* Comp. Int. and Neurosc. doi:10.1155/2017/5863512

Liu, L., Li, W., Wu, X., & Zhou, B. X. (2019). Infant cry language analysis and recognition: an experimental approach. *IEEE/CAA Journal of Automatica Sinica.* pp. 1-11. doi:. doi:10.1109/JAS.2019.1911435

Liu, L., Li, Y., & Kuo, K. (2018). Infant cry signal detection, pattern extraction and recognition. In *Proceedings of 2018 International Conference on Information and Computer Technologies (ICICT)*, DeKalb, IL, pp. 159-163. 10.1109/INFOCT.2018.8356861

Liu, M., & Zhang, D. (2016). Pairwise Constraint-Guided Sparse Learning for Feature Selection. *IEEE Transactions on Cybernetics*, *46*(1), 298–310. doi:10.1109/TCYB.2015.2401733 PMID:26151948

Lotte, F., Congedo, M., Lécuyer, A., Lamarche, F., & Arnaldi, B. (2007). A review of classification algorithms for EEG-based brain–computer interfaces. *Journal of Neural Engineering*, *4*(2), R1–R13. doi:10.1088/1741-2560/4/2/R01 PMID:17409472

Lubis, C., & Gondawijaya, F. (2019). Heart Sound Diagnose System with BFCC, MFCC, and Backpropagation Neural Network. *IOP Conference Series. Materials Science and Engineering*, *508*, 012119. doi:10.1088/1757-899X/508/1/012119

Luo, L. Z. (2007). Development of a gold nanoparticles based chemiluminescence imaging assay and its application. *Analytica Chimica Acta*, ▪▪▪, 106–111.

MacKie, R., & Doherty, V. (1991). Seven-point checklist for melanoma. *Clinical and Experimental Dermatology*, *16*(2), 151–152. doi:10.1111/j.1365-2230.1991.tb00329.x PMID:1867692

Maddirala, A. K., & Shaik, R. A. (2016). Removal of EOG Artifacts From Single Channel EEG Signals Using Combined Singular Spectrum Analysis and Adaptive Noise Canceler. *IEEE Sensors Journal*, *16*(23), 8279–8287. doi:10.1109/JSEN.2016.2560219

Madyastha, R. K., & Aazhang, B. (1994). An algorithm for training multilayer perceptrons for data classification and function interpolation. *IEEE Transactions on Circuits and Systems. I, Fundamental Theory and Applications*, *41*(12), 866–875. doi:10.1109/81.340848

Mahmudi, T., Kafieh, R., & Rabbani, H. (2014, Feb. 15-20). Comparison of macular OCTs in right and left eyes of normal people. In *Proc. SPIE 9038, Medical Imaging 2014: Biomedical Applications in Molecular, Structural, and Functional Imaging, 90381K,* San Diego, CA. doi:10.1117/12.2044046

Majumder, S., Mondal, T., & Deen, M. (2017). Wearable sensors for remote health monitoring. *Sensors, 17*(1), 130. doi:10.339017010130

Malan, N. S. & Sharma, S. (2018). Removal of Ocular Atrifacts from Single Channel EEG Signal Using DTCWT with Quantum Inspired Adaptive Threshold. *2018 2nd International Conference on Biomedical Engineering (IBIOMED)*, 94–99. doi:10.1109/IBIOMED.2018.8534915

Malan, N. S., & Sharma, S. (2019). Feature selection using regularized neighbourhood component analysis to enhance the classification performance of motor imagery signals. *Computers in Biology and Medicine*, *107*, 118–126. doi:10.1016/j.compbiomed.2019.02.009 PMID:30802693

Malladi, R., Sethian, J. A., & Vemuri, B. C. (1995). Shape modeling with front propagation: A level set approach. *IEEE T. Pattern Anal. Mac. Int.*, *17*(2), 158–175. doi:10.1109/34.368173

Manic, K. S., Naimi, I. S. I., Hasoon, F. N., & Rajinikanth, V. (2019). Jaya algorithm-assisted evaluation of tooth elements using digital bitewing radiography images. *Computational Techniques for Dental Image Analysis,* 107-128. doi:. doi:10.4018/978-1-5225-6243-6.ch005

Manz, A., Graber, N., & Widmer, H. Á. (1990). Miniaturized total chemical analysis systems: A novel concept for chemical sensing. *Sensors and Actuators. B, Chemical*, *1*(1-6), 244–248.

Markstedt, K., Mantas, A., Tournier, I., Martínez Ávila, H., Hägg, D., & Gatenholm, P. (2015). 3D bioprinting human chondrocytes with nanocellulose–alginate bioink for cartilage tissue engineering applications. *Biomacromolecules*, *16*(5), 1489–1496.

Martínez-Pérez, M. E., Hughes, A. D., Stanton, A. V., Thom, S. A., Bharath, A. A., & Parker, K. H. (1999, September). Retinal blood vessel segmentation by means of scale-space analysis and region growing. In International Conference on Medical Image Computing and Computer-Assisted Intervention (pp. 90-97). Springer, Berlin, Germany.

Massaro, S., & Pecchia, L. (2019). Heart rate variability (HRV) analysis: A methodology for organizational neuroscience. *Organizational Research Methods*, *22*(1), 354–393. doi:10.1177/1094428116681072

Matovinović, M. S. (2009). 1. Pathophysiology and Classification of Kidney Diseases. *EJIFCC*, *20*(1), 2–11. Retrieved from http://www.ncbi.nlm.nih.gov/pubmed/27683321. PMID:27683321

McGill, K. C., Lateva, Z. C., & Marateb, H. R. (2005). EMGLAB: An interactive EMG decomposition program. *Journal of Neuroscience Methods*, *149*(2), 121–133. doi:10.1016/j.jneumeth.2005.05.015 PMID:16026846

McKight, P. E. & Najab, J. (2010). Kruskal-Wallis Test. *The corsini encyclopedia ofpsychology*, 1-1.

Mellinger, J., Schalk, G., Braun, C., Preissl, H., Rosenstiel, W., Birbaumer, N., & Kübler, A. (2007). An MEG-based brain-computer interface (BCI). *NeuroImage*, *36*(3), 581–593. doi:10.1016/j.neuroimage.2007.03.019 PMID:17475511

Menzies, S. W., Ingvar, C., Crotty, K. A., & McCarthy, W. H. (1996). Frequency and morphologic characteristics of invasive melanomas lacking specific surface microscopic features. *Archives of Dermatology*, *132*(10), 1178–1182. doi:10.1001/archderm.1996.03890340038007 PMID:8859028

Milgram, P. & Kishino, F. (1994). A taxonomy of mixed reality visual displays. *IEICE Transactions on Information Systems, E77-D.*

Ming, M., Shaona, L., Haitao, M., Yuliang, M., & Yunyuan, G. (2015). Feature extraction method of motor imagery EEG based on DTCWT sample entropy. *2015 34th Chinese Control Conference (CCC)*, 3964–3968. doi:10.1109/ChiCC.2015.7260250

Mironov, V. (2005). The second international workshop on bioprinting, biopatterning and bioassembly. *Expert Opinion on Biological Therapy*, *5*(8), 1111–1115.

Mishchenko, Y., Kaya, M., Ozbay, E., & Yanar, H. (2017). Developing a 3- to 6-state EEG-based brain-computer interface for a robotic manipulator control. *bioRxiv*. doi:10.1101/171025

Mishra, V. K., Bajaj, V., & Kumar, A. (2016, February). Classification of normal, ALS, and myopathy EMG signals using ELM classifier. In *2016 2nd International Conference on Advances in Electrical, Electronics, Information, Communication and Bio-Informatics (AEEICB),* (pp. 455-459).

Mishra, V. K., Bajaj, V., Kumar, A., Sharma, D., & Singh, G. K. (2017). An efficient method for analysis of EMG signals using improved empirical mode decomposition. *AEÜ. International Journal of Electronics and Communications*, *72*, 200–209. doi:10.1016/j.aeue.2016.12.008

Moazam, F. M., Barman, S. A., Paolo, R., Andreas, H., Abdul, B., Bunyarit, U., ... Christopher, O. G. (2012). An approach to localize the retinal blood vessels using bit planes and centerline detection. *Computer Methods and Programs in Biomedicine*, *108*(2), 600–616. doi:10.1016/j.cmpb.2011.08.009 PMID:21963241

Moers, C., Möbius, B., Rosanowski, F., Nöth, E., Eysholdt, U., & Haderlein, T. (2012). Vowel- and Text-Based Cepstral Analysis of Chronic Hoarseness. *Journal of Voice*, *26*(4), 416–424. doi:10.1016/j.jvoice.2011.05.001 PMID:21940144

Mohamed, W. N. H. W., Salleh, M. N. M., & Omar, A. H. O. (2012). A comparative study of Reduced Error Pruning method in decision tree algorithms. In *Proceedings - 2012 IEEE International Conference on Control System, Computing and Engineering, ICCSCE.* (pp. 392–397). 10.1109/ICCSCE.2012.6487177

Mohamed, N. A., Zulkifley, M. A., & Hussain, A. (2014). Local binary patterns for optic disc segmentation. In *Proceedings of International Conference on Applied Computer and Applied Computational Science*, 149–153. doi:10.1109/ISCAIE.2015.7298324

Moodithaya, S., & Avadhany, S. T. (2012). Gender differences in age-related changes in cardiac autonomic nervous function. *Journal of Aging Research*. PMID:22187649

Mouser, V. H., Levato, R., Bonassar, L. J., D'Lima, D. D., Grande, D. A., Klein, T. J., & Malda, J. (2017). Three-dimensional bioprinting and its potential in the field of articular cartilage regeneration. *Cartilage*, *8*(4), 327–340.

Mura, S., Nicolas, J., & Couvreur, P. (2013). Stimuli-responsive nanocarriers for drug delivery. *Nature Materials*, *12*(11), 991.

Muthusamy, H., Polat, K., & Yaacob, S. (2015). Particle Swarm Optimization Based Feature Enhancement and Feature Selection for Improved Emotion Recognition in Speech and Glottal Signals. *PLoS One*, *10*(3). doi:10.1371/journal.pone.0120344 PMID:25799141

Nachbar, F., Stolz, W., Merkle, T., Cognetta, A. B., Vogt, T., Landthaler, M., ... Plewig, G. (1994). The ABCD rule of dermatoscopy: High prospective value in the diagnosis of doubtful melanocytic skin lesions. *Journal of the American Academy of Dermatology*, *30*(4), 551–559. doi:10.1016/S0190-9622(94)70061-3 PMID:8157780

Nagaraj, N., & Virmani, M. (2017). Is 'Information' Fundamental for a Scientific Theory of Consciousness? In *Self, Culture and Consciousness* (pp. 357–378). Singapore: Springer. doi:10.1007/978-981-10-5777-9_21

Nagel, T. (1974). What is it like to be a bat? *The Philosophical Review*, *83*(4), 435–450. doi:10.2307/2183914

Naseer, N., & Hong, K.-S. (2015). fNIRS-based brain-computer interfaces: A review. *Frontiers in Human Neuroscience*, *9*. doi:10.3389/fnhum.2015.00003

National Comprehensive Cancer Network. (2003). Breast cancer Clinical Practice Guidelines in Oncology. *Journal of the National Comprehensive Cancer Network: 1*(2), 148. doi:10.6004/jnccn.2003.0016 PMID:19768876

Navarro, A. A., Ceccaroni, L., Velickovski, F., Torrellas, S., Miralles, F., Allison, B. Z. … Faller, J. (2011). Context-Awareness as an Enhancement of Brain-Computer Interfaces. *IWAAL*. doi:10.1007/978-3-642-21303-8_30

Nicolau, S., & Marescaux, J. (2011). Augmented reality in laparoscopic surgical oncology. *Surgical Oncology*, *20*(3), 189–201. doi:10.1016/j.suronc.2011.07.002 PMID:21802281

Nie, D., Wang, L., Adeli, E., Lao, C., Lin, W., & Shen, D. (2019). 3-D Fully Convolutional Networks for Multimodal Isointense Infant Brain Image Segmentation. *IEEE Transactions on Cybernetics*, *49*(3), 1123–1136. doi:10.1109/TCYB.2018.2797905 PMID:29994385

Niemeijer, M., Staal, J. J., Ginneken, B. V., Loog, M., & Abramoff, M. D. (2004). Comparative study of retinal vessel segmentation methods on a new publicly available database. In *J. M. Fitzpatrick & M. Sonka (Eds.), S.* P. I. E. Medical Imaging, 5370, pp. 648–656. doi:10.1117/12.535349

Niemeyer, C. M. (2004). *Nanobiotechnology: concepts, applications and perspectives*. John Wiley & Sons.

Nikolic, M. (2001). *Detailed analysis of clinical electromyography signals: EMG decomposition, findings and firing pattern analysis in controls and patients with myopathy and amyotrophic lateral sclerosis* (Doctoral dissertation).

Nikolic, M., & Krarup, C. (2011). EMGTools, an adaptive and versatile tool for detailed EMG analysis. *IEEE Transactions on Biomedical Engineering*, *58*(10), 2707–2718. doi:10.1109/TBME.2010.2064773 PMID:20699205

Nisha, R., Srinivasa, K. S. R., Thanga, M. K., & Jagatha, P. (2017). Biochemical evaluation of creatinine and urea in patients with renal failure undergoing hemodialysis. *Journal of Clinical Pathology and Laboratory Medicine*, *1*(2), 1–5.

Norcia, A. M., Appelbaum, L. G., Ales, J. M., Cottereau, B. R., & Rossion, B. (2015). The steady-state visual evoked potential in vision research: A review. *Journal of Vision (Charlottesville, Va.)*, *15*(6), 4–4. doi:10.1167/15.6.4 PMID:26024451

Norstebo, C. A. (2003). Intelligent Textiles, Soft Products. *Journal of Future Materials.*

Novi, Q., Guan, C., Dat, T. H., & Xue, P. (2007). Sub-band common spatial pattern (SBCSP) for brain-computer interface. In *3rd International IEEE/EMBS Conference On Neural Engineering, 2007. CNE'07*, 204–207. Piscataway, NJ: IEEE.

Noy, A., Miller, A. E., Klare, J. E., Weeks, B. L., Woods, B. W., & DeYoreo, J. J. (2002). Fabrication of luminescent nanostructures and polymer nanowires using dip-pen nanolithography. *Nano Letters*, *2*(2), 109–112.

O'mahony, J. (2012). U.S. Patent Application No. 13/503,902.

Ocha, V., Seromenho, R., Correia, J., Mascioletti, A., Picano, A., & Goncalves, G. (2008). Wearable computing for patients with coronary diseases. *Proc. of the IEEE Int. Conf. Automation, Quality Testing, Robotics*, 3, pp. 37–42. doi:10.100710916-015-0272-9

Oizumi, M., Albantakis, L., & Tononi, G. (2014). From the phenomenology to the mechanisms of consciousness: Integrated information theory 3.0. *PLoS Computational Biology*, *10*(5). doi:10.1371/journal.pcbi.1003588 PMID:24811198

Oliveira, R. B., Papa, J. P., Pereira, A. S., & Tavares, J. M. R. (2016). Computational methods for pigmented skin lesion classification in images: Review and future trends. *Neural Computing & Applications*, 1–24.

Ostovan, A. G. (2018). Fabrication of water-compatible superparamagnetic molecularly imprinted biopolymer for clean separation of baclofen from bio-fluid samples: A mild and green approach. *Talanta*, *179*, 760–768.

Ottini, L., Palli, D., Rizzo, S., Federico, M., Bazan, V., & Russo, A. (2010). Male breast cancer. *Critical Reviews in Oncology/Hematology*, *73*(2), 141–155. doi:10.1016/j.critrevonc.2009.04.003 PMID:19427229

Pachori, R. B. (2008). Discrimination between ictal and seizure-free EEG signals using empirical mode decomposition. *Research Letters in Signal Processing*, *2008*, 14. doi:10.1155/2008/293056

Pachori, R. B., Avinash, P., Shashank, K., Sharma, R., & Acharya, U. R. (2015). Application of empirical mode decomposition for analysis of normal and diabetic RR-interval signals. *Expert Systems with Applications*, *42*(9), 4567–4581. doi:10.1016/j.eswa.2015.01.051

Pachori, R. B., Kumar, M., Avinash, P., Shashank, K., & Acharya, U. R. (2016). An improved online paradigm for screening of diabetic patients using RR-interval signals. *Journal of Mechanics in Medicine and Biology*, *16*(01). doi:10.1142/S0219519416400030

Park, H., Oh, S., Noh, Y., Kim, J. Y., & Kim, J. H. (2018). Heart rate variability as a marker of distress and recovery: The effect of brief supportive expressive group therapy with mindfulness in cancer patients. *Integrative Cancer Therapies*, *17*(3), 825–831. doi:10.1177/1534735418756192 PMID:29417836

Patidar, S., & Pachori, R. B. (2014). Classification of cardiac sound signals using constrained tunable-Q wavelet transform. *Expert Systems with Applications*, *41*(16), 7161–7170. doi:10.1016/j.eswa.2014.05.052

Patidar, S., Pachori, R. B., & Acharya, U. R. (2015). Automated diagnosis of coronary artery disease using tunable-Q wavelet transform applied on heart rate signals. *Knowledge-Based Systems*, *82*, 1–10. doi:10.1016/j.knosys.2015.02.011

Patolsky, F. Z. (2004). Electrical detection of single viruses. *Proceedings of the National Academy of Sciences of the United States of America*, *101*(39), 14017–14022.

Pattichis, C. S., & Elia, A. G. (1999). Autoregressive and cepstral analyses of motor unit action potentials. *Medical Engineering & Physics*, *21*(6-7), 405–419. doi:10.1016/S1350-4533(99)00072-7 PMID:10624737

Pease, R. F. (1981). Electron beam lithography. *Contemporary Physics*, *22*(3), 265–290.

Peng, Z. K., Jackson, M. R., Rongong, J. A., Chu, F. L., & Parkin, R. M. (2009). On the energy leakage of discrete wavelet transform. *Mechanical Systems and Signal Processing*, *23*(2), 330–343. doi:10.1016/j.ymssp.2008.05.014

Penn, A. A., & Shatz, C. J. (1999). Brain waves and brain wiring: The role of endogenous and sensory-driven neural activity in development. *Pediatric Research*, *45*(4 Pt 1), 447–458. doi:10.1203/00006450-199904010-00001 PMID:10203134

Penrose, R., & Hameroff, S. (1998). The PenroseHameroff 'Orch OR'Model of Consciousness. *Philosophical Transactions of the Royal Society of London. Series A, Mathematical and Physical Sciences*, *356*, 1869–1896.

Perez, M., Alun, H. D., Thorn, S. A., & Kim, P. H. (2007). Improvement of a retinal blood vessel segmentation method using the insight segmentation and registration toolkit (ITK). In *29th Annual International Conference of the Engineering in Medicine and Biology Society, EMBS 2007.* Piscataway, NJ: IEEE. 892-895.

Pérez-Madrigal, M. M. (2015). Insulating and semiconducting polymeric free-standing nanomembranes with biomedical applications. *Journal of Materials Chemistry. B, Materials for Biology and Medicine*, *3*(29), 5904–5932.

Pfeiffer, G. (1999). The diagnostic power of motor unit potential analysis: An objective Bayesian approach. *Muscle & Nerve: Official Journal of the American Association of Electrodiagnostic Medicine*, *22*(5), 584–591. doi:10.1002/(SICI)1097-4598(199905)22:5<584::AID-MUS6>3.0.CO;2-0 PMID:10331357

Pfurtscheller, G. & Neuper, C. (2001). Motor imagery and direct brain-computer communication. *Proceedings of the IEEE*, *89*(7), 1123–1134.

Pfurtscheller, G., Flotzinger, D., Pregenzer, M., Wolpaw, J. R., & McFarland, D. (1995). EEG-based brain computer interface (BCI). Search for optimal electrode positions and frequency components. *Medical Progress Through Technology*, *21*(3), 111–121. PMID:8776708

Pfurtscheller, G., & Lopes da Silva, F. H. (1999). Event-related EEG/MEG synchronization and desynchronization: Basic principles. *Clinical Neurophysiology*, *110*(11), 1842–1857. doi:10.1016/S1388-2457(99)00141-8 PMID:10576479

Piner, R. D., Zhu, J., Xu, F., Hong, S., & Mirkin, C. A. (1999). " Dip-pen" nanolithography. science, 283(5402), 661-663.

Piskorski, J., Guzik, P., Krauze, T., & Żurek, S. (2010). Cardiopulmonary resonance at 0.1 Hz demonstrated by averaged Lomb-Scargle periodogram. *Central European Journal of Physics*, *8*(3), 386–392.

Pokropivny, V. V. (2007). Classification of nanostructures by dimensionality and concept of surface forms engineering in nanomaterial science. *Materials Science and Engineering C*, *27*(5-8), 990–993.

Pola, T. & Vanhala, J. (2007). Textile Electrodes in ECG Measurement. In 2007 3rd International Conference on Intelligent Sensors, Sensor Networks and Information.

Porta, A., Gnecchi-Ruscone, T., Tobaldini, E., Guzzetti, S., Furlan, R., & Montano, N. (2007). Progressive decrease of heart period variability entropy-based complexity during graded head-up tilt. *Journal of Applied Physiology*, *103*(4), 1143–1149. doi:10.1152/japplphysiol.00293.2007 PMID:17569773

Porta, A., Guzzetti, S., Furlan, R., Gnecchi-Ruscone, T., Montano, N., & Malliani, A. (2007). Complexity and nonlinearity in short-term heart period variability: Comparison of methods based on local nonlinear prediction. *IEEE Transactions on Biomedical Engineering*, *54*(1), 94–106. doi:10.1109/TBME.2006.883789 PMID:17260860

Potharaju, S. P., & Sreedevi, M. (2016). An improved prediction of kidney disease using SMOTE. *Indian Journal of Science and Technology*, *9*(31). doi:10.17485/ijst/2016/v9i31/95634

Prasad, A., Choi, J., Jia, Z., Park, S., & Gartia, M. R. (2019). Nanohole array plasmonic biosensors: Emerging point-of-care applications. *Biosensors & Bioelectronics*.

Prasad, N., & Houserkova, D. (2007). The role of various modalities in breast imaging. *Biomedical Papers of the Medical Faculty of the Palacky University, Olomouc*, Czech Republic, *1519*(2), 209–218. doi:10.5507/bp.2007.036 PMID:18345253

Prinz, J. (2012). The conscious brain. Oxford, UK: Oxford University Press. doi:10.1093/acprof:oso/9780195314595.001.0001

Quinlan, J. R. (1986). Induction of Decision Trees. *Machine Learning*, *1*(1), 81–106. doi:10.1007/BF00116251

Quinlan, J. R. (1993). *C4.5: Programs for Machine Learning*. San Francisco, CA: Morgan Kaufmann Publishers.

Rabbani, H., Allingham, M. J., Mettu, P. S., Cousins, S. W., & Farsiu, S. (2015). Fully automatic segmentation of fluorescein leakage in subjects with diabetic macular edema. *Investigative Ophthalmology & Visual Science*, *56*(3), 1482–1492. doi:10.1167/iovs.14-15457 PMID:25634978

Raja, N. S. M., Kavitha, G., & Ramakrishnan, S. (2012). Analysis of vasculature in human retinal images using particle swarm optimization based Tsallis multi-level thresholding and similarity measures. *Lecture Notes in Computer Science*, *7677*, 380–387. doi:10.1007/978-3-642-35380-2_45

Rajinikanth, V., Dey, N., Kumar, R., Panneerselvam, J., & Raja, N. S. M. (2019). Fetal head periphery extraction from ultrasound image using Jaya algorithm and Chan-Vese segmentation. *Procedia Computer Science*, *152*, 66–73. doi:10.1016/j.procs.2019.05.028

Rajinikanth, V., Raja, N. S. M., Satapathy, S. C., & Fernandes, S. L. (2017). Otsu's multi-thresholding and active contour snake model to segment dermoscopy images. *Journal of Medical Imaging and Health Informatics*, *7*(8), 1837–1840. doi:10.1166/jmihi.2017.2265

Ramos, A. C., Hernández, R. G., & Vellasco, M. (2016). Feature selection methods applied to motor imagery task classification. In *2016 IEEE Latin American Conference On Computational Intelligence (LA-CCI)*, 1–6. Piscataway, NJ: IEEE.

Ramoser, H., Muller-Gerking, J., & Pfurtscheller, G. (2000). Optimal spatial filtering of single trial EEG during imagined hand movement. *IEEE Transactions on Rehabilitation Engineering*, *8*(4), 441–446. doi:10.1109/86.895946 PMID:11204034

Rantanen, J., Vuorela, T., Kukkonen, K., & Ryynänen, O. (2001). Improving human thermal comfort with smart clothing. *Proceedings of the 2001 IEEE Systems, Man and Cybernetics Conference*.10.1109/ICSMC.2001.973012

Rao, R. P. N., & Scherer, R. (2010). Brain-Computer Interfacing [In the Spotlight]. *IEEE Signal Processing Magazine*, *27*(4), 152–150. doi:10.1109/MSP.2010.936774

Rao, R. V. (2016). Jaya: A simple and new optimization algorithm for solving constrained and unconstrained optimization problems. *International Journal of Industrial Engineering Computations*, *7*, 19–34.

Rao, R. V., & More, K. C. (2017). Design optimization and analysis of selected thermal devices using self-adaptive Jaya algorithm. *Energy Conversion and Management*, *140*, 24–35. doi:10.1016/j.enconman.2017.02.068

Ravindra, B. V., Sriraam, N., & Geetha, M. (2017). Classification of non-chronic and chronic kidney disease using SVM neural networks. *International Journal of Engineering & Technology*, *7*(1.3), 191. doi:10.14419/ijet.v7i1.3.10669

Ravindra, B. V., Sriraam, N., & Geetha, M. (2018). Chronic kidney disease detection using back propagation neural network classifier. In *Proceedings of the 2018 International Conference on Communication, Computing and Internet of Things, IC3IoT 2018* (pp. 65–68). Piscataway, NJ: IEEE. 10.1109/IC3IoT.2018.8668110

Rees, A., Powell, L. C., Chinga-Carrasco, G., Gethin, D. T., Syverud, K., Hill, K. E., & Thomas, D. W. (2015). 3D bioprinting of carboxymethylated-periodate oxidized nanocellulose constructs for wound dressing applications. *BioMed Research International*.

Reisner, D. E. (2008). *Bionanotechnology: global prospects*. CRC Press.

Reuter, M. A., & Reuter, H. J. (1999). *History of Endoscopy: An Illustrated Documentation*. Stuttgart, Germany: Kohlhammer.

Richani, K., Romero, R., Kim, Y. M., Cushenberry, E., Soto, E., Han, Y. M., & Kim, C. J. (2006). Tissue microarray: An effective high-throughput method to study the placenta for clinical and research purposes. *The Journal of Maternal-Fetal & Neonatal Medicine*, *19*(8), 509–515.

Richman, J. S., & Moorman, J. R. (2000). Physiological time-series analysis using approximate entropy and sample entropy. *American Journal of Physiology. Heart and Circulatory Physiology*, *278*(6), H2039–H2049. doi:10.1152/ajpheart.2000.278.6.H2039 PMID:10843903

Rodrigues, D. G., & Weibel, N. (2017). Exploring mixed reality in specialized surgical environments. In *CHI Conference Extended Abstracts on Human Factors in Computing Systems* (pp. 2591-2598), New York, NY. 10.1145/3027063.3053273

Rokach, L., & Maimon, O. (2005). Top-Down Induction of Decision Trees Classifiers – A Survey. *IEEE Transactions on Systems, Man and Cybernetics. Part C, Applications and Reviews*, *35*(4), 476–487. doi:10.1109/TSMCC.2004.843247

Rubini, L., & Eswaran, P. (2015). Generating comparative analysis of early stage prediction of Chronic Kidney Disease. *International Journal Of Modern Engineering Research*, *5*(49), 49–55.

Ruecha, N., Rangkupan, R., Rodthongkum, N., & Chailapakul, O. (2014). Novel paper-based cholesterol biosensor using graphene/polyvinylpyrrolidone/polyaniline nanocomposite. *Biosensors & Bioelectronics*, *52*, 13–19.

Salaita, K., Wang, Y., & Mirkin, C. A. (2007). Applications of dip-pen nanolithography. *Nature Nanotechnology*, *2*(3), 145.

Saleh, M. M., & Ali, M. (2011). Retinal image analysis using curvelet transform and multistructure elements morphology by reconstruction. *IEEE Transactions on Biomedical Engineering*, *58*(5), 1183–1192. doi:10.1109/TBME.2010.2097599 PMID:21147592

Samorezov, J. E., & Alsberg, E. (2015). Spatial regulation of controlled bioactive factor delivery for bone tissue engineering. *Advanced Drug Delivery Reviews*, *84*, 45–67.

Santra, S., De Luca, A., Bhaumik, S., Ali, S. Z., Udrea, F., Gardner, J. W., ... Guha, P. K. (2015). Dip pen nanolithography-deposited zinc oxide nanorods on a CMOS MEMS platform for ethanol sensing. *RSC Advances*, *5*(59), 47609–47616.

Satapathy, S. C. & Rajinikanth, V. (2018). Jaya algorithm guided procedure to segment tumor from brain MRI. *Journal of Optimization*. doi:10.1155/2018/3738049

Satava, R. M. (1993). Virtual reality surgical simulator. *Surgical Endoscopy*, *7*(3), 203–205. doi:10.1007/BF00594110 PMID:8503081

Schalk, G., & Leuthardt, E. C. (2011). Brain-computer interfaces using electrocorticographic signals. *IEEE Reviews in Biomedical Engineering*, *4*, 140–154. doi:10.1109/RBME.2011.2172408 PMID:22273796

Schlogl, A., Kronegg, J., Huggins, J., & Mason, S. (2007). *19 evaluation criteria for bci research.* Toward Brain-Computer Interfacing.

Sengupta, N., Sahidullah, M., & Saha, G. (2016). Lung sound classification using cepstral-based statistical features. *Computers in Biology and Medicine*, *75*, 118–129. doi:10.1016/j.compbiomed.2016.05.013 PMID:27286184

Seth, A. K. (2005). Causal connectivity of evolved neural networks during behavior. *Network (Bristol, England)*, *16*(1), 35–54. doi:10.1080/09548980500238756 PMID:16350433

Seth, A. K., Dienes, Z., Cleeremans, A., Overgaard, M., & Pessoa, L. (2008). Measuring consciousness: Relating behavioural and neurophysiological approaches. *Trends in Cognitive Sciences*, *12*(8), 314–321. doi:10.1016/j.tics.2008.04.008 PMID:18606562

Seth, A. K., Izhikevich, E., Reeke, G. N., & Edelman, G. M. (2006). Theories and measures of consciousness: An extended framework. *Proceedings of the National Academy of Sciences of the United States of America*, *103*(28), 10799–10804. doi:10.1073/pnas.0604347103 PMID:16818879

Shannon, B. J. & Paliwal, K. K. (2003). A Comparative Study of Filter Bank Spacing for Speech Recognition. In *Microelectronic Engineering Research Conference 41:* 310–12. Retrieved from https://maxwell.ict.griffith.edu.au/spl/publications/papers/merc03_ben.pdf

Sharanreddy, P. K. K. (2013, March). Detection of primary brain tumor present in eeg signal using wavelet transform and neural network [Journal (Paginated)]. Retrieved from https://www.biomedscidirect.com/990/detection_of_primary_brain_tumor_present_in_eeg_signal_using_wavelet_transform_and_neural_network/articlescategories

Sharma, R. R. & Pachori, R. B. (2017b, February). A new method for non-stationary signal analysis using eigenvalue decomposition of the Hankel matrix and Hilbert transform. In *2017 4th International Conference on Signal Processing and Integrated Networks (SPIN),* (pp. 484-488). 10.1109/SPIN.2017.8049998

Sharma, R. R., Chandra, P., & Pachori, R. B. (2019a). Electromyogram signal analysis using eigenvalue decomposition of the Hankel matrix. In Machine Intelligence and Signal Analysis (pp. 671-682). doi:10.1007/978-981-13-0923-6_57

Sharma, R. R., Kumar, M., & Pachori, R. B. (2019c). Automated CAD identification system using time–frequency representation based on eigenvalue decomposition of ECG signals. In Machine Intelligence and Signal Analysis (pp. 597-608). doi:10.1007/978-981-13-0923-6_51

Sharma, R. R., Kumar, A., Pachori, R. B., & Acharya, U. R. (2019b). Accurate automated detection of congestive heart failure using eigenvalue decomposition based features extracted from HRV signals. *Biocybernetics and Biomedical Engineering*, *39*(2), 312–327. doi:10.1016/j.bbe.2018.10.001

Sharma, R. R., Kumar, M., & Pachori, R. B. (2019d). Joint time-frequency domain based CAD disease sensing system using ECG signals. *IEEE Sensors Journal*, *19*(10), 3912–3920. doi:10.1109/JSEN.2019.2894706

Sharma, R. R., & Pachori, R. B. (2017a). Time–frequency representation using IEVDHM–HT with application to classification of epileptic EEG signals. *IET Science, Measurement & Technology*, *12*(1), 72–82. doi:10.1049/iet-smt.2017.0058

Sharma, R. R., & Pachori, R. B. (2018a). Eigenvalue decomposition of Hankel matrix-based time-frequency representation for complex signals. *Circuits, Systems, and Signal Processing*, 1–17.

Sharma, R. R., & Pachori, R. B. (2018b). Improved eigenvalue decomposition-based approach for reducing cross-terms in Wigner–Ville distribution. *Circuits, Systems, and Signal Processing*, 1–21.

Sharma, R. R., & Pachori, R. B. (2018c). Baseline wander and power line interference removal from ECG signals using eigenvalue decomposition. *Biomedical Signal Processing and Control*, *45*, 33–49. doi:10.1016/j.bspc.2018.05.002

Sharma, R., Pachori, R. B., & Upadhyay, A. (2017). Automatic sleep stages classification based on iterative filtering of electroencephalogram signals. *Neural Computing & Applications*, *28*(10), 2959–2978. doi:10.100700521-017-2919-6

Sharma, S., & Patil, H. A. (2015). Combining Evidences from Bark Scale and Mel Scale Warped Features for VTLN. In *Proceedings of the 2nd International Conference on Perception and Machine Intelligence (PerMIn '15)*. ACM, New York, NY, 133-136.

Shawe-Taylor, J., & Sun, S. (2011). A review of optimization methodologies in support vector machines. *Neurocomputing*, *74*(17), 3609–3618. doi:10.1016/j.neucom.2011.06.026

Shaw, L., & Bagha, S. (2012). Online EMG signal analysis for diagnosis of neuromuscular diseases by using PCA and PNN. *International Journal of Engineering Science and Technology*, *4*(10), 4453–4459.

Sheffield, D., Krittayaphong, R., Cascio, W. E., Light, K. C., Golden, R. N., Finkel, J. B., & Sheps, D. S. (1998). Heart rate variability at rest and during mental stress in patients with coronary artery disease: Differences in patients with high and low depression scores. *International Journal of Behavioral Medicine*, *5*(1), 31–47. doi:10.120715327558ijbm0501_3 PMID:16250714

Sher, A., & Thorpy, M. (1986). Endoscopic observations of obstructive sleep apnea in children with anomalous upper airways: Predictive and therapeutic value. *International Journal of Pediatric Otorhinolaryngology*, *11*(2), 135–146. doi:10.1016/S0165-5876(86)80008-8 PMID:3744695

Shi, H., Nie, K., Dong, B., Long, M., Xu, H., & Liu, Z. (2018). Recent progress of microfluidic reactors for biomedical applications. *Chemical Engineering Journal*, *361*, 635–650.

Shree, V. T. D., Revanth, K., Raja, N. S. M., & Rajinikanth, V. (2018). A hybrid image processing approach to examine abnormality in retinal optic disc. *Procedia Computer Science*, *125*, 157–164. doi:10.1016/j.procs.2017.12.022

Shriranjani, D., Tebby, S. G., Satapathy, S. C., Dey, N., & Rajinikanth, V. (2018). Kapur's entropy and active contour-based segmentation and analysis of retinal optic disc. *Lecture Notes in Electrical Engineering*, *490*, 287–295. doi:10.1007/978-981-10-8354-9_26

Shukla, R. S., & Aggarwal, Y. (2017a). Heart Rate Variability Time-Domain Analysis in Pulmonary Metastasis to Assess Performance Status. *Indian Journal of Social Research*, *14*(2), 540–545.

Shukla, R. S., & Aggarwal, Y. (2017b). Spectral Analysis to Evaluate the Effect of Treatment on Autonomic Nervous System in Pulmonary Metastasis. *Journal of Cancer Research and Therapeutics*, 13.

Shukla, R. S., & Aggarwal, Y. (2018a). Electrocardiogram in Lung Cancer Patients Envisage as Pseudo-Myocardial Infarction and Ischemic Heart Disease. *Journal of Clinical Engineering*, *43*(1), 48–52. doi:10.1097/JCE.0000000000000252

Shukla, R. S., & Aggarwal, Y. (2018b). Heart Rate Variability in Male Breast Cancer. *Clinical Cancer Investigation*, *7*(3), 125. doi:10.4103/ccij.ccij_12_18

Shukla, R. S., & Aggarwal, Y. (2018c). Nonlinear Heart Rate Variability based Analysis and Prediction of Performance Status in Pulmonary Metastases Patients. *Biomedical Engineering: Applications, Basis and Communications*, *16*(2), 145–155.

Shukla, R. S., & Aggarwal, Y. (2018d). Time-domain heart rate variability-based computer-aided prognosis of lung cancer. *Indian Journal of Cancer*, *55*(1), 61. doi:10.4103/ijc.IJC_395_17 PMID:30147095

Shukla, R. S., & Aggarwal, Y. (2018e). Nonlinear Heart Rate Variability based artificial intelligence in lung cancer prediction. *Journal of Applied Biomedicine*, *16*(2), 145–155. doi:10.1016/j.jab.2017.12.002

Sielhorst, T., & Navab, N. (2004). An augmented reality delivery simulator for medical training. In *proceedings of Workshop on Augmented Environments for Medical Imaging-MICCAI Satellite Workshop*, 141, pp. 11–20.

Silliman, R. A., Guadagnoli, E., Weitberg, A. B., & Mor, V. (1989). Age as a predictor of diagnostic and initial treatment intensity in newly diagnosed breast cancer patients. *Journal of Gerontology*, *44*(2), M46–M50. doi:10.1093/geronj/44.2.M46 PMID:2921470

Singh, S., Prakash, C., & Ramakrishna, S. (2019). 3D Printing of Polyether-ether-ketone for Biomedical Applications. *European Polymer Journal*, *114*, 234–248.

Sivakamasundari, J., Kavitha, G., Natarajan, V., & Ramakrishnan, S. (2015). An approach to content based retinal image retrieval using papamarkos multilevel thresholding method. *J. Med. Imaging Health Inf.*, *5*(3), 527–532. doi:10.1166/jmihi.2015.1419

Smith, L., & MacNeil, S. (2011). State of the art in non-invasive imaging of cutaneous melanoma. *Skin Research and Technology*, *17*(3), 257–269. doi:10.1111/j.1600-0846.2011.00503.x PMID:21342292

Soenen, S. J. (2015). (Intra) cellular stability of inorganic nanoparticles: Effects on cytotoxicity, particle functionality, and biomedical applications. *Chemical Reviews*, ▪▪▪, 2109–2135.

Sofka, M., & Stewart, C. V. (2006). Retinal vessel centerline extraction using multiscale matched filters, confidence and edge measures. *IEEE Transactions on Medical Imaging*, *25*(12), 1531–1546. doi:10.1109/TMI.2006.884190 PMID:17167990

Song, L. & Gordon, E. (n.d.). *Phase Synchrony Rate for the Recognition of Motor Imagery in BCI*. 8.

Song, L., Gordon, E., & Gysels, E. (2006). Phase Synchrony Rate for the Recognition of Motor Imagery in Brain-Computer Interface. In Y. Weiss, B. Schölkopf, & J. C. Platt (Eds.), Advances in Neural Information Processing Systems Vol. 18, pp. 1265–1272. Retrieved from http://papers.nips.cc/paper/2849-phase-synchrony-rate-for-the-recognition-of-motor-imagery-in-brain-computer-interface.pdf

Sood, S., Kumar, M., Pachori, R. B., & Acharya, U. R. (2016). Application of empirical mode decomposition–based features for analysis of normal and CAD heart rate signals. *Journal of Mechanics in Medicine and Biology*, *16*(01). doi:10.1142/S0219519416400029

Spano, E., Di Pascoli, S., & Iannaccone, G. (2016). Low-Power Wearable ECG Monitoring System for Multiple-Patient Remote Monitoring. *IEEE Sensors Journal*, *16*(13), 5452–5462. doi:10.1109/JSEN.2016.2564995

Sreejini, K. S., & Govindan, V. K. (2015). Improved multiscale matched filter for retina vessel segmentation using PSO algorithm. *Egyptian Informatics Journal*, *16*(3), 253–260. doi:10.1016/j.eij.2015.06.004

Srinivasan, S. (1997). Wootz steel: an advanced material of the ancient world.

Sriraam, N., Natasha, V., & Kaur, H. (2011). Data Mining Techniques and Medical Decision Making for Urological Dysfunction. In Data Warehousing and Mining (pp. 2506–2516). Hershey, PA: IGI Global. doi:10.4018/978-1-59904-951-9.ch153

Sriraam, N., & Tejaswini, S. (2014). Infant Cry Detection and Pain Scale Assessment: A Pilot Study. *International Journal of Biomedical and Clinical Engineering*, *3*(1), 42–51. doi:10.4018/ijbce.2014010104

Sriraam, N., Tejaswini, S., & Chavan, A. A. (2016). Development of Portable Medical Electronic Device for Infant Cry Recognition: A Primitive Experimental Study. *International Journal of Biomedical and Clinical Engineering*, *5*(2), 53–63. doi:10.4018/IJBCE.2016070104

Staal, J. J., Abramoff, M. D., Niemeijer, M., Viergever, M. A., & Ginneken, B. V. (2004). Ridge based vessel segmentation in color images of the retina. *IEEE Transactions on Medical Imaging*, *23*(4), 501–509. doi:10.1109/TMI.2004.825627 PMID:15084075

Stapelberg, N. J., Neumann, D. L., Shum, B. H. K., McConnell, H., & Hamilton-Craig, I. (2018). The sensitivity of 38 heart rate variability measures to the addition of artifact in human and artificial 24-hr cardiac recordings. *Annals of Noninvasive Electrocardiology*, *23*(1). doi:10.1111/anec.12483 PMID:28670841

Subas, A., Alickovic, E., & Kevric, J. (2017). Diagnosis of chronic kidney disease by using random forest. In IFMBE proceedings, 62, pp. 589–594. Germany: Springer Verlag. doi:10.1007/978-981-10-4166-2_89

Subasi, A., Yilmaz, M., & Ozcalik, H. R. (2006). Classification of EMG signals using wavelet neural network. *Journal of Neuroscience Methods*, *156*(1-2), 360–367. doi:10.1016/j.jneumeth.2006.03.004 PMID:16621003

Sudhan, G. H. H., Aravind, R. G., Gowri, K., & Rajinikanth, V. (2017). Optic disc segmentation based on Otsu's thresholding and level set. In *International Conference on Computer Communication and Informatics (ICCCI)*. 10.1109/ICCCI.2017.8117688

Sultan, S., Siqueira, G., Zimmermann, T., & Mathew, A. P. (2017). 3D printing of nano-cellulosic biomaterials for medical applications. *Current Opinion in Biomedical Engineering*, *2*, 29–34.

Sur, S., & Sinha, V. K. (2009). Event-related potential: An overview. *Industrial Psychiatry Journal*, *18*(1), 70–73. doi:10.4103/0972-6748.57865 PMID:21234168

Susurla, S., Krishna Kumar, R., & Kamakoti, V. (2012). Portable Low Cost 3 Lead Wireless Wearable ECG Device. *IFMBE Proceedings*, *39*. doi:10.1007/978-3-642-29305-4_349

Suykens, J. A., & Vandewalle, J. (1999). Least squares support vector machine classifiers. *Neural Processing Letters*, *9*(3), 293–300. doi:10.1023/A:1018628609742

Tan, D., Maniruzzaman, M., & Nokhodchi, A. (2018). Advanced pharmaceutical applications of Hot-Melt Extrusion coupled with Fused Deposition Modelling (FDM) 3D printing for personalised drug delivery. *Pharmaceutics*, *10*(4), 203.

Tangermann, M., Müller, K.-R., Aertsen, A., Birbaumer, N., Braun, C., Brunner, C., ... Mueller-Putz, G. (2012). Review of the BCI competition IV. *Frontiers in Neuroscience*, *6*, 55. doi:10.3389/fnins.2012.00055 PMID:22811657

Tantaratana, S., & Thomas, J. B. (1981). A Class of Nonparametric Sequential Tests. *IEEE Transactions on Information Theory*, *27*(5), 596–606. doi:10.1109/TIT.1981.1056401

Tarvainen, M. P., Niskanen, J. P., Lipponen, J. A., Ranta-Aho, P. O., & Karjalainen, P. A. (2014). Kubios HRV–heart rate variability analysis software. *Computer Methods and Programs in Biomedicine*, *113*(1), 210–220. doi:10.1016/j.cmpb.2013.07.024 PMID:24054542

Teber, D., & Rassweiler, J. (2009). Augmented reality: A new tool to improve surgical accuracy during laparoscopic partial nephrectomy? Preliminary in vitro and in vivo results. *European Urology*, *56*(2), 332–338. doi:10.1016/j.eururo.2009.05.017 PMID:19477580

Tejaswini, S., Sriraam, N. & Pradeep, G. C. M. (2016). Recognition of infant cries using wavelet derived mel frequency feature with SVM classification. In *Proceedings of 2016 International Conference on Circuits, Controls, Communications and Computing (I4C),* Bangalore, India, pp. 1-4. 10.1109/CIMCA.2016.8053313

Tejaswini, S., Sriraam, N., & Pradeep, G. C. M. (2019). Preterm Neonates Cry Pattern Recognition Using Bark Frequency Cepstral Coefficients. In *Proceedings of 2019 1st International Conference on Advanced Technologies in Intelligent Control, Environment, Computing and Communication Engineering,* Bangalore, India.

Tejaswini, S., Sriraam, N., & Pradeep, G. C. M. Cloud-Based Framework for Pain Scale Assessment in NICU- A Primitive Study with Infant Cries. In *Proceedings of 2018 3rd International Conference on Circuits, Control, Communication and Computing (I4C),* Bangalore, India, pp. 1-4. 10.1109/CIMCA.2018.8739712

Thomas, K. P., Guan, C., Tong, L. C., & Prasad, V. A. (2008). An adaptive filter bank for motor imagery based Brain Computer Interface. In *Proceedings of Annual International Conference of the IEEE Engineering in Medicine and Biology Society*. 1104–1107. 10.1109/IEMBS.2008.4649353

Tibshirani, R. (2017). Regression shrinkage and selection via the lasso: A retrospective. *Journal of the Royal Statistical Society. Series B, Statistical Methodology*, 273–282. doi:10.1111/j.1467-9868.2011.00771.x@10.1111/(ISSN)1467-9868.TOP_SERIES_B_RESEARCH

Tiwari, J. N. (2012). Zero-dimensional, one-dimensional, two-dimensional and three-dimensional nanostructured materials for advanced electrochemical energy devices. *Progress in Materials Science*, *57*(4), 724–803.

Tomasic, I., Frljak, S., & Trobec, R. (2013). Estimating the Universal Positions of Wireless Body Electrodes for Measuring Cardiac Electrical Activity. *IEEE Transactions on Biomedical Engineering*, *60*(12), 3368–3374. doi:10.1109/TBME.2013.2276291 PMID:23925363

Tononi, G. (2004). An information integration theory of consciousness. *BMC Neuroscience*, *5*(1), 42. doi:10.1186/1471-2202-5-42 PMID:15522121

Tononi, G. (2008). Consciousness as integrated information: A provisional manifesto. *The Biological Bulletin*, *215*(3), 216–242. doi:10.2307/25470707 PMID:19098144

Tononi, G., Sporns, O., & Edelman, G. M. (1994). A measure for brain complexity: Relating functional segregation and integration in the nervous system. *Proceedings of the National Academy of Sciences of the United States of America*, *91*(11), 5033–5037. doi:10.1073/pnas.91.11.5033 PMID:8197179

Touhami, A. (2014). Biosensors and Nanobiosensors: Design and Applications. *Nanomedicine (London)*, ▪▪▪, 374–400.

Tran, K. T., & Nguyen, T. D. (2017). Lithography-based methods to manufacture biomaterials at small scales. *Journal of Science: Advanced Materials and Devices*, *2*(1), 1–14.

Trulla, L. L., Giuliani, A., Zbilut, J. P., & Webber, C. L. Jr. (1996). Recurrence quantification analysis of the logistic equation with transients. *Physics Letters. [Part A]*, *223*(4), 255–260. doi:10.1016/S0375-9601(96)00741-4

Tuduce, R. I., Cucu, H., & Burileanu, C. (2018). Why Is My Baby Crying? An In-Depth Analysis of Paralinguistic Features and Classical Machine Learning Algorithms for Baby Cry Classification. In *2018 41st International Conference on Telecommunications and Signal Processing, TSP 2018*: 1–4. 10.1109/TSP.2018.8441363

Udhayarasu, M., Ramakrishnan, K., & Periasamy, S. (2017). Assessment of chronic kidney disease using skin texture as a key parameter: For South Indian population. *Healthcare Technology Letters*, *4*(6), 223–227. doi:10.1049/htl.2016.0098 PMID:29383256

Ueno, A., Akabane, Y., Kato, T., Hoshino, H., Kataoka, S., & Ishiyama, Y. (2007). Capacitive sensing of electrocardiographic potential through cloth from the dorsal surface of the body in a supine position: A preliminary study. *IEEE Trans. Biomed. Eng.*, *54*(4), 759–766.

Vaezi, M., Black, C., Gibbs, D., Oreffo, R., Brady, M., Moshrefi-Torbati, M., & Yang, S. (2016). Characterization of new PEEK/HA composites with 3D HA network fabricated by extrusion freeforming. *Molecules (Basel, Switzerland)*, *21*(6), 687.

Vaishnavi, G. K., Jeevananthan, K., Begum, S. R., & Kamalanand, K. (2014). Geometrical analysis of schistosome egg images using distance regularized level set method for automated species identification. *J. Bioinformatics Intell. Cont*, *3*(2), 147–152. doi:10.1166/jbic.2014.1080

Valchinov, E., Antoniou, A., Rotas, K. & Pallikarakis, N. (2014). Wearable ECG System for Health and Sports Monitoring. doi:10.13140/2.1.2281.4406

Van Gulick, R. (2018). "Consciousness". *The Stanford Encyclopedia of Philosophy* (Spring 2018 Edition), Edward N. Zalta (Ed.). Retrieved from https://plato.stanford.edu/archives/spr2018/entries/consciousness/

VandenBos, G., Knapp, S., & Doe, J. (2001). Role of reference elements in the selection of resources by psychology undergraduates. Retrieved from http://jbr.org/articles.html

Vazquez, M., Carter, D., Brambilla, E., Gazdar, A., Noguchi, M., Travis, W. D., ... Henschke, C. I. (2009). Solitary and multiple resected adenocarcinomas after CT screening for lung cancer: Histopathologic features and their prognostic implications. *Lung Cancer (Amsterdam, The Netherlands)*, *64*(2), 148–154. doi:10.1016/j.lungcan.2008.08.009 PMID:18951650

Vidyashree, H. M., Maheshkumar, K., Sundareswaran, L., Sakthivel, G., Partheeban, P. K., & Rajan, R. (2019). Effect of yoga intervention on short-term heart rate variability in children with autism spectrum disorder. *International Journal of Yoga*, *12*(1), 73. doi:10.4103/ijoy.IJOY_66_17 PMID:30692787

Vijayavenkataraman, S., Lu, W. F., & Fuh, J. Y. H. (2016). 3D bioprinting of skin: A state-of-the-art review on modelling, materials, and processes. *Biofabrication*, *8*(3), 032001.

Vijayavenkataraman, S., Yan, W. C., Lu, W. F., Wang, C. H., & Fuh, J. Y. H. (2018). 3D bioprinting of tissues and organs for regenerative medicine. *Advanced Drug Delivery Reviews*, *132*, 296–332.

Virmani, M., & Nagaraj, N. (2019). A novel perturbation based compression complexity measure for networks. *Heliyon (London)*, *5*(2). doi:10.1016/j.heliyon.2019.e01181 PMID:30828654

Vlăsceanu, G. M., Iovu, H., & Ioniţă, M. (2019). Graphene inks for the 3D printing of cell culture scaffolds and related molecular arrays. *Composites. Part B, Engineering*.

von Rosenberg, W., Chanwimalueang, T., Adjei, T., Jaffer, U., Goverdovsky, V., & Mandic, D. P. (2017). Resolving ambiguities in the LF/HF ratio: LF-HF scatter plots for the categorization of mental and physical stress from HRV. *Frontiers in Physiology*, *8*, 360. doi:10.3389/fphys.2017.00360 PMID:28659811

Wang, J., Feng, Z., & Lu, N. (2017). Feature extraction by common spatial pattern in frequency domain for motor imagery tasks classification. *2017 29th Chinese Control and Decision Conference (CCDC)*, 5883–5888. Piscataway, NJ: IEEE. 10.1109/CCDC.2017.7978220

Wang, H. J. (2006). Template synthesized molecularly imprinted polymer nanotube membranes for chemical separations. *Journal of the American Chemical Society*, *128*(50), 15954–15955.

Wang, J. (2005). Carbon-nanotube based electrochemical biosensors: A review. *Electroanalysis*, *17*(1), 7–14.

Wang, L. a. (2006). Multicolor FRET silica nanoparticles by single wavelength excitation. *Nano Letters*, ▪▪▪, 84–88.

Wang, S., Rao, R. V., Chen, P., Zhang, Y., Liu, A., & Wei, L. (2017). Abnormal breast detection in mammogram images by feed-forward neural network trained by Jaya algorithm. *Fundamenta Informaticae*, *151*(1-4), 191–211. doi:10.3233/FI-2017-1487

Ward, M. A. (2011). Thermoresponsive polymers for biomedical applications. *Polymers*, *3*(3), 1215–1242.

Weaver, P. (1964). *The technique of lithography*. London: BT Batsford.

Webster, J. G. (1998). *Medical Instrumentation: Application and Design*. New York, NY: John Wiley & Sons.

Wighton, P., Lee, T. K., Lui, H., McLean, D. I., & Atkins, M. S. (2011). Generalizing common tasks in automated skin lesion diagnosis. *IEEE Transactions on Information Technology in Biomedicine*, *15*(4), 622–629. doi:10.1109/TITB.2011.2150758 PMID:21550892

Wilkinson, C. P., Ferris, F. L. III, Klein, R. E., Lee, P. P., Agardh, C. D., Davis, M., ... Verdaguer, J. T. (2003). Proposed international clinical diabetic retinopathy and diabetic macular edema disease severity scales. *Ophthalmology*, *110*(9), 1677–1682. doi:10.1016/S0161-6420(03)00475-5 PMID:13129861

Williams, L. D. (2006). *Nanotechnology demystified*. McGraw Hill Professional.

Winokur, E. S., Delano, M. K., & Sodini, C. G. (2013). A wearable cardiac monitor for long-term data acquisition and analysis. *IEEE Transactions on Biomedical Engineering*, *60*(1), 189–192. doi:10.1109/TBME.2012.2217958

Witten, H., Frank, E., Trigg, L., Hall, M., Holmes, G., & Cunningham, S. J. (1999). Weka: Practical Machine Learning Tools and Techniques with Java Implementations.

Xia, Y. a. (1998). Soft lithography. *Annual Review of Materials Science*, *28*(1), 153–184.

Xie, J. L. (2008). Putting electrospun nanofibers to work for biomedical research. *Macromolecular Rapid Communications*, *29*(22), 1775–1792.

Xu, B., & Song, A. (2008). Pattern recognition of motor imagery EEG using wavelet transform. *Journal of Biomedical Science and Engineering*, *1*(01), 64–67. doi:10.4236/jbise.2008.11010

Xu, N., Ye, X., Wei, D., Zhong, J., Chen, Y., Xu, G., & He, D. (2014). 3D artificial bones for bone repair prepared by computed tomography-guided fused deposition modeling for bone repair. *ACS Applied Materials & Interfaces*, *6*(17), 14952–14963.

Xu, P. J., Zhang, H., & Tao, X. M. (2008). Textile-structured electrodes for electrocardiogram. *Textile Progress*, *40*(4), 183–213. doi:10.1080/00405160802597479

Xu, Q. T. (2004). Fabrication of free-standing metallic pyramidal shells. *Nano Letters*, *4*(12), 2509–2511.

Xu, X., He, L., Zhu, B., Li, J., & Li, J. (2017). Advances in polymeric materials for dental applications. *Polymer Chemistry*, *8*(5), 807–823.

Yadugiri, V. T. (2010). 'Plenty of room'-fifty years after the Feynman lecture. Current Science, (00113891), 99(7).

Yang, K. C. (2010). Quantum dot-based visual in vivo imaging for oral squamous cell carcinoma in mice. *Oral Oncology*, *46*(12), 864–868.

Yang, K. Z. (2010). Graphene in mice: Ultrahigh in vivo tumor uptake and efficient photothermal therapy. *Nano Letters*, *10*(9), 3318–3323.

Yang, R., Song, A., & Xu, B. (2010). Feature extraction of motor imagery eeg based on wavelet transform and higher-order statistics. *International Journal of Wavelets, Multresolution, and Information Processing*, *8*(3), 373–384. doi:10.1142/S0219691310003535

Yang, W., Wang, K., & Zuo, W. (2012). Neighborhood Component Feature Selection for High-Dimensional Data. *JCP*, *7*(1), 161–168.

Yeragani, V. K., Sobolewski, E., Kay, J., Jampala, V. C., & Igel, G. (1997). Effect of age on long-term heart rate variability. *Cardiovascular Research*, *35*(1), 35–42. doi:10.1016/S0008-6363(97)00107-7 PMID:9302345

Yliperttula, M., Chung, B. G., Navaladi, A., Manbachi, A., & Urtti, A. (2008). High-throughput screening of cell responses to biomaterials. european journal of pharmaceutical sciences, 35(3), 151-160.

Yohe, S. T., Kopechek, J. A., Porter, T. M., Colson, Y. L., & Grinstaff, M. W. (2013). Triggered Drug Release from Superhydrophobic Meshes using High-Intensity Focused Ultrasound. *Advanced Healthcare Materials*, *2*(9), 1204–1208.

Youlden, D. R., Cramb, S. M., Dunn, N. A., Muller, J. M., Pyke, C. M., & Baade, P. D. (2012). The descriptive epidemiology of female breast cancer: An international comparison of screening, incidence, survival and mortality. *Cancer Epidemiology*, *36*(3), 237–248. doi:10.1016/j.canep.2012.02.007 PMID:22459198

Yousefi, J., & Hamilton-Wright, A. (2014). Characterizing EMG data using machine-learning tools. *Computers in Biology and Medicine*, *51*, 1–13. doi:10.1016/j.compbiomed.2014.04.018 PMID:24857941

Yuan, H., & He, B. (2014). Brain-computer interfaces using sensorimotor rhythms: Current state and future perspectives. *IEEE Transactions on Biomedical Engineering*, *61*(5), 1425–1435. doi:10.1109/TBME.2014.2312397 PMID:24759276

Yu, S., Hariram, K. P., Kumar, R., Cheang, P., & Aik, K. K. (2005). In vitro apatite formation and its growth kinetics on hydroxyapatite/polyetheretherketone biocomposites. *Biomaterials*, *26*(15), 2343–2352.

Yu, Y., Zhou, Z., Yin, E., Jiang, J., Tang, J., Liu, Y., & Hu, D. (2016). Toward brain-actuated car applications: Self-paced control with a motor imagery-based brain-computer interface. *Computers in Biology and Medicine*, *77*, 148–155. doi:10.1016/j.compbiomed.2016.08.010 PMID:27544071

Zabidi, A., Mansor, W., Lee, Y. K., & Fadzal, C. C. W. (2012). Short-time Fourier Transform analysis of EEG signal generated during imagined writing. *2012 International Conference on System Engineering and Technology (ICSET)*, 1–4. 10.1109/ICSEngT.2012.6339284

Zarschler, K. R. (2016). Ultrasmall inorganic nanoparticles: State-of-the-art and perspectives for biomedical applications. *Nanomedicine; Nanotechnology, Biology, and Medicine*, ▪▪▪, 1663–1701.

Zhang, D., Ni, N., Chen, J., Yao, Q., Shen, B., Zhang, Y., & Mo, X. (2015). Electrospun SF/PLCL nanofibrous membrane: A potential scaffold for retinal progenitor cell proliferation and differentiation. *Scientific Reports*, *5*, 14326.

Zhang, H., Chung, S. W., & Mirkin, C. A. (2003). Fabrication of sub-50-nm solid-state nanostructures on the basis of dip-pen nanolithography. *Nano Letters*, *3*(1), 43–45.

Zhang, J., Cao, Y., Qiao, M., Ai, L., Sun, K., Mi, Q., ... Wang, Q. (2018). Human motion monitoring in sports using wearable graphene-coated fiber sensors. *Sensors and Actuators A. Physica A*, *274*, 132–140.

Zhang, P., Xia, J., Wang, Z., & Guan, J. (2014). Gold nanoparticle-packed microdisks for multiplex Raman labelling of cells. *Nanoscale*, *6*(15), 8762–8768.

Zhang, Y., Nam, C. S., Zhou, G., Jin, J., Wang, X., & Cichocki, A. (2018). Temporally Constrained Sparse Group Spatial Patterns for Motor Imagery BCI. *IEEE Transactions on Cybernetics*, 1–11. doi:10.1109/TCYB.2018.2841847 PMID:29994667

Zhang, Yu., Zhou, G., Jin, J., Zhang, Y., Wang, X., & Cichocki, A. (2017). Sparse Bayesian multiway canonical correlation analysis for EEG pattern recognition. *Neurocomputing*, *225*, 103–110. doi:10.1016/j.neucom.2016.11.008

Zhou, G., Zhao, Q., Zhang, Y., Adalı, T., Xie, S., & Cichocki, A. (2016). Linked Component Analysis From Matrices to High-Order Tensors: Applications to Biomedical Data. *Proceedings of the IEEE*, *104*(2), 310–331. doi:10.1109/JPROC.2015.2474704

Zhu, Y., Xu, K., Xu, C., Zhang, J., Ji, J., Zheng, X., ... Tian, M. (2016). PET Mapping for Brain-Computer Interface Stimulation of the Ventroposterior Medial Nucleus of the Thalamus in Rats with Implanted Electrodes. *Journal of Nuclear Medicine: Official Publication, Society of Nuclear Medicine*, *57*(7), 1141–1145. doi:10.2967/jnumed.115.171868 PMID:26917709

Zou, C., Qin, Y., Sun, C., Li, W., & Chen, W. (2017). Motion artefact removal based on periodical property for ECG monitoring with wearable systems. *Pervasive and Mobile Computing*, *40*, 267–278.

About the Contributors

N. Sriraam received M.Tech degree (with distinction) in Biomedical Engineering from Manipal Institute of Technology(MIT), Manipal, India, in 2000, and the Ph.D. degree in Information Technology from the Multimedia University, Cyberjaya, Malaysia, in the area of biomedical signal processing, in 2007. He is currently working as Professor and Head, Department of Medical Electronics, Ramaiah Institute of Technology, Bangalore, India. He is the author or coauthor of 150 articles published in journals and has been involved in several sponsored research projects. His research interests include biomedical signal processing, data mining, and neural networks. He is the editor–in-chief of International Journal of Biomedical and Clinical Engineering (IJBCE),USA, and is also reviewing panel member for Journals such as IEEE Transactions, IEEE Electronics letters, and Elsevier Publications. Dr. Sriraam is Senior Member of IEEE and IEEE Engineering in Medicine and Biology Society (EMBS), life member of Telemedicine Society of India and member of Medical Computer Society of India. Currently, he is serving as Chairman of IEEE EMBS Chapter, Bangalore Section India.

* * *

Yogender Aggarwal is working as an Assistant professor in Bioengineering department, Birla Institute of Technology, Mesra, Ranchi, Jharkhand. He completed his Doctorate from BIT Mesra in 2011, and MSc in Biomedical Instrumentation from BIT Mesra in 2005. He earned a BASc in Instrumentation Hons from Delhi University in 2002.

Uma Arun received a BE degree in Electronics and Communication Engineering from ACCET, Madurai Kamaraj University, in 1988, and MS degree in Electronics and Controls from BITS, Pilani, in 1996. She is working towards her Ph.D in Vishveswaraya Technological University, Belgaum. She is working as Assistant Professor in Medical Electronics Department, MSRIT, Bangalore. She has 24 years of teaching experience and her area of interest is biomedical applications.

Elmer Jeto Gomes Ataide was born in 1993 in Goa, India. He received his BSc. degree in Medicine with a specialization in Health Information Administration from Manipal Academy of Higher Education, Karnataka, India, in 2014. He completed his MSc. degree Health Informatics with a specialization in Healthcare IT Management at the same university in 2016. He worked as a research assistant for one year at the Diabetic Foot Clinic, Kasturba Medical College Hospital and carried out his research on non-invasive glucose detection, measuring core body temperature changes. He is pursuing his PhD in Medical Engineering at Otto-von-Guericke University Magdeburg, Germany. His research interests include Medical imaging, Machine Learning, Augmented Reality in surgical suites and Computer Aided Diagnosis.

Axel Boese is chair manager and senior researcher at the INKA chair at OVG University. He is expert in medical device development and clinical application with more than nine years of experience. He has several developments, publications, and patents in the field of image-guided therapies. Dr. Boese is certified investigator for clinical studies and medical device testing and GCP, Member of VDE and DGBMT and of the DIN Standardisation committee 063-01-02 AA and Co-founder of the company M3DP.

Marco Filax received his Master of Science in 2013 at the Otto von Guericke University. He works as a research assistant at the Chair of Software Engineering. His research interests include, but are not limited to, pattern recognition, computer vision, pervasive cameras, formal verification techniques, and requirement analysis.

Michael Friebe is a German citizen with expertise in diagnostic imaging and image-guided therapies, as founder/innovator/CEO/investor, and scientist. After a B.Sc. in Electrical Engineering, he spent five years in San Francisco as a Research and Design Engineer at an MRI and Ultrasound device manufacturer. In that time, he graduated with an M.Sc. in Technology Management from Golden Gate University, San Francisco, and back in Germany obtained his PhD in Medical Physics. Dr. Friebe is a research fellow of TUM, Munich, an adjunct professor at the Queensland University of Technology in Brisbane, and a professor of Image-Guided Therapies at Otto-von-Guericke-University in Magdeburg, Germany. He is a listed inventor of more than 85 patents, author of 200 papers, board member of four medical technology start-up companies, and an investment partner of a MedTec investment fund. From 2016 to 2018, he was a Distinguished Lecturer of the IEEE EMBS teaching innovation generation and MedTec entrepreneurship.

Holger Fritzsche is a research assistant at the chair of catheter technologies and image-guided therapies under the direction of Prof. Michael Friebe at the Otto-von-Guericke-University Magdeburg. His research focus is in addition to biomechanics/hemodynamics on imaging, intervention, and endoscopic systems. For the PhD program, he heads a university-based, start-up laboratory for innovation generation and technical transfer of medical technologies in minimal invasive therapies with the aim of creating a network node between industry, medicine, and university teaching.

M Esther Hannah is a Professor with the department of information technology, St. Joseph's College of Engineering. Her research interests include machine learning, cognitive science, artificial intelligence, and Deep learning.

Pınar Çakır Hatır is an assistant professor in the Department of Biomedical Engineering at Istanbul Arel University and her research interests focus on development of functional polymeric materials and their applications in biomedical engineering. She holds a Ph.D. in Biotechnology/Polymer Chemistry at Sorbonne Universities, University of Technology of Compiègne (Compiègne, France) and a M.Sc. in Organic Chemistry at Bogazici University (Istanbul, Turkey). During her PhD, she was a research member of Marie Curie Research Training Networks, FP7; NASCENT (Nanomaterials for Application in Sensors, Catalysis and Emerging Technologies) and IRMED (Intelligent Recognition Materials for Extraction and Detection). She has 15-plus years of experience in running research projects in different fields ranging from drug delivery, separation, nanostructures to molecularly imprinted polymers. Currently, she has two national projects and a EuroNanoMed project under Horizon 2020. Also, she is one of two management committee members of COST Action (CA16215) from Turkey.

Sheryl John is a motivating and talented professor and academic advisor driven to inspire students to pursue academic and personal excellence. She strives to create a challenging and engaging learning environment so her students become life-long researchers and learners. John has an exceptional track record of research success with multiple published articles.

Palani Thanaraj K. has completed his Ph.D. in the field of Biomedical Engineering involving applications of Machine Learning in the detection of epilepsy. In his research work, he has used EEG and MRI data for non-invasive epilepsy detection. He has published the outcome of his research in reputed journals indexed in SCI and SCOPUS. Moreover, he has guided undergraduate and postgraduate students in the fields of Machine Learning, Deep Learning, Image Processing, and soft computing techniques.

Mohit Kumar received the B.Tech. degree in electronics and communication engineering from Uttar Pradesh Technical University, Lucknow, India, in 2009, and the M.E. degree in electronic instrumentation and control engineering from Thapar University, Patiala, India, in 2013. He has completed the Ph.D. degree in electrical engineering from Indian Institute of Technology Indore, Indore, India, in 2019. His research interest is in the area of biomedical signal processing.

E. Muthu Kumaran received his B.E, M.E, and Ph.D. Degrees in Electronics and Communication Engineering from Anna University, Chennai, India. He has more than 12 years of teaching and research experiences in reputed colleges and universities. He is working as an Assistant Professor in the Department of Electronics and Communication Engineering at Dr. B. R. Ambedkar Institute of Technology (Govt.), Port Blair. His major research interests are Signal/Image Processing, Soft Computing, and Embedded System. He has undertaken several Government-sponsored major research projects and seminar grants. He has published many International/National Books and Journals in reputed publications.

Nitesh Singh Malan joined School of Biomedical Engineering, Indian Institute of Technology (Banaras Hindu University), India, in July 2016, as a PhD student. He received his Master's in technology in Biomedical Engineering from Motilal Nehru National Institute of Technology Allahabad, India, and Bachelor's in Technology from JSS Academy of Technical Education, Noida, India. His current area of research is Brain-Computer Interface and he has two publications in the same field.

Nithin Nagaraj has a Bachelors degree in Electrical and Electronics Engineering from National Institute of Technology Karnataka (NITK, Surathkal, 1999), Master's degree in Electrical Engineering from Rensselaer Polytechnic Institute (RPI), Troy, New York (2001), and PhD from National Institute of Advanced Studies, Bengaluru (NIAS, 2010). He is Associate Professor at Consciousness Studies Programme, NIAS. His research areas are Complexity Theories of Consciousness, modeling information flow in brain networks, causality testing and brain-inspired learning algorithms. He has co-authored more than 15 international journal publications, several national & international conference papers, and is also the co-inventor of two US Patents. He has co-edited the volume 'Self, Culture and Consciousness: Interdisciplinary Convergences on Knowing and Being' published by Springer Nature in March 2018.

Ram Bilas Pachori was born in Morena, India, in 1979. He received the B.E. degree with honours in Electronics and Communication Engineering from Rajiv Gandhi Technological University, Bhopal, India, in 2001, the M.Tech. and Ph.D. degrees in Electrical Engineering from Indian Institute of Technology (IIT) Kanpur,

Kanpur, India, in 2003 and 2008, respectively. He worked as a Postdoctoral Fellow at Charles Delaunay Institute, University of Technology of Troyes, Troyes, France, 2007-2008. He served as an Assistant Professor at Communication Research Center, International Institute of Information Technology, Hyderabad, India, 2008-2009. He served as an Assistant Professor at Discipline of Electrical Engineering, IIT Indore, Indore, India, 2009-2013. He worked as an Associate Professor at Discipline of Electrical Engineering, IIT Indore, Indore, India, 2013-2017, where presently he has been working as a Professor since 2017. He is also an Associated Faculty with Discipline of Biosciences & Biomedical Engineering at IIT Indore. Pachori is also a Visiting Professor at School of Medicine, Faculty of Health and Medical Sciences, Taylor´s University, Subang Jaya, Malaysia, since December 2018. He worked as a Visiting Scholar at Intelligent Systems Research Center, Ulster University, Northern Ireland, UK, during December 2014. He is an Associate Editor of Electronics Letters, Biomedical Signal Processing and Control Journal and an Editor of IETE Technical Review Journal. He is a senior member of IEEE and a Fellow of IETE. He has more than 160 publications which include journal papers, conference papers, books, and book chapters. His publications have around 4,200 citations, h index of 34, and i10 index of 77 (Google Scholar, May 2019). Pachori has served on review boards for more than 90 scientific journals and served for scientific committees of various national and international conferences. His research interests are in the areas of biomedical signal processing, non-stationary signal processing, speech signal processing, signal processing for communications, computer-aided medical diagnosis, and signal processing for mechanical systems.

G. C. M. Pradeep is working as Professor in the Dept of Neonatalogy, M. S. Ramaiah Medical College and Hospitals, Bengaluru, India.

V. Rajinikanth is Professor, Department of EIE, St. Joseph's College of Engineering, Chennai, Tamilnadu, India. He received his Ph.D, titled 'Heuristic algorithm based system identification and controller design' in 2013 from Anna University, TN, India. He has published over 60 papers in the field of heuristic algorithm applications. His research interest is heuristic algorithm-assisted medical image and signal processing.

Shreeniwas Raut has worked as a Medical Oncologist at HCG Cancer & Research Institute since October, 2016. He completed his DM, Medical Oncology (GCRI, Ahmedabad) in 2014, MD, Medicine (LTMMC Mumbai, MUHS) in 2009, and MBBS (BJMC, Pune) in 2004.

B. V. Ravindra received his Master's Degree in Software Engineering from BITS Pilani. His research interests include application of machine learning techniques and Image processing in biomedical field.

T. Y. Satheesha is working as an associate professor in ECE Department at Nagarjuna College of Engineering and Technology (NCET), Bangalore, Karnataka, India. He received a doctoral degree in 2017 from Jawaharlal Nehru Technological University Anantapur, Andrapradesh, India. He completed his master's degree with distinction in 2010 from BMS College of Engineering, Bangalore, Karnataka, India. His current research interest is Biomedical Image Processing. He has applied for Post Doc in Science and Engineering Research Board – National Post Doctorate Fellow (SERB-NPDF) through GITAM University, Bangalore. He has delivered and organized many technical/non-technical and placement-related talks. He attended 20 workshops. He published over 15 Journals and 25 national and international conference papers. He secured many best paper awards for national/international conferences and journals and was honored by Karnataka Science and Technology Academy (KSTA) Dept. of Science and Technology, Govt. of Karnataka, for his wonder special talk and also contribution towards society for created awareness in urban, rural, women, children, and youth for Human Rights Education. Recently, he was awarded IEAE-Research Excellence Award 2017 for excellent research work, and he has Secured Young Achiever Award 2017 for his research work submitted to IEAE. He is an Editor, Reviewer, and Jury for many conferences and journals. He was a judge for many co-curricular activities. Presently, he is an International Electrical and Electronics Engineering (IEEE) member for Society on Social Implications of Technology (SSIT) (student branch) Bangalore. He is an Editorial member of International Journal of Medical Imaging at Science (PG) Publishing Group and a professional with editorial board membership for IEAE. Moreover, he is a Reviewer for Advances in Science, Technology and Engineering Systems Journal (ASTESJ). He also has given many LIVE TV shows on astrology and astrophysics on many channels.

Rishi Raj Sharma received the M.Tech. degree from Atal Bihari Vajpayee-Indian Institute of Information Technology and Management, Gwalior, India, and the Ph.D. degree from the Indian Institute of Technology Indore, India. He was an Assistant Professor with the Faculty of Engineering and Technology, Raja Balwant Singh College, Agra, India. He also served as a Research Scientist with the National Brain Research Centre, Gurgaon, India. He is an Assistant Professor with the Faculty of Communication Engineering, Military College of Telecommunication Engineering, Mhow, India. His area of research covers time-frequency analysis, signal processing, and its applications in various bio-medical fields, especially neurological signals, muscle signals, and heart signals.

Reema Shukla has completed her PhD from Bio-Engineering department at Birla Institute of Technology, Mesra. Currently, working in Bioengineering department at School of Bioengineering Sciences and Research, MITADT University, Pune. She completed her M.Tech. (Electronics Department) from MPSTME, NMIMS University, Mumbai, and B.E. from Biomedical Department, Thadomal Shahani College of Engineering, Mumbai, Maharashtra. She previously worked in several academic and corporate organizations.

Navjot Singh is pursuing his B.E Degree at Dr. B. R. Ambedkar Institute of Technology, Port Blair. His areas of interest include Signal/Image Processing and embedded system. He has participated in various technical symposiums, seminars, and paper presentations.

Seema Singh got her B.Tech (Electronics and Communication Engineering) degree form Jamia Millia Islamia, a Central University, Delhi, in 2002. Her M.Tech degree is in Electronics branch from Sir MVIT, Bangalore, in 2007. She is Gold medalist and VTU rank holder in M.Tech degree. She was awarded the PhD degree from JNTU, Hyderabad, in 2015 in the area of Neural Networks and Flight control systems. She is working as Associate Professor in Dept. of Electronics and Communication Engineering, BMSIT&M, since 2010. She has authored one book chapter, and 25 publications in reputed International Journals and International/National Conferences. She has received an award for guiding best project of the year from KSCST during 2015. Her research interest lies in the field of anomaly detection, neural networks, image processing, Control Systems, and biomedical engineering. She has given several expert talks on Artificial Neural Networks and its Applications and chaired many sessions of conferences. Her research work is mainly dedicated to application of neural networks in varied fields with undergraduate, postgraduate, and PhD scholars. She has one patent filed in 2018, which dealt with application of neural network in image processing field.

Rakesh Sinha is a Professor at Bio-Engineering Department, Birla Institute of Technology, Mesra, Ranchi.

A. Swarnalatha has received her B.E. degree in Electronics and telecommunication in 1994 from Dr. B A Marathwada University, Aurangabad, and M.E. degree in 2004 from Sathyabama University, Chennai. She completed her doctorate degree from Anna University, Chennai, in 2014. She has 21 years of teaching experience and her areas of interest include VLSI Design, Soft computing, Reconfigurable architectures, wireless communication and image processing. She is a reviewer with Elsevier journals and has about 20 publications in International Journals.

S. Tejaswini received the B.E. degree in Medical electronics (ML) from Sri Krishna Institute of Technology, Bangalore, India, in 2010, and M.Tech degree (First Class with distinction) in Biomedical Signal Processing and Instrumentation from R V College of Engineering, Karnataka, India, in 2012. She is pursuing her Ph.D at Department of Medical Electronics, M. S. Ramaiah Institute of Technology, Bangalore, India, under the guidance of Dr. N. Sriraam. Her main area of Interest is biomedical Signal Processing. She is working as Assistant Professor, Medical Electronics, at M. S. Ramaiah Institute of Technology, Bangalore, India.

Index

www.ingramcontent.com/pod-product-compliance
Lightning Source LLC
LaVergne TN
LVHW081522300926
849161LV00006B/1267
* 9 7 8 1 7 9 9 8 0 3 2 6 3 *